FOCUS ON COLORECTAL CANCER RESEARCH

HORIZONS IN CANCER RESEARCH

Volume 1: Prostate Cancer
John N. Lucas (Editor)
ISBN 1-59454-100-0

Volume 2: Trends in Ovarian Cancer Research
A. P. Bardos (Editor)
ISBN 1-59454-023-3

Volume 3: Percutaneous Cryotherapy of Renal Cell Carcinoma under an Open MRI System
Junta Harada, Kazuo Miyasaka and Sajio Sumida (Editors)
ISBN 1-59454-169-8

Volume 4: Focus on Colorectal Cancer Research
Julia D. Martinez (Editor)
ISBN 1-59454-101-9

FOCUS ON COLORECTAL CANCER RESEARCH

JULIA D. MARTINEZ
EDITOR

Nova Biomedical Books
New York

Production Coordinator: Donna Dennis
Editorial Production Manager: Donna Dennis
Senior Production Editor: Susan Boriotti
Office Manager: Annette Hellinger
Graphics: Andrea Charles, Magdalena Nuñez and Annemarie VanDeWater
Editorial Production: Marius Andronie, Maya Columbus, Keti Datunashvili, Andrew Kallio, Vladimir Klestov, Lorna Loperfido, Joann Overton and Rusudan Razmadze
Circulation: Ave Maria Gonzalez, Vera Popovic, Luis Aviles, Alexandra Columbus, Raymond Davis, Cathy DeGregory, Melissa Diaz, Marlene Nuñez, Jeannie Pappas, Lauren Perl and Katie Sutherland

Library of Congress Cataloging-in-Publication Data
Available Upon Request

ISBN: 1-59454-101-9

An Imprint of Nova Science Publishers, Inc.
400 Oser Ave, Suite 1600
Hauppauge, New York 11788-3619
Tel. 631-231-7269 Fax 631-231-8175
e-mail: Novascience@earthlink.net
Web Site: http://www.novapublishers.com

Printed in the United States of America

CONTENTS

PREFACE

In Western countries, cancer of the large intestine and rectum (colorectal cancer) is the second most common type of cancer and the second leading cause of cancer death (after lung cancer). The incidence of colorectal cancer begins to rise at age 40 and peaks between ages 60 and 75. Cancer of the large intestine (colon cancer) is more common in women; rectal cancer is more common in men. About 5 percent of the people with colon or rectal cancer have more than one cancer of the colorectum at the same time. People with a family history of colon cancer have a higher risk of developing the cancer themselves. A family history of familial polyposis or a similar disease also increases the risk of colon cancer. People with ulcerative colitis or Crohn's disease have a higher risk of developing cancer. The risk is related to the person's age when the condition developed and the length of time the person has had the condition.

Diet plays some role in the risk of colon cancer, but exactly how it affects risk is unknown. Throughout the world, people at highest risk tend to live in cities and eat a diet typical of affluent Westerners. Such a diet is low in fiber and high in animal protein, fats, and refined carbohydrates such as sugar. Risk seems to be reduced by a diet high in calcium, vitamin D, and vegetables such as brussels sprouts, cabbage, and broccoli. Taking an aspirin every other day also seems to reduce the risk of colon cancer.

Colorectal cancer is the third leading cause of cancer related death in both men and woman in industrialized countries. Major advances have been made to understand the molecular events leading to the formation of adenomatous polyps and cancer. Most colorectal cancers are sporadic, but a significant proportion (5-6 %) has a clear genetic background. It is now widely accepted that colorectal carcinogenesis is a multistep process involving the inactivation and activation of a variety of well defined tumor suppressor genes, oncogenes and DNA mismatch repair genes. Over the past recent years, evidence has accumulated indicating that apart from mutations or allelic losses, generally considered as genetic alterations, epigenetic alterations through aberrant promoter methylation and histone modification play a major role in the evolution and progression of colon cancer. In this article we summarize the current knowledge of the molecular pathogenesis of common hereditary syndromes and sporadic forms of colorectal cancer. Novel molecular diagnostic tools for early diagnosis and prevention of colorectal cancer are discussed in chapter I.

The principal goal of chapter II was to assess how physical activity performed in different life periods is associated with the risk of colorectal cancer, since it is unclear whether activity performed in early or later life are real determinants of risk reduction. In total 239 incident cases of colorectal cancer confirmed by histopathology and 239 controls, matched to cases by age (+/- 5 years) and gender, were enrolled. Controls were chosen from amongst patients with no history of cancer from the same hospital and admitted for treatment for non-neoplastic conditions unrelated to digestive tract diseases. Data on occupational and recreational physical activity were collected in standardized interviews for the ages 20 through 30, 40, 50, and 60 years. Besides lifestyle and socio-demographic characteristics, such as education, occupation, and lifetime smoking, the usual dietary pattern for 148 beverage and food items was assessed within a food frequency questionnaire. Median values of total physical activity based on MET-hours/week were consistently lower in cases than in controls at each age. In multivariate conditional logistic regression, the highest quartile of total physical activity compared with the lowest quartile yielded odds ratios below one for each age and for total lifetime. The adjusted odds ratio (OR) for total lifetime was 0.53 (95% confidence interval (CI): 0.30-0.94) for the highest quartile. In the age-specific analyses, the risk reduction was significant only for age 30 (OR = 0.45; CI: 0.25 – 0.79). The relevant confounding effects by body mass index, total energy intake, total fiber intake, lifetime smoking, and alcohol intake were not observed. These data underline the protective role of physical activity in colorectal cancer etiology. The authors' finding on a more pronounced effect in young adulthood around age 30 might have implications for health education.

Epidemiological studies show that populations that rely on a plant-based diet have lower risks for common forms of cancer, suggesting that a strong relationship exists between diet and cancer. Phytochemicals, which are nonnutritive constituents of plants possessing health-protective effects, may provide protection specifically against colorectal cancer (CRC). While diet is very complex, research has identified certain foods and herbs that have some great potential to prevent CRC. Several possible mechanisms of action may explain the cancer preventive aspects of plant-based foods. Specifically, antioxidants from green tea, isothiocyanates from cruciferous vegetables, isoflavones in soy, and flavonoids such as those found in onions and turmeric, have potential anti-cancer effects. Chapter III will also examine the potential cancer preventive effects of herbal supplements including garlic, ginseng, and ginger. The evidence for these food products and herbals in terms of their phytochemical components as well as the proposed mechanisms of their anti-tumor activities will be discussed.

Colorectal cancer risk is determined by a combination of environmental factors and genetic predisposition. Recent evidence which is discussed in chapter IV suggests that dietary and related factors such as physical activity and body size may influence colorectal cancer risk through their effects on the serum concentration of insulin-like growth factor-I (IGF-I) and insulin-like growth factor binding protein (IGFBP)-3, two members of the growth hormone (GH)/IGF-I axis. The GH/IGF-I axis is involved in both human development as well as the maintenance of normal function and homeostasis in most cells of the body. In addition to their classical role as endocrine hormones, its members regulate a wide range of biological functions such as cell proliferation, differentiation and apoptosis through paracrine and autocrine mechanisms. This is particularly evident in its critical role as a regulator of rapidly renewing epithelial cell populations such as those found in the colon. Here its appropriate expression is responsible for the ordered migration of differentiating cells from the bottom towards the top of the colonic crypt and their eventual demise through apoptosis. During cancer development this complex network regulating tissue homeostasis breaks down, with inappropriate expression of the GH/IGF-I axis making an important contribution. The increased understanding of the molecular mechanisms and signalling pathways regulated by the GH/IGF-I axis has started to provide significant insights into the aetiology, prevention and therapy for this cancer.

Several studies have demonstrated that fermented milk consumption decrease the incidence of colorectal cancer. Using a chemically induced murine colon cancer model it was reported that conventional yogurt inhibits tumour development. In this model, the inflammatory immune response caused by the carcinogen (DMH) showed a great increase in IgG+ B cells, CD8+ T lymphocytes and in proinflammatory cytokines (TNFα and IFNγ). Yogurt feeding inhibited tumour development by decreasing the inflammatory immune response and increasing the number of IgA+ cells, CD4+ T lymphocytes, cytokines such as IL-10 and decreasing NO radicals. Yogurt also induced the apoptosis mechanisms. The local immune stimulation produced by yogurt feeding increased monocytes/macrophages population and the cytokines release in the nodular tissue and in the Peyer's patches suggesting that these cells could be responsible for IFNγ and TNFα production. The enhancement of IL-10 found would favour the regulation of the immune response, not only in the inhibition model of the tumour growth, but also when yogurt is given long term. The immune mechanisms involved by yogurt to decrease the inflammatory immune response caused by the carcinogen were different to those observed with an antiinflammatory drug (indomethacin). Indomethacin did not increase immune infiltrative cell activity in the large intestine and the cytokine levels were diminished. Nitric oxide synthase enzyme determinations showed that in mice fed with yogurt, the IFNγ enhancement was not related to inflammation, but to an immunomodulation. We demonstrated that the only single yogurt supplementation was unable to inhibit tumour development in the initiation stage, however it inhibited the tumour growth (promption and progression) when it was administered cyclically after tumour induction. Cellular apoptosis increase observed could explain the importance for the TNFα levels found in the mice fed long term with yogurt. The normal microflora has an important function in the intestinal inflammatory process preceding tumour development, lactic acid bacteria present in yogurt play a role in this process since it has been shown that these bacteria and fermented milk products act on the microbial enzyme activities associated with colon carcinogenesis. Chapter V will show that yogurt can inhibit the promotion and progression of chemically induced colon cancer in mice through its antiinflammatory effect, cell apoptosis and by its immunomodulating properties.

Epidemiological, experimental, and clinical studies have demonstrated that colon carcinogenesis might be prevented by nonsteroidal anti-inflammatory drugs (NSAID) as discussed in chapter VI. Although there are some controversies, recent studies have revealed that NSAID suppresses colon carcinogenesis at adenoma stage where cyclooxygenase-2, a major molecular target in this action, is mainly expressed in interstitial cells but not in tumor cells. Therefore, it is unlikely that NSAID prevents colon cancer formation through modulating the functions of tumor cells. A more possible assumption is that NSAID suppresses colon carcinogenesis through the inhibition of prostaglandin formation. However, at present mechanisms by which how prostaglandins promote colon carcinogenesis have not been elucidated yet. Since prostaglandins act through both membrane receptors and nuclear receptors such as peroxisome proliferator receptor γ or δ, one of the focuses in this area is to investigate their roles in colon carcinogenesis.

The recognition of flat colorectal lesions and the use of chromoscopy as a diagnostic tool in colonoscopy has followed a similar evolution to gastric and early oesophageal cancers. Hence, concepts and diagnostic techniques that were used only for malignancies of the stomach and oesophagus have now been applied in colorectal cancer. The first case of a depressed lesion was reported in 1977, but until 1994, when a flat adenoma cohort and classification was reported, flat and depressed lesions were thought to be a unique Japanese phenomena (phantom carcinoma or Akita disease). Studies from Western groups now prove this to be incorrect. For the detection of large polyps and advanced colorectal cancers, chromoendoscopy and magnification colonoscopy is not required. The strength of the techniques are essentially in identification of flat and diminutive colorectal lesions whose detection with conventional colonoscopy is sub-optimal. Current data proposes flat adenomas may account for in excess of 30% of all colorectal lesions. In addition, malignant potential conferred in this group may be significantly higher compared to conventional colorectal polypoid lesions. Magnification colonoscopy complemented by mucosal dye spraying may therefore be a helpful diagnostic tool. Most flat colorectal lesions are small and have an innocent appearance at initial colonoscopy. Macroscopic non-magnified views commonly reveal only subtle architectural deviation, such as a modest colour change (discolour and faint redness) or a loss of the vascular net. The use of stains such as indigo carmine in addition to magnification colonoscopy can offer a quick and simple diagnostic tool in this group. Chapter VII explores new colonoscopic diagnostic and therapeutic techniques now available in Western practice, previously developed by Japanese groups. The authors discuss the controversies surrounding the diagnosis and therapeutic strategies involved in flat and depressed colorectal lesions and explore the concept of 'virtual biopsy' techniques as applicable to high-magnification chromoscopic colonoscopy. Finally, new and evolving diagnostic colonoscopic techniques using autofluorescence are discussed.

Colorectal cancer is a common disease with high rate of mortality and very well understood genetics. The majority of patients are diagnosed in an advanced stage of the disease, thus requiring chemotherapy. Chapter VIII reports that prognosis and treatment modality for advanced colorectal cancer depends on the tumor stage, since the accumulation of molecular alterations has been commonly associated with poor prognosis and treatment failure. Although there is evidence of benefit of chemotherapy in adjuvant and metastatic settings, its use still remains unsatisfactory because of intrinsic or acquired drug resistance. The most commonly used protocols in advanced colorectal carcinoma include the antimetabolite 5-fluorouracil (5-FU). Several effective alternative treatment options became available for patients with colorectal cancer who relapse after a 5-FU-based chemotherapy. The introduction of irinotecan and oxaliplatin to the therapy with 5-FU/leucovorin has contributed to increase therapeutic options and to improve response rates and survival. The development of oral agents broadened the treatment options available for patients with this disease. Based on the diversity of molecular behavior of advanced colorectal cancer, a number of new agents entered clinical trials. Among others, cyclooxygenase-2 inhibitors, vascular endothelial growth inhibitors and epidermal growth factor inhibitors, are under investigation. Furthermore, the knowledge of the genetics characteristics can be useful to identify prognostic differences, tumor molecular staging and patient stratification, leading to elect a better treatment modality.

The application of laparoscopic techniques for curative resection of colorectal cancer is controversial, mainly owing to reports of cancer recurrence at the port site wounds. Despite research efforts of clinical studies and animal models, neither the actual rate nor the mechanisms causing port site metastasis are known. In chapte IX, the authors gathered data from clinical series of laparoscopic surgery for colorectal cancer, having more then 50 patients each. The port site recurrence in 3901 patients participated in these series was approximately 0.67%. Although the methods and patient selection in these studies varies, this numbers may be comparable to the incidence reported for other malignancies, and in laparotomies for colorectal cancer. Chapter IX reviews the technical aspects relative to laparoscopic resection of colorectal cancer, and summarizes the research regarding the potential causes for port site metastasis, and suggested protective measures. It also suggests that wound recurrence may possibly be a result of an unfortunate learning curve, rather then an inherited concern. The final results of the large randomized studies will hopefully solve this question in the near future.

A new trial design for a surgical outcome trial with an immune modulator was developed by consensus of an international study group. Granulocyte-colony stimulating factor (G-CSF, filgrastim) was tested in a randomized, controlled trial for prevention of postoperative infectious complications and a sub-optimum recovery from operation in patients with colorectal cancer and increased perioperative risk (ASA 3 and 4). The rationale for the trial and the design of the randomized, placebo controlled, double-blinded trial (n = 40 patients for each group) is described in chapter X. This prototype trial includes the following elements:

- The study population was restricted to patients with high risk (ASA 3 and 4) and left sided surgical resection of colorectal cancer.
- Clinic modeling randomized trials (CMRTs) in rodents were used to help to define trial conditions.
- Patients were allocated by random to the control or treatment group (n = 40/group). Two antibiotics (A = cefuroxime/metronidazole and B = ofloxacin/metronidazole) were balanced, randomized in a 2 x 2 design (G-CSF/placebo x antibiotic A/B) in the trial. The double blinding strategy of the trial was assessed by psychometric indices.
- A new endpoint construct (integrated outcome concept) was evaluated with quality of life (EORTC-QLQ-C30 and QLQ-C38 cancer module) and a recovery index (Mc Peek index) were used as primary endpoints. Qualitative analysis of clinical relevance was performed by both patients and doctors.
- A confirmatory statistical model with quality of life as the first primary endpoint in the hierarchic test procedure is used. Statistical analysis uses an area under the curve (AUC) model for improvement of quality of life at discharge from hospital, two and six months after operation. The second primary endpoint is the McPeek index.

- The management of postoperative complications was directed by an evidence based guideline.

A new trial design for preoperative prophylaxis and postoperative recovery was developed and used to avoid previous methodological failures. The trial was performed in three centers within two years plus an additional half year for follow up. At present it can be concluded that the trial protocol is feasible and can therefore be used to test other immune-modulators in complex clinical scenarios. Data analysis will demonstrate the effect of G-CSF on the different endpoints.

Cancer is a genetic disease. Most cancer-causing mutations are somatic, occurring in the affected tissue during the course of carcinogenesis. However, most cancers also have an hereditary component that is caused by predisposing mutations that affect the germline, are heritable and contribute to the initiation of carcinogenesis. Colorectal cancer is probably the condition for which the most is known about the genes affected by cancer-causing mutations, their normal functions and their carcinogenic effects when mutated. Hereditary colorectal cancer syndromes are classified according to the presence of unusually large number of adenomatous or hamartomatous polyps. The polyposis syndromes include Familial Adenomatous Polyposis and its variants. The hamartomatous polyposis syndromes include juvenile polyposis, Peutz-Jeghers syndrome, and Cowden syndrome. More common than any of the polyposis syndromes is the Hereditary Non-Polyposis Colorectal Cancer. Chapter XI addresses the molecular basis of these syndromes with particular emphasis to the recent advances in this rapidly progressive field and the applications of such knowledge in developing new diagnostic, preventive and therapeutic strategies.

In: Focus on Colorectal Cancer Research
Editor: Julia D. Martinez, pp. 1-23
ISBN #1-59454-101-9

Chapter I

Molecular Pathogenesis of Colorectal Cancer: Implications for Molecular Diagnosis

Christian N. Arnold, Hubert E. Blum and Fritz von Weizsäcker
University of Freiburg, Department of Medicine, Freiburg, Germany

Abstract

Colorectal cancer is the third leading cause of cancer related death in both men and woman in industrialized countries. Major advances have been made to understand the molecular events leading to the formation of adenomatous polyps and cancer. Most colorectal cancers are sporadic, but a significant proportion (5-6 %) has a clear genetic background. It is now widely accepted that colorectal carcinogenesis is a multistep process involving the inactivation and activation of a variety of well defined tumor suppressor genes, oncogenes and DNA mismatch repair genes. Over the past recent years, evidence has accumulated indicating that apart from mutations or allelic losses, generally considered as genetic alterations, epigenetic alterations through aberrant promoter methylation and histone modification play a major role in the evolution and progression of colon cancer. In this article we summarize the current knowledge of the molecular pathogenesis of common hereditary syndromes and sporadic forms of colorectal cancer. Novel molecular diagnostic tools for early diagnosis and prevention of colorectal cancer are discussed.

Introduction

Colorectal neoplasia is one of the most common malignancies in the Western world. The lifetime risk of colorectal cancer in the general population is 5-6 % [1]. About 50% of the population will develop a colon tumor – generally an adenomatous polyp- by the age of 70. About one tenth of these will proceed to malignant cancer [2]. Over the past 15 years it has been demonstrated that colorectal cancer is a multistep genetic disease. Epidemiologic studies have suggested that environmental factors support the development of colon cancer

[3]. This assumption is supported by geographic variations in the prevalence of colon cancer worldwide. Low fiber and high fat diet is believed to be associated with a higher risk of developing colon cancer in Western countries [4]. Further, red meat is associated with a higher colon cancer risk. Dietary factors may promote colorectal carcinogenesis by altering intestinal bacterial flora, slowing gastrointestinal transit time and recycling of bile acids However, up to today it is not well understood how these environmental factors promote cancer formation [5].

Interestingly, some individuals are more prone to acquire colorectal cancer than others. It has been shown, that about 25 % of colon cancer patients have a familial background and 15% have a strong family history with a first or second degree relative involved [2]. Those individuals have at least a 2-fold increased risk to develop colon cancer compared to the general population. The relative risk to acquire colorectal cancer correlates with the number of affected individuals, young age and level of relatedness to the affected individuals. Up to 5-6 % of colon cancers are considered to be inherited syndromes, most commonly familial adenomatous polyposis (FAP) or hereditary non-polyposis colorectal cancer (HNPCC) [6]. For both syndromes disease causing mutations have been identified. FAP is caused by germline mutations of the tumor suppressor gene *adenomatous polyposis coli (APC)* [7, 8]. *APC* alterations are seen in most colorectal cancers, either familial or sporadic [5]. HNPCC is caused by mutations in DNA mismatch repair genes, of which most commonly *hMLH1* and *hMSH2* are affected [6]. Less common hereditary colorectal cancer syndromes are the polyposis syndromes juvenile polyposis coli (JPS) syndrome, Cowden's disease (CD) and the Bannayan-Riley-Ruvalcaba (BRR) syndrome, all of which are characterized by the formation of harmatomatous juvenile polyps with typical histological criteria. The Peutz-Jeghers syndrome (PJS) is defined by the occurrence of hamartomatous polyps throughout the gastrointestinal tract and melanocytic macules of the lips, buccal mucosa and digits. For all of these syndromes disease causing genes have been identified **(Table 1)** [9]. The latter tumor syndromes are discussed in more detail elsewhere.

Table 1: Hereditary disorders predisposing to colorectal cancer

syndrome	**gene**
Familial adenomatous polyposis (FAP)	*APC*
Hereditary non-polyposis colorectal cancer (HNPCC)	*hMLH1, hMSH2, hMSH6, PMS1, PMS2, hMLH3, EXO1*
Peutz-Jeghers syndrome (PJS)	*STK11*
Juvenile polyposis (JPS)	*MADH4/BMPR1A*
Cowden's disease (CD)	*PTEN/MMAC1*
Bannayan-Ruvalcaba syndrome (BRS)	*PTEN*

In general, colon carcinoma results from the cummulative effect of multiple sequential genetic alterations (multistep carcinogenesis) which can be acquired as in sporadic forms or be inherited as in genetic tumor syndromes. The genetic alterations leading to tumor formation can be used for screening, early diagnosis and staging. Numerous genetic alterations can be specifically identified and used as molecular markers.

1. Familial Adenomatous Polyposis

Clinical Features

FAP is an autosomal dominantly inherited disease which affects 1 out of 7000 individuals. The penetrance of the disease is almost 100%. Typically, by the second and third decade of life hundreds to thousands of adenomatous polyps develop in the large bowel. These tumors are not malignant *per se*, but in case of an inactivating event of the second allele they will inevitably progress to invasive cancer. FAP has a penetrance of almost 100%, and it is recommended to have the colon surgically removed by the age of 30. In addition, patients with FAP frequently develop extracolonic manifestations in the course of the disease, such as retinal lesions, osteomas, duodenal or ampullary polyps, desmoids of the skin or brain tumors.

Molecular Pathogenesis

By linkage analyses, the APC locus was mapped to chromosome 5q. Further molecular studies demonstrated a strong linkage to markers close to chromosome 5q21. In 1991 the disease causing *APC* gene was identified [7, 8]. The APC protein interacts with the intracellular protein β-catenin, which, when activated, proceeds to the nucleus and stimulates cell proliferation by transcriptional activation of *c-myc*, cyclin D1, TCF/LEF or the peroxisome-proliferator-activated receptor delta (PPARδ)[10]. β–catenin levels also influence cell adhesion. Once β-catenin levels rise, cell proliferation is activated which finally leads to adenoma formation. In concert with other factors, intact APC inactivates cellular proliferation by the degradation of β-catenin through ubiquitination and degradation through the proteasome pathway [11]. In case of an inactivating mutation, APC-mediated β-catenin degradation is inhibited and nuclear β-catenin levels increase.

Approximately 30% of FAP patients are negative for APC mutations [12]. It has been stated, that a significant proportion of FAP in APC negative individuals might be caused by bi-allelic mutations of the *MYH* gene [13]. In these cases, FAP might indeed be an autosomal recessive disorder caused by somatic mutations in *MYH*, which encodes a glycosylase, is involved in base excision repair (BER) and primarily targets oxidative DNA damage. Colorectal tumors from *MYH* patients show an excess of G>T transversion mutations in the *APC* gene because of the inability to remove lesions induced by the base 8-oxo-guanine. There is currently no evidence, that *MYH* mutations play a pathogenetic role outside *MYH* associated polyposis. However, it is yet not clear how *MYH* mutations induce the formation of intestinal polyposis.

Interestingly, the number of polyps in FAP is determined by the location of the germline mutation within the *APC* open reading frame. It was soon recognized, that FAP patients do not show uniform clinical features but rather present with different phenotypes [14]. In many cases, this difference is defined by the inactivating mutation. In most cases, the mutation of the *APC* gene results in a C-terminal truncation of the protein. A mutation between codons 1250 and 1464 will lead to the most severe form of the disease with a high number of polyps and early age of manifestation. Mutations within exon 3, however, present with an attenuated phenotype [15]. These patients develop polyps later in life and the penetrance of the disease is lower. Retinal lesions (congenital hypertrophy of the retinal pigment epithelium, CHRPE) are associated with truncating mutations between codons 463 and 1387 **(Fig. 1).**

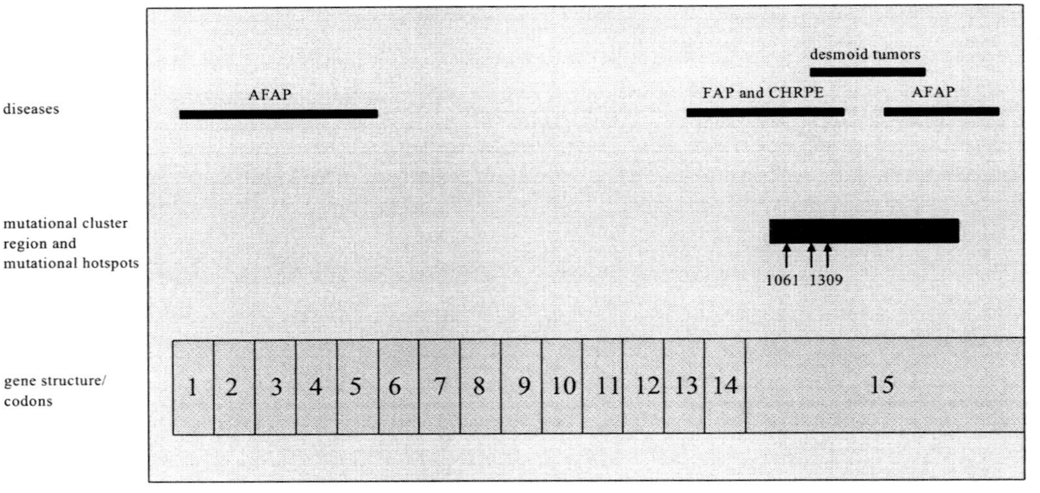

Fig. 1: *APC* gene structure._The lower bar indicates the genes with exons 1 to 15. The mutation cluster regions spans parts of exon 15, mutational hotspots are indicated by arrows. Disease phenotypes correlate with mutations indifferent regions of the *APC* gene. AFAP (attenuated familial adenomatous polyposis); CHRPE(congenital hypertrophy of the retinal pigment epithelium).

The *APC* gene also serves as a "modifier gene" in colorectal cancer susceptibility. In case of the *I1307K* mutation, isoleucin is converted to lysine at position 1307 [16]. This polymorphism converts an AAATAAAA sequence to a relatively unstable microsatellite A^8 sequence which creates a region of hypermutability and induces "slipping" of DNA polymerase. The *I1307K* mutations also causes a predisposition to sporadic mutations at more distant sites of the gene which then might lead to further structure abnormalities of the gene. This alteration has been identified in 6% of Ashkenazy Jews, and it is associated with a 2 - 3 fold increased risk to develop colorectal cancer but does not cause the formation of adenomatous polyps *per se*.

Molecular Diagnosis

The clinical diagnosis can be confirmed by the molecular analysis of the affecting germline mutation. A large proportion of these alterations can be detected by the *in vitro* transcription-translation test, also called the *in vitro* protein truncation test [17], which is commercially available. Once a truncated APC protein has been found, the size of the protein will give hints to the suspected location of the mutation and sequence analysis will be performed. Sequence analysis is successful in more than 90% of those cases initially screened by the above mentioned test. Once a disease causing mutation is known, affected family members or relatives at risk can be easily screened for the presence of this mutation after careful genetic counselling.

2. Hereditary Non-Polyposis Colorectal Cancer

Clinical Features

HNPCC is an autosomal dominant disorder clinically characterized by the early onset of colorectal cancer and extracolonic manifestations in multiple members of a family without increased total number of colorectal polyps. HNPCC affects predominantly the proximal colon and is characterized by an early age of onset. Synchronous and metachronous tumor formation, especially in the setting of a colorectal cancer in the proximal colon, suggest the diagnosis of HNPCC. Besides their location, tumors of the HNPCC spectrum have typical pathological features like lymphocytic infiltration, high mucinous content and poor differentiation. Typically, HNPCC patients develop tumors without detectable preceding adenomas. This is due to an accelerated adenoma-carcinoma sequence in HNPCC. Therefore, HNPCC is phenotypically different to FAP with respect to number and location of the polyps. Besides their higher risk for malignancies of the colon and rectum, individuals with HNPCC also frequently acquire tumors at extracolonic sites, such as endometrial, ovarian, urinary, pancreas, gastric, small bowel or brain cancers. The penetrance of the disease is about 80% but colorectal cancers caused by the HNPCC syndrome in general have a better prognosis, similar to microsatellite instability high (MSI-H) sporadic colorectal cancers (see below).

Molecular Pathogenesis

In the early 1990s it was recognized, that some colorectal cancers had a high number of deletion or insertion mutations at short simple repetitive sequences called microsatellites [18]. Microsatellite sequences are widely spread throughout the genome and are routinely used for linkage analyses. Within a short period of time it was found, that 12-15% of all colorectal cancers display the replication error (RER) or microsatellite instability (MSI) phenotype [19]. These tumors feature thousands of deletion or insertion mutations, occurring in coding and non-coding areas of the genome. In patients with HNPCC, linkage analyses soon correlated the syndrome to loci on chromosomes 2p and 3p21-23. It was then recognized that the disease causing genes belonged to the DNA mismatch repair system and were homologues to the bacterial MutL and MutS complexes. They were consequently termed *hMLH1* and *hMSH2* [20]. Later, several additional genes were identified, called *hPMS1, hPMS2, hMSH3, hMSH6, hMLH3* and *EXO1*. The human DNA mismatch-repair system requires the concerted action of several proteins, which form complexes to achieve specific functions [21]. The mutSα complex, formed by *hMSH2* and *hMSH6*, has a high affinity to single base pair mismatches. By binding to a mismatch, the mutL complex, formed by *hMLH1* and *hPMS2*, is recruited and the DNA repair machinery is activated. In case of larger deletion or insertion mutations (also called "loop-out" mispairing) in repetitive sequences, the mutSβ-complex, formed by *hMSH2* and *hMSH3*, is involved, also by recruiting the mutL-complex to permit distinction between the mutated and the authentic sequence, which eventually leads to the repair of the defective DNA strand.

The most common involved genes in HNPCC are *hMLH1* and *hMSH2*. These two genes account for 90% of all known mutations in HNPCC families. Germline mutations have also less commonly been found in *hPMS2, hPMS1, hMSH6*, and recently also in *EXO1* [22] and *hMLH3* [23], though the clinical significance of mutations in the latter two genes remains to be established. Interestingly, mutations in *hMHS6* result in only a partial deficiency of mismatch repair and low levels of MSI (MSI-low phenotype) [24] They account for an attenuated HNPCC phenotype with a later age of onset and incomplete penetrance. However, there seems to be an elevated risk of endometrial cancer in female carriers [25] In case of *hMLH1* and *hMSH2* mutations, high level MSI (MSI-H) is typically observed. The level of MSI is usually assessed by the use of five microsatellite markers from a standard panel of markers defined by the National Cancer Institute in 1998 [26]. MSI-H is present when two of five markers are unstable. The MSI-L phenotype is present when only one out of five markers is unstable.

The consequence of a defective DNA mismatch-repair system is the acquisition of multiple mutations in coding and non-coding sequences. These mutations most commonly occur in microsatellite sequences. Most of these sequences occur in non-coding areas of the genome and mutations in these sequences are of no apparent relevance but rather represent the genetic fingerprint of these malignancies. However, many genes harbour microsatellite sequences in their coding regions and they are prone to mutations in patients with the MSI phenotype. These so called target genes include growth factors (TGF beta-receptor II, IGF-II-receptor), regulator of the cell cycle and apoptosis (E2F4, BAX), and even the mismatch repair genes *hMSH3* and *hMSH6* themselves [20]. There is a growing list of genes found to be involved in patients with the MSI phenotype **(Table 2)**. It is generally believed, that transformation to malignancy is associated with mutations of these target genes [27].

Table 2: Target genes in malignancies of the MSI phenotype

marker	repeat
TGFβRII	$(A)_{10}$
IGFIIR	$(G)_8$
BAX	$(G)_8$
hMSH3	$(A)_8$
hMSH6	$(C)_8$
hMLH3	$(A)_{10}$
MBD4	$(A)_{10}$
PTEN	$(A)_6$
WISP3	$(A)_9$
hRAD50	$(A)_9$
RIZ	$(A)_9$
Caspase-5	$(A)_{10}$
hGARE	$(T)_8$

Molecular Diagnosis

Diagnosis of HNPCC relies on family history which should meet the Amsterdam or Bethesda criteria **(Table 3).** Once an individual is identified or suspected to have HNPCC, genetic counselling and testing will be performed. Testing for HNPCC is complicated by the fact, that there are several DNA mismatch repair genes that can be involved. Patients who meet the Amsterdam or Bethesda criteria or have a strong familiar colorectal cancer risk are first screened for MSI **(Fig. 2)**. However, in the case of a MSI-H cancer it must always be considered that approximately 15% of sporadic colon cancers also have this phenotype (see below). In case of a MSI-H malignancy, the individual at risk will be searched for a pathogenic mutation by single strand confirmation polymorphism (SSCP) and DNA sequencing in the most commonly involved DNA mismatch repair genes *hMSH2* and *hMLH1*. Mutations in these two mismatch repair genes account for approximately 35% and 60% of genetically characterized HNPCC cases [28]. The mutations that occur in both genes are small insertions, deletions or base substitutions resulting in frameshift, truncation or missense mutations. A growing number of disease causing mutations have been identified which can be seen in detail on the ICG-Hereditary Nonpolyposis Colon Cancer web site (*http://www.nfdht.nl*). Genetic testing for the *hMLH1* and *hMSH2* genes is commercially available in selected laboratories.

Table 3: Clinical criteria for the diagnosis of HNPCC

Amsterdam criteria:	
1.	At least 3 affected relatives with verified colorectal cancer
2.	At least two successive generations affected
3.	At least one is a first degree relative of the other two
4.	One involved individual is at <50 years of age
5.	FAP is excluded
Modified Amsterdam criteria:	
	Same as Amsterdam criteria except that extra colonic HNPCC associated malignancies are included.
Bethesda criteria:	
1.	Individuals with cancer in families that meet the Amsterdam criteria.
2.	Individuals with two HNPCC-related cancers including synchronous and metachronous colorectal cancers or associated extra colonic cancers.
3.	Individuals with colorectal cancer and a first degree relative with colorectal cancer and/or HNPCC-related extra colonic cancer and/or a colorectal adenoma; one of the cancers diagnosed at age less than 45, the adenoma at age less than 40.
4.	Individuals with colorectal cancer or endometrial cancer diagnosed at age less than 45.
5.	Individuals with right-sided colorectal cancer with an undifferentiated pattern (solid/cribriform) or histopathological characteristics diagnosed at age less than 45.
6.	Individuals with signet ring cell type colorectal cancer diagnosed at age less than 45.
7.	Individuals with adenomas diagnosed at age less than 40.

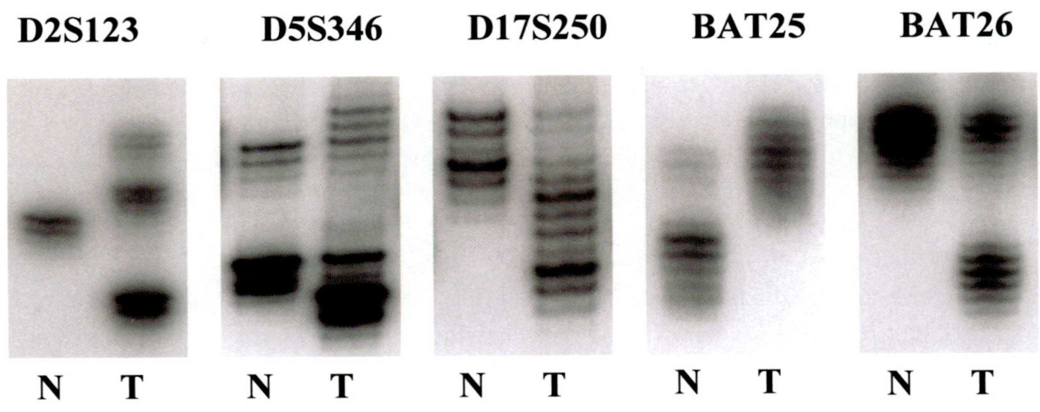

Fig. 2: MSI analysis using five recommended markers. Normal tissue (N) is compared with tumor tissue (T) of the same individual. All tumors show different allele sizes represented by insertion or deletion mutations in the microsatellite sequences of the respective markers.

Another approach to screen for HNPCC is the immunohistochemical staining for the mismatch repair genes in the tumor which will identify the defective mismatch repair protein **(Fig. 3)**. Pathogenic mutations in a mismatch repair gene usually lead to the absence of detectable protein. However, some missense mutations still result in the formation of a defective protein that can be detected by immunohistochemistry. Once the search for the disease causing mutation was successful, family members at risk can be directly screened for this mutation and close clinical surveillance for cancer will be the consequence.

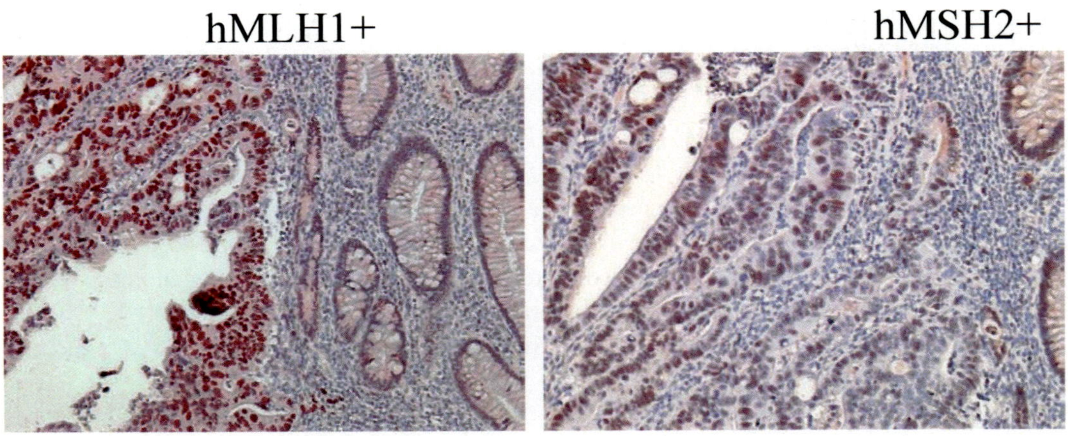

Fig. 3: hMLH1 and hMSH2 expression analysis. Representative expression analysis performed by immunohistochemistry in tumors expressing hMLH1 and hMSH2.

Unlike the APC gene, mutations in the mismatch repair genes do not frequently result in truncated proteins, but rather represent missense mutations or other variants like mutations in splice sites. The inability to detect *hMSH2* and *hMLH1* mutation in half of the patients with HNPCC implies that genetic screening techniques by now are far from perfect and have a fairly low specificity (<50%). In addition, so far unidentified genes might exist. The development of reliable genetic testing still remains a challenge.

Recently, a new testing approach has been published [29]. A wild-type allele might be able to mask a mutant allele in the process of sequencing. To avoid this problem, the conversion technique has been developed. This procedure converts diploid to haploid cells resulting in differential analysis of the maternal and paternal allele.

3. Sporadic Colorectal Cancer

Non-hereditary colorectal cancer belongs to the most common malignancies worldwide. Its characteristic is the step-wise progression from normal colonic epithelium to neoplastic growth associated with sequential molecular abnormalities in each step [5]. In the early 1990s it was elegantly shown that colorectal tumors arise as the result of activated oncogenes and inactivated tumor suppressor genes [30]. It was soon believed that the acquisition of numerous such alterations eventually lead to the formation of colon cancer.

Historic Background and Molecular Pathogenesis

Adenoma-Carcinoma-Sequence

In 1988 the use of restriction fragment polymorphism (RFLP) analysis allowed to characterize the frequency and location of chromosomal losses in colorectal cancers [31]. It was shown, that in most cases of sporadic colon cancers several chromosomal segments were deleted. When compared to normal tissue, one chromosomal allele was lost, termed "loss of heterozygosity" (LOH). It was shown that specific chromosomal loci showed high frequencies of allelic losses as on chromosomes 17p, 18q and 5q [30]. It was then demonstrated that the essential gene on 17p was the *p53* tumor suppressor gene. In colorectal cancer 75% had undergone LOH at this locus and in most cases the residual allele had been inactivated by a mutational event. In the late 1980s a further candidate gene on chromosome 18q called "*deleted in colorectal carcinoma*" gene (*DCC*) was identified. Up to 70% of colon cancers have been shown to carry mutations at this site. It is believed that the second allele is generally inactivated by LOH. Mutations of the *DCC* gene are also found in 50% of advanced adenomas of the colon [30]. The presence of 18q alterations has been proven as a prognostic marker for survival [32]. Tumors are usually grouped into stages depending on their size and progression. Generally, stage II colon cancers have a better overall survival than stage III malignancies. However, in the scenario of stage II cancers with *DCC* inactivation the outcome appears to be equivalent to stage III colorectal cancers [33]. Tumors of the same stage have a worse outcome once one 18q allele is deleted.

In individuals with colon cancers allelic deletions of chromosome 5q, which carries the *APC* gene (see above), have been observed in up to 50% of cases and in about 30% of adenomas, respectively [31, 34].

Besides alterations in tumor suppressor genes, activating mutations of the oncogene *k-ras* contribute to the molecular pathogenesis of colorectal cancer. The oncogene *k-ras* on chromosome 12 encodes a protein which transforms extracellular growth signals to the nucleus and influences processes of signal transduction. Mutations of *k-ras* are found in 50% of large polyps and colorectal cancer [31, 35]. Mutations are in general gene-activating missense mutations and result in continuous growth signals. Missense mutations are found predominantly in codons 12, 13 and 61. It has been demonstrated, that mutations in *k-ras* correlate with the size of the lesions and progression of dysplasia. In adenomas of small size (<2cm) *k-ras* mutations are found in 14% whereas 33% of the larger adenomas (>2cm) carry these alterations. In only moderately dysplastic adenomas *k-ras* lesions are found in 33% whereas highly dysplastic lesions are mutated in up to 50% [30]. *K-ras* mutations have also been screened in their usefulness as a molecular and prognostic marker. As tumor DNA is shed in the stool it can be specifically extracted and amplified by PCR. Mutations of *k-ras* in the stool corresponded to the alterations found in the tumor [36]. The analyses of DNA extracted from the stool detected almost 90% of all tumors carrying *k-ras* mutations. However, the sensitivity of this method was only 33% and has to be increased significantly to serve as a valid test for routine use in the clinical setting. The main problem remains that *k-ras* muations are not specific for colorectal cancer and can also be found in dysplastic lesions of the pancreas and the bile epithelium.

All of these alterations usually occur in the early steps of colorectal neoplasia and a high number of tumors are altered either by a mutation or allelic loss. It was in the early 1990s when the stepwise model of colorectal carcinogenesis was first described in which each pathogenic step is accompanied by specific genetic alterations finally leading to the formation of tumors in the colon [30]. It is now believed that not so much the sequence of these alterations but rather the accumulation of these genetic modifications is driving cancer growth in the colon.

Microsatellite Instability

Tumors evolving through inactivating mutations of certain tumor suppressor genes, activating mutations of oncogenes and allelic losses belong to the "chromosomal instability" (CIN) or "suppressor" pathway [37]. Although this model is considered virtually as a dogma in tumor biology, we now know that there are multiple mechanisms of tumor development in the colon. While looking for LOH events using microsatellite markers, a second – and completely unrelated - type of genomic instability was detected by three independent research groups. This type of hyper-mutability, termed MSI, was linked to 12-15% of all colorectal tumors, and more than 90% of the cancers in HNPCC [19, 38, 39]. Recognition of the implications of MSI led to the identification of the genes responsible for HNPCC (or Lynch syndrome) and insights into a novel mechanism of tumorigenesis in colon cancer. Mutations in seven different genes (*hMSH2, hMSH6, hMLH1, hPMS1, hPMS2, EXO1* and *hMLH3*) have now been associated with the syndrome (see HNPCC). Tumors characterized by MSI are believed to evolve through the "mutator" pathway [37].

Over the past few years, *hMLH1* has gained greater importance, as it was recognized that this gene was also not expressed in most of the sporadic colon cancers with MSI-H, which comprises about 75% of the entire MSI group (or 12-15 % of all colon cancers). MSI-H in a tumor indicates that the DNA MMR system has been inactivated. This requires bi-allelic loss of either *hMSH2* or *hMLH1* (which are the "major" DNA MMR genes), or a combination of losses of the other, "minor" genes. Gene inactivation can occur through several mechanisms, including point mutations, insertion or deletion mutations that create frameshifts, or large scale chromosomal deletions or rearrangements. In HNPCC, it is not unusual to find a germline mutation in either *hMSH2* or *hMLH1* in combination with a LOH event at the paired allele, completing the two-hit model of gene inactivation in the tumor.

In 1998, evidence begun to accumulate that *hMLH1* was inactivated by epigenetic modification of its promoter [40, 41]. In general, genes can be inactivated by an epigenetic mechanism whereby the gene promoter undergoes transcriptional silencing by the hypermethylation of CpG islands (i.e., clusters of cytosine residues followed by a guanosine) in the gene promoter [42]. The regulation of this process is not clearly understood, but the covalent attachment of a methyl group to the cytosines in CpG sequences (which are greatly over-represented in gene promoters) apparently impairs the ability of transactivating factors to bind and turn on gene expression. This is a common mechanism by which cells regulate gene expression, and by which genes are silenced during the inactivation of one of the X chromosomes.

Different Molecular Pathways

We now believe that there exist additional molecular pathways in colorectal tumorigenesis besides the "suppressor" and the "mutator" pathway [43]. While analysing 209 high risk stage II and stage III sporadic colon cancers we found that a proportion of 14% were classified as MSI-H while the remainder was MSI-L or microsatellite stable (MSS). However, while 51% of cancers showed characteristics of the "suppressor" pathway defined by LOH, in 3.4% of the investigated tumors characteristics of both the "suppressor" and the "mutator" pathway (LOH and MSI-H) were found, and a high percentage of 38% of all tumors did not demonstrate characteristics of either pathway of genomic instability (**Fig. 4**). This data suggests that some colorectal cancers are defined by an overlap of the "suppressor" and the "mutator" pathway. However, we showed for the first time that a significant proportion of colon cancers might progress through further not yet defined molecular mechanisms of genomic instability (**Fig. 5**).

Epigenetic Gene Silencing

The mechanism of epigenetic gene silencing has been found to inactivate several tumor suppressor genes in a variety of tumors [44], and it has now been shown that hypermethylation of the promoter region in the *hMLH1* gene leads to a lack of expression of its protein and accounts for MSI in non-hereditary colorectal cancers [40]. It was reported that both alleles of *hMLH1* were hypermethylated in five out of six MSI colon cancer cell lines that lacked identifiable mismatch repair gene mutations [41]. Proof of principle was provided by an experiment in which the demethylating agent 2-deoxy-5-azacytidine reversibly restored the expression of both *hMLH1* alleles as well as functional mismatch repair activity to these cells. This distinct pathway of colorectal tumorigenesis - involving transcriptional silencing of selected genes in cancers – has been termed the CpG island methylator phenotype (CIMP) [45], and is distinct from age related (type A) methylation, which is observed in gene promoters as a function of age.

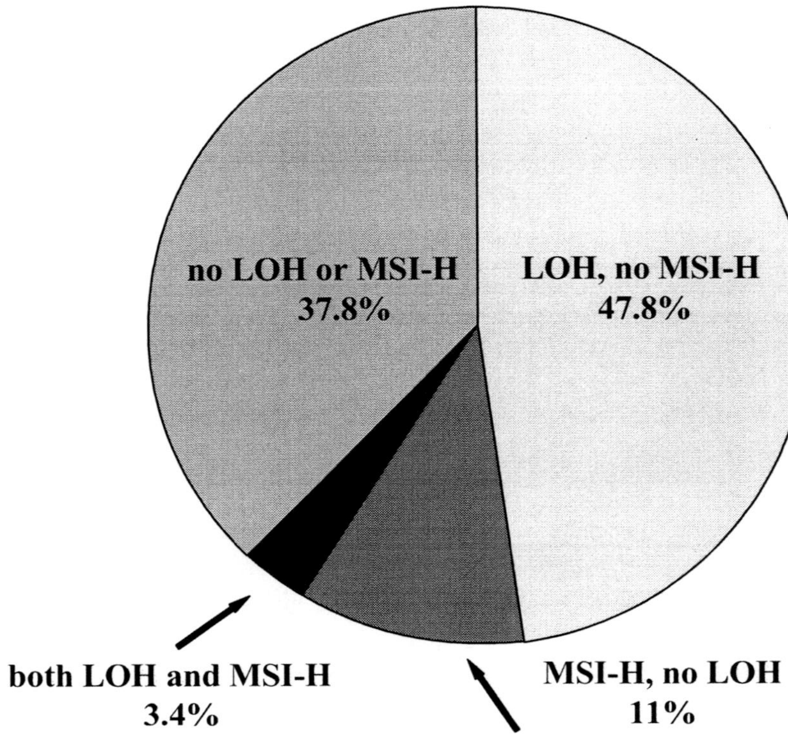

Fig. 4: Exclusiveness and overlap among subsets of genomic instability. Summary of genomic instability patterns for 209 sporadic colon cancers. Tumors were screened for allelic losses (LOH) and MSI.

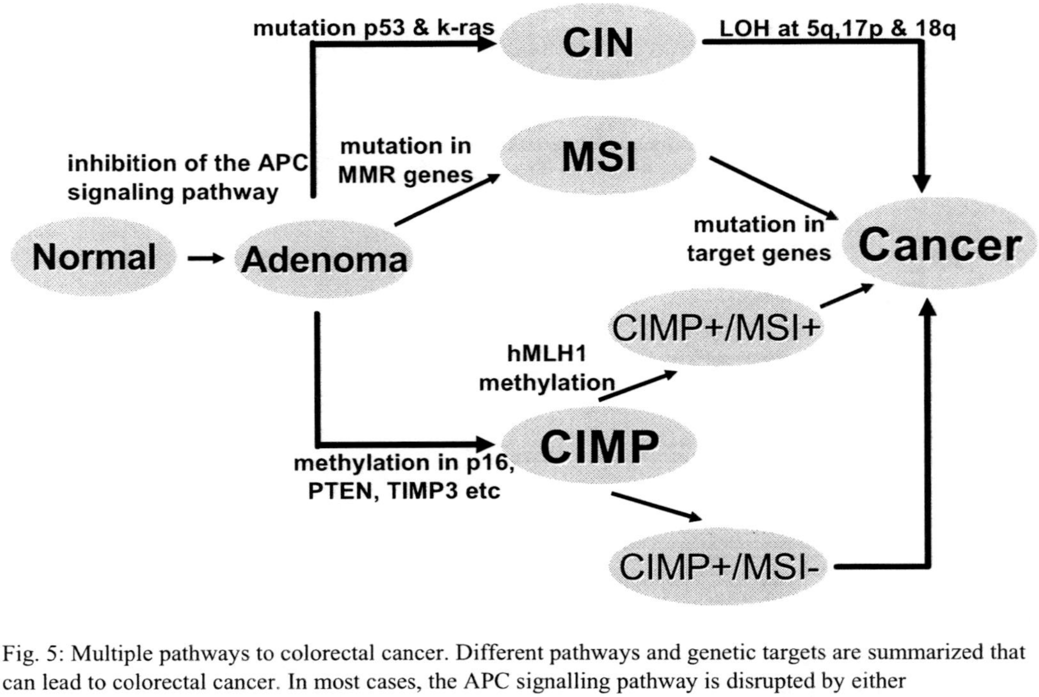

Fig. 5: Multiple pathways to colorectal cancer. Different pathways and genetic targets are summarized that can lead to colorectal cancer. In most cases, the APC signalling pathway is disrupted by either mutations/deletions of the APC gene. Tumor formation can proceed through the CIN pathway, characterized

by multiple mutations and allelic losses of tumor suppressor genes and *k-ras*. Alternatively, mutations of MMR genes lead to the MSI phenotype as in the familial syndrome HNPCC. A further mechanism of tumor formation can be caused through the CpG island methylator phenotype (CIMP) which silences genes through promoter methylation. CIMP can either progress through silencing the *hMLH1* gene among others causing the MSI phenotype (CIMP+/MSI+). Alternatively, a variety of tumor suppressor genes apart from *hMLH1* can be silenced through promoter methylation (CIMP+/MSI-).

These new findings have focused the attention on the contributions of epigenetics to tumorigenesis, and there is growing evidence that epigenetically-mediated gene silencing can selectively produce loss of key functions in cancer (**Table 4**). An increasing number of cancer genes is being recognized with dense methylation in normally unmethylated promoter CpG islands [46].

Table 4: Genes hypermethylated in cancer

function	gene
cell cycle control	*Rb, p16 (INK4α), p15, p73, RARβ2*
DNA repair	*hMLH1, O^6MGMT, GSTP1, BRCA1*
apoptosis	*DAP-kinase, $p14^{ARF}$. APAF1, caspase-8, TMS1, PTEN*
cell adhesion and invasion	*E-cadherin, VHL, APC, TIMP3, thrombospondin1, HPP1*
growth factors	*estrogene receptor, androgene receptor, RASSF1A, endothelin-B-receptor*

New Hypothesis – The Serrated Pathway

Recently an alternative model of colorectal cancer pathogenesis has been proposed [51]. The so-called "serrated" pathway is assumed to be driven by inhibition of apoptosis and subsequent epigenetic inactivation of components of the DNA repair system. The earliest of such microscopic lesions of dysplasia called "aberrant crypt foci" (ACF) showed *k-ras* alterations in 68% [52]. In addition, none of the dysplastic lesions investigated had evidence of either *APC* or *β-catenin* inactivation. These data implicate that neither *k-ras* nor the *APC* pathway is necessarily involved in the initiation of colorectal cancer. It has been stated that the inhibition of apoptosis followed by the epigenetic inactivation of DNA repair mechanisms accounts for a significant proportion in hyperplastic polyps and serrated adenomas [51]. It has been shown that methylation of *hMLH1* was observed in some ACF and hyperplastic polyps indicating that silencing of the mismatch repair gene is an early event [53, 54].

Similarly, some data indicate a "serrated" pathway for MSI-L unstable cancers. These lesions tend to have alterations on chromosome 1p, *k-ras* mutations [51] and epigenetic silencing of the O^6-methylguanin-DNA-methyltransferase (O^6-MGMT) gene by promoter hypermethylation [55]. The function of this gene is to remove mutagenic methyl adducts from guanine nucleotides. In addition, these lesions have the typical features of serrated adenomas [56]. It is speculated that the down-regulation of the apoptosis receptor Fas (CD95) leads to loss of apoptosis in the lesions of the "serrated" pathway [57]. Furthermore, *k-ras* mutations are known to inhibit Fas expression [58]. It may be assumed that the disruption of apoptosis has a permissive role of further inactivation of the DNA repair system. This hypothesis needs to be confirmed, however.

Molecular/Genetic Profiles and Therapeutic Strategies

Sporadic colon tumors evolving through the "mutator" pathway are in general MSI-H through aberrant promoter methylation of *hMLH1* [40]. It has been shown that these cases tend to have a better prognosis in terms of overall survival compared to MSS tumors [26]. However, when treated with 5-Fluorouracil (5-FU) based chemotherapy it has been published recently that these tumors do not respond to treatment as well as MSS tumors [47]. There even seems to be a trend towards a poorer treatment response and survival in MSI-H tumors when subjected to 5-FU based chemotherapy which still remains the standard treatment regimen in colorectal cancers. We have shown in *in-vitro* studies that MSI-H colorectal cancer cell lines which are deficient in mismatch repair by either mutational inactivation or promoter hypermethylation of the *hMLH1* gene are resistant to 5-FU treatment compared to mismatch repair proficient cell lines by mechanisms which are currently not clearly understood [48, 49]. However, the insertion of an intact *hMLH1* gene by transfer of chromosome 3 restored mismatch repair function and rendered the cells sensible to 5-FU treatment. The same result was obtained by treatment with the DNA demethylating agent 2-deoxy-5-azacytidine in cells which were mismatch repair deficient through promoter hypermethylation of *hMLH1*. Through demethylation of the *hMLH1* gene these cells re-expressed *hMLH1* transcripts and protein after 24 hour treatment with the demethylating agent and regained sensitivity to 5-FU treatment (**Fig. 6**). This finding could open an elegant future treatment option for MSI-H sporadic colorectal cancers to first start a "sensitizing" treatment with a demethylating agent followed by a conventional treatment regimen.

These findings demonstrate the importance of future molecular characterisation of colorectal cancer especially in the setting of different sensitivity to chemotherapeutic agents. We conducted a study to optimize the characterisation of colorectal cancers evolving through the "mutator" pathway [50]. These tumors are currently defined by microsatellite analysis by the use of five consensus microsatellite markers which were defined on a conference of MSI in colorectal cancer of the National Cancer Institute (NCI) in 1998 [26]. We compared the ability of standard microsatellite analysis, *hMLH1* expression performed by immunohistochemistry and *hMLH1* promoter hypermethylation. A total of 27 MSI-H colorectal cancers were investigated. We found, that by simply using expression analysis or the promoter methylation study of the *hMLH1* gene, a significant number of MSI-H cancers might be missed compared to conventional microsatellite testing (**Table 5**). These findings suggest that both additional assays are not sufficiently reliable to detect all cancers undergoing the "mutator" pathway, or that there might exist additional mechanisms in the molecular pathogenesis of MSI-H cancers besides *hMLH1* inactivation.

Table 5: Correlation of MMR gene expression and methylation status in MSI-H cancers

Tumors	methylated	unmethylated	total
lack of hMLH1 expression	14 (93%)	1 (7%)	15
hMLH1 expression	5 (42%)	7 (58%)	12
total	19 (70%)	8 (30%)	27

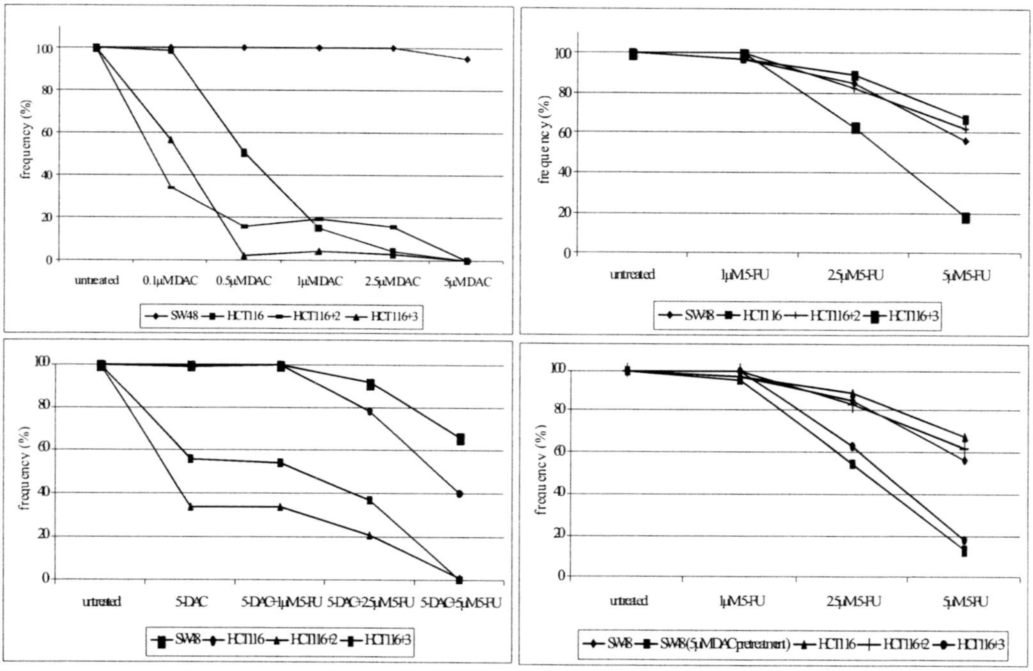

Fig. 6: 5-FU susceptibility of colorectal cancer cell lines. a) The colorectal cancer cell lines SW48, HCT116, HCT116+chr2 and HCT116+chr3 cells were cultivated in growth medium or exposed to 5 aza-dC for 24 h. The cell line SW48 is mismatch repair (MMR) deficient through promoter methylation of *hMLH1*, HCT116 is MMR deficient through biallelic deletion of *hMLH1*, HCT116 + chr3 is MMR proficient through chromosomal transfer containing the intact *hMLH1* gene, and HCT116+chr2 was used as a control cell line. Medium was exchanged and cells were allowed to form colonies over a period of 10-12 days. 5-DAC treatment alone did not cause a significant decrease in the growth of SW48 cells. On the contrary, 5-DAC caused a significant decrease in colony formation of HCT116 cells which was even stronger in the chromosome-transferred derivatives HCT116+chr2 and HCT116+chr3 b) Cells were continuously exposed to increasing concentrations of 5-FU over 10-12 days. After administration of 2.5 µM 5-FU, HCT116+chr3 cells responded with a 40% decrease in colony formation compared to 11% in HCT116, 17% in HCT116+chr2 and 15% in SW48 cells, respectively. HCT116+chr3 cells showed an 82% reduction in the clonal surviving fraction after 5 µM treatment, compared to a 33% reduction in HCT116, 38% in HCT116+chr2 and 44% in SW48 cells confirming the *in vitro* resistance of MMR deficient cell lines to 5-FU. c) Cells were pretreated with 0.1 µM 5-aza-dC for 24 h and then continuously exposed to various concentrations of 5-FU. Combined treatment showed synergistic cytotoxicity in all cell lines d) SW48 cells were pretreated with 5 µM 5 aza-dC for 24 h and then exposed to different doses of 5-FU (1µM, 2.5 µM, and 5 µM). HCT116, HCT116+ch2 and HCT116+ch3 cells were only treated with 5-FU. As expected, low dose 5-DAC treatment combined with 5-FU did not potentiate a decrease in colony forming ability in SW48 cells. However, growth curves were identical for SW48 and HCT116+chr3 cells after pretreatment with 5 µM 5-DAC and subsequent 5-FU treatment for SW48 cells and 5-FU treatment only for HCT116+chr3 cells, demonstrating that re-expression of *hMLH1* by promoter demethylation sensitizes SW48 cells to 5-FU chemotherapy *in vitro*.

4. Molecular Tests for Cancer Diagnosis and Prognosis

Insights in the molecular defects in colorectal cancer have not only elucidated the pathogenic role of such lesions but also facilitated molecular tools for early diagnosis, screening and prevention. Screening effectiveness depends in large parts on the accessibility and screening tools themselves. Several methods to search for colorectal cancer have been available for some time and have proved their efficacy in a number of controlled trials [59]. Screening strategies in stool-based tests have been performed for a long time, but have had only a modest effect in reducing the incidence of colorectal cancer due to low compliance, insufficient sensitivity and specificity as in fecal occult blood testing [60, 61].

Single Gene Tests

Much focus has been placed on molecular DNA-based stool tests which promise a much more accurate alternative than conventional methods of colorectal cancer screening. It has been shown that tumor DNA is stable in stool, can be extracted and further subjected to amplification by polymerase chain reaction (PCR) to screen for genetic alterations. The earliest of such studies concentrated on the detection of *k-ras* mutations [36]. This test is highly feasible and sensitive, because tumor *k-ras* mutations are easily detected in the stool and mainly occur at mutational "hot spots" such as codons 12 and 13. Its main limitation is the low sensitivity, as *k-ras* mutations occur only in up to 30-50% of colorectal cancers.

Another single gene study tested *APC* mutations in fecal DNA from patients with colorectal carcinoma [62]. Using the approach of digital protein truncation, the investigators identified *APC* alterations in 26 of 46 subjects with neoplasia (57%) and in none of the controls.

The same laboratory studied the microsatellite marker BAT26 in the feces of patients with proximal sporadic colorectal cancer [63]. Using a digital-PCR-based method they found that 18 of 46 investigated cancers had microsatellite alterations. Identical mutations could be identified in the stool in 17 out of these 18 cases. However, as stated in the above sections, genetic alterations in colorectal cancer are highly heterogeneous and multiple rather than single genes should be targeted to design a highly sensitive assay.

Multiple Gene Testing

A few such studies have been published (**Table 6**). Dong et al. used a panel of three genetic targets – *p53, k-ras,* and the microsatellite marker BAT-26 – to detect tumor associated alterations in the feces from patients with colorectal carcinoma [64]. The three alterations, which cover to some extend the "suppressor" and the "mutator" pathway, were able to detect 36 out of 51 (71%) patients with colorectal cancer.

Table 6: Multi targeted DNA-based stool tests for the detection of colorectal cancer

study	cases	DNA markers	sensitivity	specificity
Ahlquist 2000 [64]	22 cancers 11 adenomas 28 controls	*k-ras, p53, APC* *BAT 26, long-DNA*	91% (20/22) 82% (9/11)	93% (26/28)
Dong 2001 [63]	51 cancers	*k-ras, p53, BAT26*	71% (36/51)	not done
Calistri 2003 [65]	56 cancers 38 controls	*k-ras, p53, APC,* *5 MSI loci, long DNA*	51% (27/56) 59% (*long-DNA, k-ras and p53*)	97% (37/38)

A study conducted by Ahlquist et al. targeted mutations on *k-ras, APC* and *p53* as well as the MSI marker BAT-26 [65]. In addition, long DNA, which is exfoliated by nonapoptotic dysplastic colonocytes into the stool and is less degraded than DNA from healthy colonic mucosa, served as a molecular target. From the selected genes, "hot spot" mutations on the *k-ras, APC* and *p53* genes were targeted. The sensitivity of this study was 91% for colon cancers and 82% for adenomas. Specificity was 93%, increasing to 100% when *k-ras* was excluded.

Recently, a study by Calistri et al. was published investigating *p53* exons 5-8, *k-ras* exons 1-2, four fragments of *APC* exon 15, and 5 microsatelite loci in the feces and tumors of patients with colorectal cancers and healthy subjects, respectively [66]. Moreover, long DNA was evaluated for four exons of both *p53* and *APC*. The most frequent alterations in the tumors were *k-ras* (34%), *p53* (34%), MSI (13%) and *APC* mutations (13%). The most frequent mutational events in the stool were the detection of long DNA (51%), *k-ras* (11%), *p53* and MSI (6%) and *APC* (2%), respectively. Both *K-ras* and *p53* increased the sensitivity of long DNA to detect tumor cells to 59%. Interestingly, multiple molecular abnormalities in the feces of tumor patients were rarely found. Molecular alterations were not observed in the stool of healthy individuals except for one case with long-DNA demonstrating the high specificity of this assay.

DNA-based stool tests have the potential to achieve meaningful results compared to conventional colorectal cancer screening methods. Moreover, compared to fecal occult blood tests, DNA-based assay also have the potential to detect asymptomatic adenomas, most of which do not bleed or blood loss is intermittent [65]. However, apart from the already high specificity, sensitivity of these assays has to be improved to serve as a valid and reliable screening approach. DNA-based stool tests are currently developed but not yet commercially available.

Molecular Markers and Prognosis

Molecular markers have also been used to predict survival and response to chemotherapy. MSI-H cancers are generally believed to have a better overall prognosis in terms of disease free and overall survival when compared to MSS cancers [26]. The latter cancers tend to have a worse outcome once alterations on chromosome 18q are detected in stage III colorectal cancers [33]. Similarly, MSI-H cancers have a worse prognosis once mutations of the target gene TGFβ-RII are present. It has been shown, that in the *in-vitro* setting MSI-H colorectal cancer cell lines do not respond to 5-FU based chemotherapy, different to mismatch repair proficient cell lines [42, 49]. These findings have been confirmed in a retrospective study, showing that a) untreated MSI-H cancers have a better outcome than MSS cancers and b) 5-FU based chemotherapy does not improve the outcome of MSI-H colorectal cancers but rather deteriorates survival compared to MSS cancers [47]. MSI analysis may serve as a predictive factor in the future and might influence treatment strategies. This has been confirmed recently by a study investigating the tumor response to irinotecan [67]. Patients with MSI-H cancers responded significantly better than MSI-L or MSS tumors indicating that this treatment appears to be more suitable for colorectal cancers originating from the "mutator" pathway.

Another approach has been chosen by the laboratory group of B. Vogelstein [68]. They studied the role of chromosomal imbalances in 180 colorectal cancer patients with no evidence of lymph-node involvement or distant metastases. DNA from the tumors was tested for imbalances of chromosomes 8p and 18q by digital single-nucleotide polymorphisms (SNP). They found, that patients whose tumors retained alleles of both chromosomes had a 100% five year survival, compared to 74% of the cases whose tumors retained only one allele of 8p or 18q, and 58% of those who had allelic imbalances on both chromosomes, respectively. Most importantly, these findings were independent of tumor stage. Similar results were obtained by Barratt et al, showing that retention of heterozygosity at one or more 17p or 18p sites was associated with a benefit from adjuvant 5-FU chemotherapy [69].

In summary, the molecular characterisation of colorectal tumorigenesis has opened a wide spectrum of screening tools for early diagnosis and prevention of colorectal cancer. Several molecular markers have been defined and are currently under investigation to choose adequate treatment regimens and to predict survival. In general, molecular screening tests have to be compared with conventional screening methods and validated in prospective trials. Techniques have to be improved and methods need be cost-effective to serve as accessible tools for the practicing clinician.

REFERENCES

[1] Terdiman, J. P., Conrad, P. G., and Sleisenger, M. H. Genetic testing in hereditary colorectal cancer: indications and procedures. *Am.J.Gastroenterol., 94*: 2344-2356, 1999.

[2] Johns, L. E. and Houlston, R. S. A systematic review and meta-analysis of familial colorectal cancer risk. *Am.J.Gastroenterol.*, *96*: 2992-3003, 2001.

[3] Doll, R. and Peto, R. The causes of cancer: quantitative estimates of avoidable risks of cancer in the United States today. *J.Natl.Cancer Inst.*, *66*: 1191-1308, 1981.

[4] Potter, J. D. Nutrition and colorectal cancer. *Cancer Causes Control*, *7*: 127-146, 1996.

[5] Kinzler, K. W. and Vogelstein, B. Lessons from hereditary colorectal cancer. *Cell*, *87*: 159-170, 1996.

[6] Marra, G. and Boland, C. R. Hereditary nonpolyposis colorectal cancer: the syndrome, the genes, and historical perspectives. *J.Natl.Cancer Inst., 87*: 1114-1125, 1995.

[7] Groden, J., Thliveris, A., Samowitz, W., Carlson, M., Gelbert, L., Albertsen, H., Joslyn, G., Stevens, J., Spirio, L., Robertson, M., and . Identification and characterization of the familial adenomatous polyposis coli gene. *Cell, 66*: 589-600, 1991.

[8] Kinzler, K. W., Nilbert, M. C., Vogelstein, B., Bryan, T. M., Levy, D. B., Smith, K. J., Preisinger, A. C., Hamilton, S. R., Hedge, P., Markham, A., and . Identification of a gene located at chromosome 5q21 that is mutated in colorectal cancers. *Science, 251*: 1366-1370, 1991.

[9] Lynch, H. T. and Lynch, J. F. Genetics of colonic cancer. *Digestion, 59*: 481-492, 1998.

[10] Fearnhead, N. S., Britton, M. P., and Bodmer, W. F. The ABC of APC. *Hum.Mol.Genet., 10*: 721-733, 2001.

[11] Oving, I. M. and Clevers, H. C. Molecular causes of colon cancer. *Eur.J.Clin.Invest, 32*: 448-457, 2002.

[12] Burt, R. W. Colon cancer screening. *Gastroenterology, 119*: 837-853, 2000.

[13] Sieber, O. M., Lipton, L., Crabtree, M., Heinimann, K., Fidalgo, P., Phillips, R. K., Bisgaard, M. L., Orntoft, T. F., Aaltonen, L. A., Hodgson, S. V., Thomas, H. J., and Tomlinson, I. P. Multiple colorectal adenomas, classic adenomatous polyposis, and germ-line mutations in MYH. *N.Engl.J.Med., 348*: 791-799, 2003.

[14] Brensinger, J. D., Laken, S. J., Luce, M. C., Powell, S. M., Vance, G. H., Ahnen, D. J., Petersen, G. M., Hamilton, S. R., and Giardiello, F. M. Variable phenotype of familial adenomatous polyposis in pedigrees with 3' mutation in the APC gene. *Gut, 43*: 548-552, 1998.

[15] Spirio, L., Olschwang, S., Groden, J., Robertson, M., Samowitz, W., Joslyn, G., Gelbert, L., Thliveris, A., Carlson, M., Otterud, B., and . Alleles of the APC gene: an attenuated form of familial polyposis. *Cell, 75*: 951-957, 1993.

[16] Laken, S. J., Petersen, G. M., Gruber, S. B., Oddoux, C., Ostrer, H., Giardiello, F. M., Hamilton, S. R., Hampel, H., Markowitz, A., Klimstra, D., Jhanwar, S., Winawer, S., Offit, K., Luce, M. C., Kinzler, K. W., and Vogelstein, B. Familial colorectal cancer in Ashkenazim due to a hypermutable tract in APC. *Nat.Genet., 17*: 79-83, 1997.

[17] Giardiello, F. M., Brensinger, J. D., Petersen, G. M., Luce, M. C., Hylind, L. M., Bacon, J. A., Booker, S. V., Parker, R. D., and Hamilton, S. R. The use and interpretation of commercial APC gene testing for familial adenomatous polyposis. *N.Engl.J.Med., 336*: 823-827, 1997.

[18] Peinado, M. A., Malkhosyan, S., Velazquez, A., and Perucho, M. Isolation and characterization of allelic losses and gains in colorectal tumors by arbitrarily primed polymerase chain reaction. *Proc.Natl.Acad.Sci.U.S.A, 89*: 10065-10069, 1992.

[19] Ionov, Y., Peinado, M. A., Malkhosyan, S., Shibata, D., and Perucho, M. Ubiquitous somatic mutations in simple repeated sequences reveal a new mechanism for colonic carcinogenesis. *Nature, 363*: 558-561, 1993.

[20] Lynch, H. T. and de la, C. A. Hereditary colorectal cancer. *N.Engl.J.Med., 348*: 919-932, 2003.

[21] Peltomaki, P. DNA mismatch repair and cancer. *Mutat.Res., 488*: 77-85, 2001.

[22] Wu, Y., Berends, M. J., Post, J. G., Mensink, R. G., Verlind, E., van der, S. T., Kempinga, C., Sijmons, R. H., van der Zee, A. G., Hollema, H., Kleibeuker, J. H., Buys, C. H., and Hofstra, R. M. Germline mutations of EXO1 gene in patients with hereditary nonpolyposis colorectal cancer (HNPCC) and atypical HNPCC forms. *Gastroenterology*, *120*: 1580-1587, 2001.

[23] Wu, Y., Berends, M. J., Sijmons, R. H., Mensink, R. G., Verlind, E., Kooi, K. A., van der, S. T., Kempinga, C., dDer Zee, A. G., Hollema, H., Buys, C. H., Kleibeuker, J. H., and Hofstra, R. M. A role for MLH3 in hereditary nonpolyposis colorectal cancer. *Nat.Genet.*, *29*: 137-138, 2001.

[24] Kolodner, R. D., Tytell, J. D., Schmeits, J. L., Kane, M. F., Gupta, R. D., Weger, J., Wahlberg, S., Fox, E. A., Peel, D., Ziogas, A., Garber, J. E., Syngal, S., Anton-Culver, H., and Li, F. P. Germ-line msh6 mutations in colorectal cancer families. *Cancer Res.*, *59*: 5068-5074, 1999.

[25] Wijnen, J., de Leeuw, W., Vasen, H., van der, K. H., Moller, P., Stormorken, A., Meijers-Heijboer, H., Lindhout, D., Menko, F., Vossen, S., Moslein, G., Tops, C., Brocker-Vriends, A., Wu, Y., Hofstra, R., Sijmons, R., Cornelisse, C., Morreau, H., and Fodde, R. Familial endometrial cancer in female carriers of MSH6 germline mutations. *Nat.Genet.*, *23*: 142-144, 1999.

[26] Boland, C. R., Thibodeau, S. N., Hamilton, S. R., Sidransky, D., Eshleman, J. R., Burt, R. W., Meltzer, S. J., Rodriguez-Bigas, M. A., Fodde, R., Ranzani, G. N., and Srivastava, S. A National Cancer Institute Workshop on Microsatellite Instability for cancer detection and familial predisposition: development of international criteria for the determination of microsatellite instability in colorectal cancer. *Cancer Res.*, *58*: 5248-5257, 1998.

[27] Calvert, P. M. and Frucht, H. The genetics of colorectal cancer. *Ann.Intern.Med.*, *137*: 603-612, 2002.

[28] Grady, W. M. Genetic testing for high-risk colon cancer patients. *Gastroenterology*, *124*: 1574-1594, 2003.

[29] Yan, H., Papadopoulos, N., Marra, G., Perrera, C., Jiricny, J., Boland, C. R., Lynch, H. T., Chadwick, R. B., de la, C. A., Berg, K., Eshleman, J. R., Yuan, W., Markowitz, S., Laken, S. J., Lengauer, C., Kinzler, K. W., and Vogelstein, B. Conversion of diploidy to haploidy. *Nature*, *403*: 723-724, 2000.

[30] Fearon, E. R. and Vogelstein, B. A genetic model for colorectal tumorigenesis. *Cell*, *61*: 759-767, 1990.

[31] Vogelstein, B., Fearon, E. R., Hamilton, S. R., Kern, S. E., Preisinger, A. C., Leppert, M., Nakamura, Y., White, R., Smits, A. M., and Bos, J. L. Genetic alterations during colorectal-tumor development. *N.Engl.J.Med.*, *319*: 525-532, 1988.

[32] Jen, J., Kim, H., Piantadosi, S., Liu, Z. F., Levitt, R. C., Sistonen, P., Kinzler, K. W., Vogelstein, B., and Hamilton, S. R. Allelic loss of chromosome 18q and prognosis in colorectal cancer. *N.Engl.J.Med.*, *331*: 213-221, 1994.

[33] Watanabe, T., Wu, T. T., Catalano, P. J., Ueki, T., Satriano, R., Haller, D. G., Benson, A. B., III, and Hamilton, S. R. Molecular predictors of survival after adjuvant chemotherapy for colon cancer. *N.Engl.J.Med.*, *344*: 1196-1206, 2001.

[34] Sasaki, M., Okamoto, M., Sato, C., Sugio, K., Soejima, J., Iwama, T., Ikeuchi, T., Tonomura, A., Miyaki, M., and Sasazuki, T. Loss of constitutional heterozygosity in colorectal tumors from patients with familial polyposis coli and those with nonpolyposis colorectal carcinoma. *Cancer Res.*, *49*: 4402-4406, 1989.

[35] Bos, J. L., Fearon, E. R., Hamilton, S. R., Verlaan-de Vries, M., van Boom, J. H., van der Eb, A. J., and Vogelstein, B. Prevalence of ras gene mutations in human colorectal cancers. *Nature*, *327*: 293-297, 1987.

[36] Sidransky, D., Tokino, T., Hamilton, S. R., Kinzler, K. W., Levin, B., Frost, P., and Vogelstein, B. Identification of ras oncogene mutations in the stool of patients with curable colorectal tumors. *Science*, *256*: 102-105, 1992.

[37] Lengauer, C., Kinzler, K. W., and Vogelstein, B. Genetic instabilities in human cancers. *Nature*, *396*: 643-649, 1998.

[38] Aaltonen, L. A., Peltomaki, P., Leach, F. S., Sistonen, P., Pylkkanen, L., Mecklin, J. P., Jarvinen, H., Powell, S. M., Jen, J., Hamilton, S. R., and . Clues to the pathogenesis of familial colorectal cancer. *Science*, *260*: 812-816, 1993.

[39] Thibodeau, S. N., Bren, G., and Schaid, D. Microsatellite instability in cancer of the proximal colon. *Science*, *260*: 816-819, 1993.

[40] Herman, J. G., Umar, A., Polyak, K., Graff, J. R., Ahuja, N., Issa, J. P., Markowitz, S., Willson, J. K., Hamilton, S. R., Kinzler, K. W., Kane, M. F., Kolodner, R. D., Vogelstein, B., Kunkel, T. A., and Baylin, S. B. Incidence and functional consequences of hMLH1 promoter hypermethylation in colorectal carcinoma. *Proc. Natl. Acad. Sci. U.S.A*, *95*: 6870-6875, 1998.

[41] Kane, M. F., Loda, M., Gaida, G. M., Lipman, J., Mishra, R., Goldman, H., Jessup, J. M., and Kolodner, R. Methylation of the hMLH1 promoter correlates with lack of expression of hMLH1 in sporadic colon tumors and mismatch repair-defective human tumor cell lines. *Cancer Res.*, *57*: 808-811, 1997.

[42] Arnold, C., Usadel, H., and Blum, H. E. Epigenetics: significance for tumor genesis and clinical features. *Dtsch.Med.Wochenschr.*, *127*: 1701-1703, 2002.

[43] Goel, A., Arnold, C. N., Niedzwiecki, D., Chang, D. K., Ricciardiello, L., Carethers, J. M., Dowell, J. M., Wasserman, L., Compton, C., Mayer, R. J., Bertagnolli, M. M., and Boland, C. R. Characterization of sporadic colon cancer by patterns of genomic instability. *Cancer Res.*, *63*: 1608-1614, 2003.

[44] Esteller, M., Corn, P. G., Baylin, S. B., and Herman, J. G. A gene hypermethylation profile of human cancer. *Cancer Res.*, *61*: 3225-3229, 2001.

[45] Toyota, M., Ahuja, N., Ohe-Toyota, M., Herman, J. G., Baylin, S. B., and Issa, J. P. CpG island methylator phenotype in colorectal cancer. *Proc.Natl.Acad.Sci.U.S.A*, *96*: 8681-8686, 1999.

[46] Esteller, M. Epigenetic lesions causing genetic lesions in human cancer: promoter hypermethylation of DNA repair genes. *Eur.J.Cancer*, *36*: 2294-2300, 2000.

[47] Ribic, C. M., Sargent, D. J., Moore, M. J., Thibodeau, S. N., French, A. J., Goldberg, R. M., Hamilton, S. R., Laurent-Puig, P., Gryfe, R., Shepherd, L. E., Tu, D., Redston, M., and Gallinger, S. Tumor microsatellite-instability status as a predictor of benefit from fluorouracil-based adjuvant chemotherapy for colon cancer. *N.Engl.J.Med.*, *349*: 247-257, 2003.

[48] Arnold, C. N., Goel, A., and Boland, C. R. Role of hMLH1 promoter hypermethylation in drug resistance to 5-fluorouracil in colorectal cancer cell lines. *Int.J.Cancer, 106*: 66-73, 2003.

[49] Carethers, J. M., Chauhan, D. P., Fink, D., Nebel, S., Bresalier, R. S., Howell, S. B., and Boland, C. R. Mismatch repair proficiency and in vitro response to 5-fluorouracil. *Gastroenterology, 117*: 123-131, 1999.

[50] Arnold, C. N., Goel, A., Compton, C., Marcus, V., Niedzwiecki, D., Dowell, J. M., Wasserman, L., Inoue, T., Mayer, R. J., Bertagnolli, M. M., and Boland, C. R. Evaluation of microsatellite instability, hMLH1 expression and hMLH1 promoter hypermethylation in defining the MSI phenotype of colorectal cancer. *Canc.Biol.Therapy, 3*: 2004, accepted for publication

[51] Jass, J. R., Whitehall, V. L., Young, J., and Leggett, B. A. Emerging concepts in colorectal neoplasia. *Gastroenterology, 123*: 862-876, 2002.

[52] Takayama, T., Ohi, M., Hayashi, T., Miyanishi, K., Nobuoka, A., Nakajima, T., Satoh, T., Takimoto, R., Kato, J., Sakamaki, S., and Niitsu, Y. Analysis of K-ras, APC, and beta-catenin in aberrant crypt foci in sporadic adenoma, cancer, and familial adenomatous polyposis. *Gastroenterology, 121*: 599-611, 2001.

[53] Hawkins, N. J. and Ward, R. L. Sporadic colorectal cancers with microsatellite instability and their possible origin in hyperplastic polyps and serrated adenomas. *J.Natl.Cancer Inst., 93*: 1307-1313, 2001.

[54] Jass, J. R., Young, J., and Leggett, B. A. Hyperplastic polyps and DNA microsatellite unstable cancers of the colorectum. *Histopathology, 37*: 295-301, 2000.

[55] Whitehall, V. L., Walsh, M. D., Young, J., Leggett, B. A., and Jass, J. R. Methylation of O-6-methylguanine DNA methyltransferase characterizes a subset of colorectal cancer with low-level DNA microsatellite instability. *Cancer Res., 61*: 827-830, 2001.

[56] Jass, J. R., Biden, K. G., Cummings, M. C., Simms, L. A., Walsh, M., Schoch, E., Meltzer, S. J., Wright, C., Searle, J., Young, J., and Leggett, B. A. Characterisation of a subtype of colorectal cancer combining features of the suppressor and mild mutator pathways. *J.Clin.Pathol., 52*: 455-460, 1999.

[57] Tateyama, H., Li, W., Takahashi, E., Miura, Y., Sugiura, H., and Eimoto, T. Apoptosis index and apoptosis-related antigen expression in serrated adenoma of the colorectum: the saw-toothed structure may be related to inhibition of apoptosis. *Am.J.Surg.Pathol., 26*: 249-256, 2002.

[58] Fenton, R. G., Hixon, J. A., Wright, P. W., Brooks, A. D., and Sayers, T. J. Inhibition of Fas (CD95) expression and Fas-mediated apoptosis by oncogenic Ras. *Cancer Res., 58*: 3391-3400, 1998.

[59] Ransohoff, D. F. and Sandler, R. S. Clinical practice. Screening for colorectal cancer. *N.Engl.J.Med., 346*: 40-44, 2002.

[60] Mandel, J. S., Bond, J. H., Church, T. R., Snover, D. C., Bradley, G. M., Schuman, L. M., and Ederer, F. Reducing mortality from colorectal cancer by screening for fecal occult blood. Minnesota Colon Cancer Control Study. *N.Engl.J.Med., 328*: 1365-1371, 1993.

[61] Mandel, J. S., Church, T. R., Ederer, F., and Bond, J. H. Colorectal cancer mortality: effectiveness of biennial screening for fecal occult blood. *J.Natl.Cancer Inst., 91*: 434-437, 1999.

[62] Traverso, G., Shuber, A., Levin, B., Johnson, C., Olsson, L., Schoetz, DJ., Hamilton, S. R., Boynton, K., Kinzler, K. W., and Vogelstein, B. Detection of APC mutations in fecal DNA from patients with colorectal tumors. *N.Engl.J.Med., 346*: 311-320, 2002.

[63] Traverso, G., Shuber, A., Olsson, L., Levin, B., Johnson, C., Hamilton, S. R., Boynton, K., Kinzler, K. W., and Vogelstein, B. Detection of proximal colorectal cancers through analysis of faecal DNA. *Lancet, 359*: 403-404, 2002.

[64] Dong, S. M., Traverso, G., Johnson, C., Geng, L., Favis, R., Boynton, K., Hibi, K., Goodman, S. N., D'Allessio, M., Paty, P., Hamilton, S. R., Sidransky, D., Barany, F., Levin, B., Shuber, A., Kinzler, K. W., Vogelstein, B., and Jen, J. Detecting colorectal cancer in stool with the use of multiple genetic targets. *J.Natl.Cancer Inst., 93*: 858-865, 2001.

[65] Ahlquist, D. A., Skoletsky, J. E., Boynton, K. A., Harrington, J. J., Mahoney, D. W., Pierceall, W. E., Thibodeau, S. N., and Shuber, A. P. Colorectal cancer screening by detection of altered human DNA in stool: feasibility of a multitarget assay panel. *Gastroenterology, 119*: 1219-1227, 2000.

[66] Calistri, D., Rengucci, C., Bocchini, R., Saragoni, L., Zloi, W., and Amadori, D. Fecal multiple molecular tests to detect colorectal cancer in stool. *Clin.Gastro.Hepatol.*, 1: 377-383, 2003.

[67] Fallik, D., Borrini, F., Boige, V., Viguier, J., Jacob, S., Miquel, C., Sabourin, J. C., Ducreux, M., and Praz, F. Microsatellite instability is a predictive factor of the tumor response to irinotecan in patients with advanced colorectal cancer. *Cancer Res., 63*: 5738-5744, 2003.

[68] Zhou, W., Goodman, S. N., Galizia, G., Lieto, E., Ferraraccio, F., Pignatelli, C., Purdie, C. A., Piris, J., Morris, R., Harrison, D. J., Paty, P. B., Culliford, A., Romans, K. E., Montgomery, E. A., Choti, M. A., Kinzler, K. W., and Vogelstein, B. Counting alleles to predict recurrence of early-stage colorectal cancers. *Lancet, 359*: 219-225, 2002.

[69] Barratt, P. L., Seymour, M. T., Stenning, S. P., Georgiades, I., Walker, C., Birbeck, K., and Quirke, P. DNA markers predicting benefit from adjuvant fluorouracil in patients with colon cancer: a molecular study. *Lancet, 360*: 1381-91, 2002.

In: Focus on Colorectal Cancer Research
Editor: Julia D. Martinez, pp. 25-40
ISBN #1-59454-101-9

Chapter II

PROTECTIVE EFFECT OF PHYSICAL ACTIVITY ON THE OCCURRENCE OF COLORECTAL CANCER

Wieslaw Jedrychowski[1,*], Karen Steindorf[2], Martina Schmidt[2], Juergen Wahrendorf[2] and Agnieszka Penar[1]

[1]Chair of Epidemiology and Preventive Medicine, Jagiellonian University, Coll. Med. 7, Kopernika street, Krakow, Poland.

[2]Unit of Environmental Epidemiology, German Cancer Research Center, Im Neuenheimer Feld 280, Heidelberg, Germany.

ABSTRACT

Background

The principal goal of our study was to assess how physical activity performed in different life periods is associated with the risk of colorectal cancer, since it is unclear whether activity performed in early or later life are real determinants of risk reduction.

Methods

In total 239 incident cases of colorectal cancer confirmed by histopathology and 239 controls, matched to cases by age (+/- 5 years) and gender, were enrolled. Controls were chosen from amongst patients with no history of cancer from the same hospital and admitted for treatment for non-neoplastic conditions unrelated to digestive tract diseases. Data on occupational and recreational physical activity were collected in standardized interviews for the ages 20 through 30, 40, 50, and 60 years. Besides lifestyle and socio-demographic characteristics, such as education, occupation, and lifetime smoking, the

* Address corresponds to: Wieslaw Jedrychowski, Chair of Epidemiology and Preventive Medicine, Jagiellonian University, Coll. Med. 7, Kopernika street, Krakow, Poland. Tel: +48-12-423-1003, Fax +48-12-422-8795, E-mail: myjedryc@cyf-kr.edu.pl

usual dietary pattern for 148 beverage and food items was assessed within a food frequency questionnaire.

Results

Median values of total physical activity based on MET-hours/week were consistently lower in cases than in controls at each age. In multivariate conditional logistic regression, the highest quartile of total physical activity compared with the lowest quartile yielded odds ratios below one for each age and for total lifetime. The adjusted odds ratio (OR) for total lifetime was 0.53 (95% confidence interval (CI): 0.30-0.94) for the highest quartile. In the age-specific analyses, the risk reduction was significant only for age 30 (OR = 0.45; CI: 0.25 – 0.79). We did not observe relevant confounding effects by body mass index, total energy intake, total fiber intake, lifetime smoking, and alcohol intake.

Conclusion

These data underline the protective role of physical activity in colorectal cancer etiology. Our finding on a more pronounced effect in young adulthood around age 30 might have implications for health education.

Key words: colorectal cancer, physical activity, case-control study

INTRODUCTION

Colorectal cancer is one of the leading causes of death from malignancies in most of western countries. Although a genetic component in the etiology of colon cancer is well established, wide differences in cancer rates between countries and changes in rates among migrants point to diet and western lifestyle as potentially important factors. Dietary factors that may explain most of the variation in rates among countries have yet not been proven, but evidence suggest that diet high in fruits and vegetables may be protective against the risk of this cancer. Among the specific factors in fruits and vegetables that have been examined in relation to cancer, present data most strongly support a benefit of higher folic acid consumption in reducing risk of colon cancer.

Since it was first suggested by Huseman et al. in 1980 [1] and Garabrant et al. in 1984 [2] that a sedentary occupation for males was a risk factor for colon cancer, interest in physical activity as a means for the primary prevention of colorectal cancer grew rapidly and provided a good body of evidence. Both retrospective case-control studies and prospective cohort studies consistently indicated a protective effect for physical activity in relation to colon cancer, in both men and women. Although the methods for assessing physical activity for both occupational and recreational activity were different and sometimes very simple and different study designs and population groups were used, a consistent reduction in risk has worldwide been demonstrated [3]. Occupational studies have examined usual lifetime occupation, while most other studies have examined activity levels two to three years prior to diagnosis. There were few attempts to distinguish the role of different types of activities (occupational vs. leisure time activity) in the colon cancer etiology. While physical activity in leisure time is very often intensive (sport) but performed over short periods of time and irregular, occupational activity is normally less intensive but systematic and performed for long periods. The lifetime period at which physical activity may have its greatest impact was not considered in most of the studies either.

Physical activity could be associated with cancer risk either indirectly through other correlated factors (confounding) or through real biological mechanisms. Up to now there is no good understanding of the biological role of physical activity in colorectal cancer as physical activity may be a marker of a healthy lifestyle. To convert the scientific evidence into public health policy guidelines we should better understand the etiological role of physical activity in colon cancer embedded in a multifactorial causation web. To fill up these gaps in our knowledge, more data must be accumulated on the risk reduction resulting from specific types of physical activity and its pattern over various life periods.

Our study aimed to assess detailed data on lifetime recreational and occupational physical activity in combination with a detailed assessment of dietary and other lifestyle factors. The principal goal of our study was to assess how physical activity performed in different life periods is associated with risk of colorectal cancer, since it is unclear whether risk reductions are more determined by activity performed in early or in later life.

Material and Methods

The hospital-based case-control study of colorectal cancer was carried out between January 2000 and November 2003 in Krakow, Poland. In total 239 incident cases of colorectal cancer confirmed by histopathology were enrolled from the First Surgical Clinic of the University Hospital in Krakow. Controls were chosen from amongst patients with no history of cancer from the same hospital and admitted for treatment for acute non-neoplastic conditions unrelated to digestive tract diseases, matched to cases by age (+/- 5 years) and gender. Of these, 58.8% were admitted for cardiovascular diseases, 12.2% for respiratory disorders, 9.5% for traumas (mostly fractures), 8.1% for diseases of the musculoskeletal system, 6.6% for blood diseases, 2.6% for endocrinological disorders, and 2.2% for acute surgical conditions. Trained interviewers used a standardized questionnaire to interview both the cases and controls. The section of the questionnaire on lifestyle included information on socio-demographic characteristics, such as education and occupation, lifetime smoking and alcohol drinking habits, occupational and leisure activity, and personal medical history.

An interviewer-administered food frequency questionnaire (FFQ) combined with an assessment of quantity of foods eaten was used to assess the usual dietary pattern for 148 beverage and food items. For each food or beverage item, a commonly used unit or portion size was specified, and participants were asked how often, on average, they consumed that amount of each food during one year. A computer program was used to calculate the nutrient content of the specified portion, using composition values from the Polish Institute of Nutrition [4-7]. The data on frequency and amount of various alcohol beverages were used to calculate the total consumption of pure alcohol in grams per day. The dietary interview focused on the reference period that was defined as one year prior to 5 years before diagnosis for cases or prior to the corresponding date of hospital admission for the controls.

The dietary part of the questionnaire included detailed information on dietary habits relating to the following food groups: cereals, milk, bread, fat used for bread, processed meats and fish, milk products and eggs, fresh fruits (summer/autumn), fresh fruits (winter/spring), meats (beef, pork), chicken, kind of fat used for baking and frying, salads and fresh and cooked vegetables, potatoes (mashed/baked), rice or pasta, soups, sweets, baked goods, etc.

Physical activity from occupational and recreational activities was assessed over whole lifetime, starting from age 20 through 30, 40, 50, and 60 years. Occupational physical activity data were ascertained during interview and the level was assessed by the interviewee and not by interviewer. Occupational physical activity was divided into four categories: no occupational activity or light work in sitting position, work in standing position, moderate occupational work, and heavy manual work being performed on most days in a week. For leisure time physical activity participants reported the average time per week spent in each age for the following activities: walking or hiking, bicycling, gardening, practicing sport or household activities. Leisure time activities were assessed for summer and winter separately. The reported time spent at each activity per week was multiplied by its typical energy expenditure requirements expressed in metabolic equivalents (METs) [8-10] and added together to yield an MET-hours per week score.

Statistical Analysis

Beyond standard descriptive statistics, conditional logistic regression models were used to estimate odds ratios and the corresponding 95% confidence intervals of colorectal cancer. In addition to univariate models, multiple regression analyses were applied to allow for adjustment. As potential confounding variables we investigated body mass index (<25, 25-<30, ≥30), total energy intake, fiber intake, calcium intake, alcohol intake, and smoking habits (lifetime pack-years). For most calculations the physical activity variables in MET-hours/week were categorized into quartiles. Quartiles were derived from the distribution in the control group. Linear trends were tested by entering the exposure variables as continuous variables in the models. Total physical activity was analyzed for each age separately, as well as for the whole lifetime where the individual mean value of total physical activity over all reported ages was calculated. The statistical software package SAS (version 8) was used, predominantly the procedure PROC PHREG.

Table 1: Characteristics and potential colorectal cancer risk factors for cases and controls in a case-control study of colorectal cancer in Poland, 2000-2003

	Cases (N=239)		Controls (N=239)		OR*	95% CI*
	N	%	N	%		
Gender:						
Males	129	53.97	129	53.97	-†	-
Females	110	46.03	110	46.03	-	-
Age:						
< 45 years	30	12.55	27	11.30	-†	-
45 – 54	60	25.10	69	28.87	-	-
55 – 64	91	38.08	82	34.31	-	-
≥ 65	58	24.27	61	25.52	-	-
Education:						
None/Primary/Vocational	94	39.33	130	54.39	1.0	-
Technical/Secondary	76	31.80	70	29.29	1.52	0.99-2.32
Bachelor/University	69	28.87	39	16.32	2.46	1.53-3.95
Smoking:						
Never smokers	113	47.28	90	37.66	1.0	-
Ex-smokers	65	27.20	63	26.36	0.76	0.47-1.23
Current smokers	61	25.52	86	35.98	0.51	0.32-0.81
Total energy intake [kcal/day] ‡:						
≤ 1665	46	19.25	60	25.10	1.0	-
> 1665 - 2151	65	27.20	60	25.10	1.42	0.84-2.39
> 2151 - 2911	78	32.64	60	25.10	1.70	1.00-2.89
> 2911	50	20.92	59	24.69	1.10	0.61-1.98
Total fibre intake [g/day] ‡:						
≤ 3.49	52	21.76	60	25.10	1.0	-
> 3.49 – 4.33	53	22.18	60	25.10	1.02	0.60-1.72
> 4.33 – 5.88	78	32.64	60	25.10	1.50	0.91-2.48
> 5.88	56	23.43	59	24.69	1.09	0.64-1.84
Alcohol intake [g/day] ‡:						
≤ 0.39	42	17.57	60	25.10	1.0	-
> 0.39 – 0.77	54	22.59	60	25.10	1.33	0.77-2.29
> 0.77 – 3.55	72	30.13	60	25.10	1.85	1.08-3.17
> 3.55	71	29.71	59	24.69	2.04	1.12-3.74
Body Mass Index						
Underweight or normal weight	65	27.20	73	37.63	1.0	-
Overweight	110	46.03	73	37.63	1.68	1.07-2.64
Obese	64	26.78	48	24.74	1.49	0.90-2.46
Missing	0	0	45	-		

* OR, odds ratio; CI, confidence interval.

† Matching variable.

‡ In quartiles based on controls.

RESULTS

The material included 239 cases and an equal number of controls matched to cases by age and gender. In each group there were 129 males and 110 females. For the whole population, ages ranged from 19 to 74 years. The mean age was 56.47 years (standard deviation (sd): 9.56) for the cases and 56.68 years (sd: 10.04) for the controls. Table 1 presents the cross-tabulation of cases and controls by age, education, smoking habit, total energy intake, total fiber intake and alcohol. Colorectal cancer cases displayed a higher education level, reported about the same amount of energy and fiber intake, but slightly higher alcohol intake than controls. Among colorectal cancer cases there was a higher proportion of persons with overweight (46.0% vs. 37.6 %).

In table 2 the distribution of total physical activity based on MET-hours/week in cases and controls at different ages is presented. Both cases and controls showed a decreasing trend in physical activity with age. Median values of total physical activity were consistently lower in cases than in controls for each age group.

Table 2: Distribution of total physical activity in cases and controls at different ages based on MET*-hours/week assessed in a case-control study of colorectal cancer in Poland, 2000-2003

Characteristics	Cases (N=239)			Controls (N=239)		
	n[†]	Median	Q1*; Q3*	n	Median	Q1; Q3
Lifetime activity	238	104.9	55.4; 173.8	193	123.5	74.3; 200.0
Physical activity by age						
Age 20	238	121.0	50.0; 204.5	193	141.6	63.5; 214.5
Age 30	236	109.8	52.5; 179.0	189	150.6	78.0; 220.0
Age 40	214	105.0	48.0; 180.0	171	138.3	60.0; 214.0
Age 50	154	78.38	42.0; 144.0	108	117.8	40.0; 202.8

* MET, metabolic equivalent; Q1, 1st quartile; Q3, 3rd quartile.
[†] Number of persons who reached that age and had non-missing values.

Table 3 gives the odds ratios for colorectal cancer and level of total physical activity in MET-hours per week for each age and for the whole lifetime. For the highest quartile of total physical activity odds ratio estimates are below one for all ages as well as for total lifetime. Multivariate adjusted odds ratios (OR) of colorectal cancer for quartiles of total lifetime physical activity (from low to high) were 1.0, 0.67 (95% CI: 0.39 – 1.16), 0.70 (95% CI: 0.40 – 1.20), and 0.53 (95% CI: 0.30 – 0.94). In the age-specific analyses, the risk reduction was significant only for age group 30, where the adjusted risk estimate for the highest quartile of physical activity was OR= 0.45 (95% confidence interval (CI): 0.25 – 0.79). For moderate high levels of physical activity ORs were also significantly lower at age 30 (OR=0.55, 95% CI: 0.32 – 0.95). The multivariate model yielded virtually the same results as the univariate model indicating no confounding effects of body mass index, total energy intake, total fiber intake, lifetime smoking, and alcohol intake.

Table 3: Univariate and multivariate odds ratios and 95% confidence intervals for colorectal cancer for total physical activity in MET*-hours/week at different ages. Case-control study of colorectal cancer in Poland, 2000-2003

Characteristics Quartiles † of physical activity	Cases (N=239)	Controls (N=239)	Unadjusted ‡		Multivariate adjusted ᑫ	
			OR*	95% CI*	OR	95% CI
Lifetime						
1 (low)	82	49	1.0	-	1.0	-
2	57	48	0.71	0.42-1.20	0.67	0.39-1.16
3	58	48	0.72	0.43-1.22	0.70	0.40-1.20
4 (high)	41	48	0.52	0.30-0.89	0.53	0.30-0.94
p-value for trend				0.08		0.10
Age 20						
1 (low)	75	49	1.0	-	1.0	-
2	64	48	0.86	0.51-1.45	0.87	0.50-1.48
3	52	48	0.71	0.42-1.21	0.70	0.40-1.21
4 (high)	47	48	0.63	0.37-1.08	0.68	0.38-1.20
p-value for trend				0.33		0.43
Age 30						
1 (low)	93	48	1.0	-	1.0	-
2	51	47	0.56	0.33-0.95	0.55	0.32-0.96
3	53	47	0.59	0.35-0.99	0.55	0.32-0.95
4 (high)	39	47	0.43	0.25-0.74	0.45	0.25-0.79
p-value for trend				0.01		0.01
Age 40						
1 (low)	64	44	1.0	-	1.0	-
2	60	42	0.98	0.57-1.71	0.85	0.48-1.52
3	52	43	0.83	0.48-1.45	0.78	0.43-1.40
4 (high)	38	42	0.62	0.35-1.11	0.58	0.32-1.07
p-value for trend				0.11		0.11
Age 50						
1 (low)	38	28	1.0	-	1.0	-
2	51	26	1.47	0.74-2.93	1.38	0.67-2.86
3	40	27	1.15	0.57-2.30	1.05	0.50-2.19
4 (high)	25	27	0.72	0.35-1.50	0.81	0.36-1.78
p-value for trend				0.43		0.58

* MET, metabolic equivalent; OR, odds ratio; CI, confidence interval.

† Quartiles based on controls, values are presented in table 2.

‡ Models adjusted for matching variables age and gender.

ᑫ Models additionally adjusted for BMI (<25, 25-<30, ≥30), total energy intake, fiber intake, smoking in pack-years, and alcohol consumption.

Discussion

These results confirm our first case-control colorectal cancer study conducted in the period 1998-1999 [55] which showed a twofold reduction in the risk of colorectal cancer among patients with higher physical activity, either in occupational or recreational hours, after adjustment for confounding effects of dietary factors (figure 1). Our first study has demonstrated that the adjusted risk of colorectal cancer was reduced by half in those persons who were active in leisure time (OR = 0.45, 95% CI: 0.24 – 0.84). The effect of occupational physical activity was about the same order of magnitude in terms of risk reduction (OR = 0.61; 95% CI: 0.29 – 1.29) and both activities combined acted as independent protective factors. Combined effects of high activity in working hours and in leisure time appeared to be in agreement with a multiplicative model on the relative risk scale. As neither moderate occupational physical activity nor moderate leisure time activity was associated with significant risk reduction, it could be deduced that vigorous physical activity might be necessary to reduce the risk. It is worthwhile to note that in our first study, for the assessment of physical activity we used self-reported levels of physical effort demanded in the occupational setting, and for the appraisal of physical activity in leisure time, recreational sedentary time expressed by the number of hours spent daily on watching TV was applied.

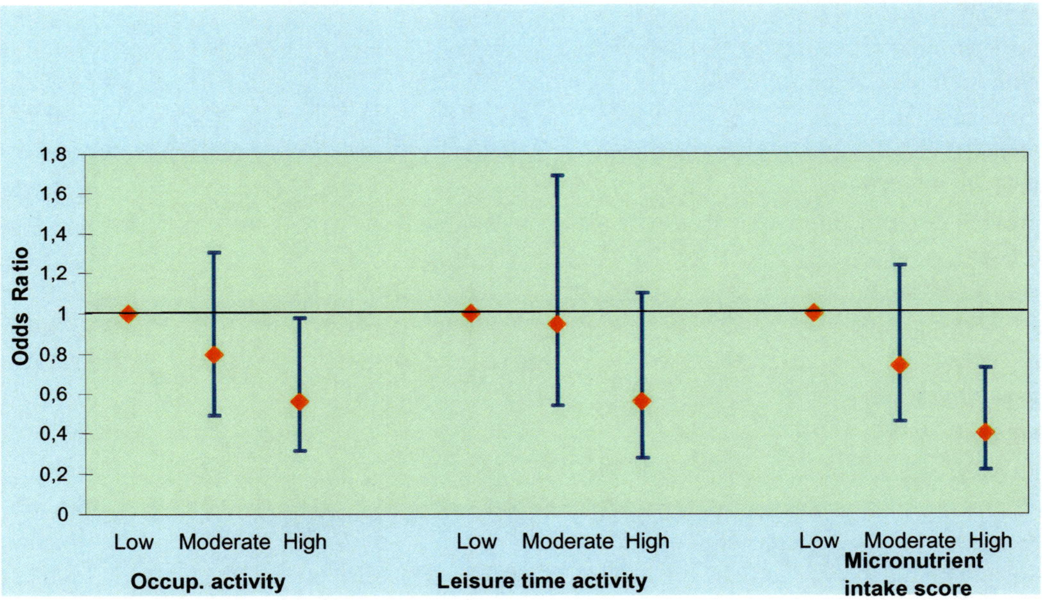

* Adjusted by education and total energy intake

Figure 1. Physical activity in occupation and leisure time and micronutrient intake (Odds Ratios and 95%-CI from multivariate* logistic model)

In our second case-control study presented here we used a much more detailed assessment of leisure time and occupational physical activity at different ages. This assessment allowed for derivation of metabolic equivalents (METs). This study confirms the consistent inverse relation between physical activity and colorectal cancer and provides more substance for the evidence in favour of a protective effect at higher levels of physical activity. Possible confounding effects of nutrition appeared to be of minor importance. On the basis of our two case-control hospital-based studies we may conclude that the results of our both studies support the hypothesis that a high level of physical activity either in occupational setting or in leisure time can result in a protective effect against colorectal cancer and that this effect is independent of nutrient intake. The study presented here suggests that the significant protective effect is more related to physical efforts in young adulthood around age 30. For 75% of our cases this refers to a period more than 20 years before the cancer diagnosis. This may have important practical implications for health education and primary prevention.

Combining colon cancer and rectal cancer together could dilute risk estimates since many authors deny the protective effect of physical effort on rectal cancer. However, there are data supporting the evidence that the beneficial effect of physical activity in terms of reduced risk was similar to that observed for colon cancer [26, 36, 54, 56, 57]. One of these studies is the study by Slattery et al. [57] who examined the association between physical activity and rectal cancer and compared this association to the one obtained for colon cancer. Data were collected using identical methods to recruit and interview cases and controls to eliminate the possibility of associations being the result of different physical activity questionnaires. The sample size of 925 cases and 1 205 controls was adequate to precisely estimate associations for men and women. The authors concluded that vigorous physical activity was associated with reduced risk of rectal cancer in both men and women (OR=0.60; 95% CI: 0.44-0.81 for men and OR=0.59; 95% CI: 0.40 - 0.86 for women). Among men, moderate levels of physical activity also were associated with reduced risk of rectal cancer (OR=0.70, 95% CI: 0.51-0.97). Participation in vigorous activity over the past 20 years conferred the greatest protection for both men and women (OR=0.55, 95% CI: 0.39-0.78 for men; OR=0.44; 95% CI: 0.30-0.67 for women). These data support strongly the evidence that the reduced risk was similar to that observed for colon cancer.

Our results of colorectal cancer are in agreement with most of the studies conducted on the protective effect of physical activity against colorectal cancer. Some of the studies have examined only colon cancer, and others have included colorectal cancers. The association held true for both men and women. Up to now, out of the 49 studies on colorectal cancer and physical activity [11-58] conducted world-wide 19 have not demonstrated a significant and clear reduction in risk of cancer among the most physically active study participants. Of particular interest is that in both cohort and case-control studies, an association was found when lifelong levels of physical activity were measured, while in studies which measured relatively recent physical activity only, the relationship was either weak or absent. There was a large variation in risk reduction estimates from different studies (in the range of 20-70%), and the average reduction was 40–50%.

Although the methods for assessing physical activity have varied among studies and have often been very simple, a considerable reduction in risk was observed in different study designs, population groups and for both occupational and recreational activity. Furthermore, a consistent dose-response relation was found in 19 studies that examined the trend in risk.

Generally, the association was strong and appears not to be confounded by diet, body mass index, and other risk factors that have been examined and controlled for in these analyses.

On the whole, study results point out that intense activity rather than its moderate level may be protective against colorectal cancer. Although it is possible that intense activity leads to better stimulation of biological reactions in comparison with moderate levels of activity, however, study participants may report intense physical activity in a much better way. Although long-term physical activity appears to be a significant predictor of colorectal cancer risk, however, it is not clear whether more active persons report their activity more accurately, or whether long-term physical activity increases protection over a long period of time. In fact, data support the better long-term recall of intense activities than of moderate activities [59], and this eventually could attenuate the risk estimation of moderate physical effort due to misclassification bias. An appraisal of cases and controls on eventual lessen ability to exercise because of illness suggests that cases do not report lower levels of past activities as a result of the tumor itself [60].

The studies have differed in types and the number of confounding variables considered for adjustment of observed association between colorectal cancer and physical activity. The studies that adjusted for factors such as body size, diet, age, cigarette smoking have not shown that this relationship was confounded to a great extent. Having in mind the strength and consistency of the relationship between colorectal cancer and physical effort, it seems not likely that confounding could change much of the established association. Interestingly, studies evaluating effect modification have shown that physical activity may most importantly reduce risk of colon cancer if a high-energy intake, a high glycaemic index or large body size are present [50].

As mentioned earlier, a great variation in risk reduction of colorectal cancer due to physical activity could result from various methods used in these studies. Some study populations have included occupational, some other hospital-based or population-based samples. Moreover, physical activity has been defined as occupational activity, ranging from a job title to a detailed lifetime history of actual occupational activities. Recreational activity ranged from simple assessments to detailed descriptions of physical efforts recorded for different types of activities. Sometimes data on physical activity have been extracted from existing records or have been based on interview-administered questionnaires. The time period for physical activity assessment has ranged from current activity to an attempt in assessing the lifetime physical activity. Mostly, there was a limited standardization of the methodology used for assessing physical activity; therefore some of the discrepancy in the study results is attributable to the large variations in the measurement of the exposures. Another possible explanation for the large variation across studies is the different definition of types of activity that have been performed by the study participants.

The primary postulated biological mechanism is that physical activity reduces intestinal transit time, and subsequently shortens the duration of contact between the colon mucosa and cancer promoting colon contents. The beneficial effect of exercise on colon motility has been demonstrated in experiments in animal models [61] and in humans [62]. Enhancing intestinal transit time may also indirectly affect the risk of colon cancer by lowering secondary bile acid concentration or by increasing fecal short chain fatty acids [62]. The studies on the effect of physical activity and colon transit time are consistent with results of the recent epidemiologic study showing that moderate physical activity and fiber intake are associated with substantial reductions in the prevalence of constipation [63]. Dukas and colleagues found that women who reported daily physical activity had a lower prevalence ratio (PR) of constipation (PR= 0.56; 95% CI: 0.44 - 0.70). Women with high fiber intake were less likely to experience constipation (PR = 0.64; 95% CI: 0.57 - 0.73) than women with the lowest fiber intake. The prevalence ratio for constipation for women who reported both daily physical activity and were in highest quintile of fiber intake was 0.32 (95% CI: 0.20-0.54) compared with those with physical activity less than once weekly and those who were in the lowest quintile of fiber intake.

Other mechanisms related to colon cancer risk, such as specific food intake (high amount of fat, alcohol or low amounts of fiber and vitamins), or an increase in body mass index, insulin resistance, prostaglandin and triglycerides levels can be changed favorably by physical activity. It was also postulated that exercise might specifically prevent cancer development through a reduction in abdominal fat mass, which might be implicated in carcinogenesis [64].

It was suggested that immune function is stimulated by physical training, which results in increase in the number and activity of macrophages, natural killer cells and lymphokine-activated killer cells and their regulating cytokines, and increased mitogen-induced lymphocyte proliferation rates [65, 66]. However, an immune function is likely to have a beneficial effect late in the cancer stage, after colorectal carcinoma cells have already been formed, and at a time when the tumor becomes invasive. Moreover, epidemiologic data suggest that the physical activity needs to act for many years to have an effect. This makes a hypothesis on immune depression an unlikely mechanism, since there is no evidence suggesting that patients with colorectal cancer did have an immune deficiency many years preceding the occurrence of cancer. On the other side, there is no evidence that physical activity affects risk for cancers of the immune system.

We found that the effect of physical activity was not related to possible inter-correlated factors such as dietary and alcohol intake and smoking habits that may either act as confounders or be part of a causal pathway between physical activity and cancer risk. However, genetic inclination for physical activity and genetic susceptibility may also be involved in the carcinogenic process. Genetic factors influence body build, physical functions, and may modify an individual's risk for certain types of cancer.

The body of evidence for the presumed mechanisms is being accumulated, and more data and research is needed to determine which mechanisms are responsible for risk of colorectal cancer. This task would not be easy as some of the postulated mechanisms are interrelated, therefore new research should help in defining the possible causal pathways that may be necessary and sufficient to reduce the colorectal cancer risk. Studies on these mechanisms should be carried out in humans and on animal models including not only colorectal cancer as the health end outcome but also measuring the impact of physical activity on intermediate stages and various markers of colorectal cancer incidence.

Since the convincing evidence for a protective role of physical activity in cancer etiology is growing rapidly, there is a requirement for moving from observational epidemiological studies to intervention controlled trials. Given the strength of the risk reductions confirmed in observational studies on colon cancer, the potential for cancer prevention with increased physical activity levels is very promising. Further progress in this field can be made not only by better understanding of the underlying biological mechanisms, more precise assessment methods of physical activity, and by additional observational epidemiological studies that would avoid deficient methodology in previous studies. To explore in a better way the potential of promoting physical activity as a prevention measure at the population level, we need to perform more observations in diverse populations with different gradients and distinct levels of physical activity. However, before we formulate concrete exercise recommendations for cancer prevention programs addressed to the population at large, evidence is needed from controlled trials of exercise interventions in the population. We expect that the experimental intervention trials would provide relevant information on effectiveness of different types of physical activity, its intensity, duration, and frequency and at which time period(s) in life the physical activity programs are most likely to produce beneficial results in cancer risk prevention programs.

ACKNOWLEDMENTS

The project and the field study was supported financially by a grant from the Polish Committee for Research (NR.6 P05D 002 20), principal investigator of the study: Prof. Wieslaw Jedrychowski M.D., Ph.D. (Chair of Epidemiology and Preventive Medicine, Jagiellonian University in Poland). The German-Polish Association and German Cancer Research Center in Heidelberg financially supported this part of analysis of the data. Food Frequency Questionnaire together with the computer software used in the study for calculation of nutrients was an adapted version of the German Food Questionnaire, kindly provided by Dr Heiner Boeing (Institute for Human Nutrition in Potsdam).

REFERENCES

[1] Huseman B, Neubauer MG, Duhne C. Sitzende Taetigkeit und Rektum-Sigma-Karzinom (in German). *Onkologie* 1980; 3: 168-171.

[2] Garabrant DH, Peters JM, Mack TM, Bernstein L. Job activity and colon cancer risk. *Am J Epidemiol* 1984; 119: 1005–1014.

[3] Vainio H, Bianchini F, eds. *IARC handbook of cancer prevention*. Vol. 6. Weight control and physical activity. Chap 5, Cancer-preventive effects. Lyon, France, IARC Press, 2002.

[4] Łoś-Kuczera M (ed.). *Food products. Composition and nutritive value*. Institute of Food and Nutrition, Publ 54, Warszawa 1990.

[5] Nadolna I, Kunachowicz H, Iwanow K. *Dishes. Composition and nutritive value,* Institute of Food and Nutrition, Publ 65, Warszawa 1994.

[6] Kunachowicz H, Nadolna I, Przygoda B, Iwanow K. *Food composition tables*. Institute of Food and Nutrition, Publ 85, Warszawa 1998.

[7] Nadolna I, Przygoda B, Troszczyńska A, Kunachowicz H. *Food composition tables. Vitamins*. Institute of Food and Nutrition, Publ 99, Warszawa 2000.

[8] Ainsworth BE, Haskell WL, Leon AS, Jacobs DR, Montoye HJ, Sallis JF, Paffenberger RS. Compendium of physical activities: classification of energy costs of human physical activities. *Med Sci Sports Exerc* 1993; 25: 71-80.

[9] Ainsworth BE, Sternfeld B, Slattery ML, Daguise V, Zahm SH. Physical activity and breast cancer: evaluation of physical activity assessment methods. *Cancer* 1998; 83 (3 suppl): 611-620.

[10] Ainsworth BE, Haskell WL, Whit MC, Irwin ML, Swartz AM, Strath SJ, O'Brien WL, Basseit DR, Schmitz KH, Emplaincourt PO, Jacobs DR, Leon A. Compendium of physical activities: an update of activity codes and MET intensities. *Med Sci Sports Exerc* 2000; 32: S498-S504.

[11] Vena JE, Graham S, Zielezny M, Swanson MK, Barnes RE, Nolan J. Lifetime occupational exercise and colon cancer. *Am J Epidemiol* 1985; 122: 357–365.

[12] Gerhardsson M, Norell SE, Kiviranta H, Pedersen NL, Ahlbom A. Sedentary jobs and colon cancer. *Am J Epidemiol* 1986; 123: 775–780.

[13] Paffenbarger RS, Hyde RT, Wing AL. Physical activity and incidence of cancer in diverse populations: a preliminary report. *Am J Clin Nutr* 1987; 45: 312–317.

[14] Wu AH, Paganini-Hill A, Ross RK, Henderson BE. Alcohol, physical activity and other risk factors for colorectal cancer: a prospective study. *Br J Cancer* 1987; 55: 687–694.

[15] Vena JE, Graham S, Zielezny M, Brasure J, Swanson MK. Occupational exercise and risk of cancer. *Am J Clin Nutr* 1987; 45: 318–327.

[16] Gerhardsson M, Floderus B, Norell SE. Physical activity and colon cancer risk. *Int J Epidemiol* 1988; 17: 743–746.

[17] Slattery ML, Schumacher MC, Smith KR, West DW, Abd-Elghany N. Physical activity, diet, and risk of colon cancer in Utah. *Am J Epidemiol* 1988; 128: 989–999.

[18] Hsing AW, McLaughlin JK, Chow W-H, Schuman LM, Chien HTC, Gridley G, Bjelke E, Wacholder S, Blot WJ. Risk factors for colorectal cancer in a prospective study among U.S. white men. *Int J Cancer* 1988; 77:549–553.

[19] Peters RK, Garabrant DH, Yu MC, Mack TM. A case-control study of occupational and dietary factors in colorectal cancer in young men by subsite. *Cancer Res* 1989; 49: 5459–5468.

[20] Fredriksson M, Bengtsson NO, Hardell L, Axelson O. Colon cancer, physical activity, and occupational exposures. A case-control study. *Cancer* 1989; 63: 1838–1842.

[21] Brownson RC, Zahm SH, Chang JC, Blair A. Occupational risk of colon cancer. An analysis by anatomic subsite. *Am J Epidemiol* 1989; 130: 675–687.

[22] Albanes D, Blair A, Taylor PR. Physical activity and risk of cancer in the NHANES I population. *Am J Public Health* 1989; 79: 744-750.

[23] Marti B, Minder CE. Physische Berufsaktivitaet und Kolonkarzinommortalitaet bei Schweizer Maennern 1979–1982 (in German). *Soz Praeventivmed* 1989; 34: 30–37, 1989.

[24] Severson RK, Nomura AM, Grove JS, Stemmermann GN. A prospective analysis of physical activity and cancer. *Am J Epidemiol* 1989; 130: 522–529.

[25] Kune G, Kune S, Watson L. Body weight and physical activity as predictors of colorectal cancer risk. *Nutr Cancer* 1990; 13: 9–17.

[26] Kato I, Tominaga S, Ikari AA. case-control study of male colorectal cancer in Aichi Prefecture, Japan: with special reference to occupational activity level, drinking habits and family history. *Jpn J Cancer Res* 1990; 81*:* 115–121.

[27] Benito E, Obrador A, Stiggelbout A, Bosch FX, Mulet M, Munoz N, Kaldor J. A population-based case-control study of colorectal cancer in Majorca. I. Dietary factors. *Int J Cancer* 1990; 45*:* 69–76.

[28] Ballard-Barbash R, Schatzkin A, Albanes D, Schiffman MH, Kreger BE, Kannel WB, Anderson KM, Helsel WE. Physical activity and risk of large bowel cancer in the Framingham Study. *Cancer Res* 1990; 50*:* 3610–3613.

[29] Gerhardsson de Verdier M, Steineck G, Hagman U, Rieger A, Norell SE. Physical activity and colon cancer: a case-referent study in Stockholm. *Int J Cancer* 1990; 46*:* 985–989.

[30] Whittemore AS, Wu-Williams AH, Lee M, Zheng S, Gallagher RP, Jiao DA, Zhou L, Wang XH, Chen K, Jung D, The C-Z, Chengde L, Yao XJ, Paffenbarger RS Jr, Henderson BE. Diet, physical activity and colorectal cancer among Chinese in North America and China. *J Natl Cancer Inst* 1990; 82*:* 915–926.

[31] Brownson RC, Chang JC, Davis JR, Smith CA. Physical activity on the job and cancer in Missouri. *Am J Pub Health* 1991;81*:* 639–642.

[32] Lee IM, Paffenberger RS, Hsieh C. Physical activity and risk of developing colorectal cancer among college alumni. *Am J Epidemiol* 1991; 83: 1324-1329.

[33] Thun MJ, Calle EE, Namboodiri MM, Flanders WD, Coates RJ, Byers T, Boffetta P, Garfinkel L, Heath CW. Risk factors for fatal colon cancer in a large prospective study. *J Natl Cancer Inst* 1992; 84: 1491-1500.

[34] Markowitz S, Morabia A, Garibaldi K, Wynder E. Effect of occupational and recreational activity on the risk of colorectal cancer among males: a case-control study. *Int J Epidemiol* 1992; 21*:* 1057–1062.

[35] Arbman G, Axelson O, Fredriksson M, Nilsson E, Sjodahl R. Do occupational factors influence the risk of colon and rectal cancer in different ways? *Cancer* (Phila.) 1993; 72: 2543–2549.

[36] Fraser G, Pearce N. Occupational physical activity and risk of cancer of the colon and rectum in New Zealand males. *Cancer Causes Control* 1993; 4*:* 45–50.

[37] Chow WH, Dosemeci M, Zheng W, Vetter R, McLaughlin JK, Gao YT, Blot WJ. Physical activity and occupational risk of colon cancer in Shanghai, China. *Int J Epidemiol* 1993; *22:* 23–29.

[38] Bostick R, Potter J, Kushi L, Steinmetz KA, McKenzie DR, Gapstur SM, Folsom AR. Sugar, meat, fat intake, and non-dietary risk factors for colon cancer incidence in Iowa women (United States). *Cancer Causes Control* 1994; 5: 38–52.

[39] Chow WH, Malker HS, Hsing AW, McLaughlin JK, Weiner JA, Stone BJ, Ericsson JL, Blot WJ. Occupational risks for colon cancer in Sweden. *J Occup Med* 1994; 36: 647–651.

[40] Lee IM, Paffenbarger RS Jr. Physical activity and its relation to cancer risk: a prospective study of college alumni. *Med Sci Sports Exercise* 1994; 26*:* 831–837.

[41] Marcus PM, Newcomb PA, Storer BE. Early adulthood physical activity and colon cancer risk among Wisconsin women. *Cancer Epidemiol Biomark Prev* 1994; 3: 641–644.

[42] Longnecker M, Gerhardsson de Verdier M, Frumkin H, Carpenter C. A case-control study of physical activity in relation to risk of cancer of the right colon and rectum. *Int J Epidemiol* 1995; 24: 42–50.

[43] Steenland K, Nowlin S, Palu S. Cancer incidence in the National Health and Nutrition Survey I follow-up data: diabetes, cholesterol, pulse and physical activity. *Cancer Epidemiol Biomark Prev* 1995; 4: 807–811.

[44] Giovannucci E, Ascherio A, Rimm EB, Colditz GA, Stampfer MJ, Willett WC. Physical activity, obesity, and risk of colon cancer and adenoma in men. *Ann Intern Med* 1995; 122: 327–334.

[45] Thune I, Lund E. Physical activity and risk of colorectal cancer in men and women. *Br J Cancer* 1996; 73: 1134–1140.

[46] White E, Jacobs EJ, Daling J. Physical activity in relation to colon cancer in middle-aged men and women. *Am J Epidemiol* 1996;144: 42–50.

[47] Martinez ME, Giovannucci E, Spiegelman D, Hunter DJ, Willett WC., Colditz GA. Leisure-time physical activity, body size, and colon cancer in women. *J Natl Cancer Inst* 1997; 89: 948–955.

[48] Lee IM, Manson JE, Ajani U, Paffenbarger RS Jr, Hennekens CH, Buring JE. Physical activity and risk of colon cancer: the Physicians'Health Study (United States). *Cancer Causes Control* 1997; 8: 568–574.

[49] Le Marchand L, Wilkens LR, Kolonel LN, Hankin JH, Lyu LC. Associations of sedentary lifestyle, obesity, smoking, alcohol use, and diabetes with the risk of colorectal cancer. *Cancer Res* 1997; 57: 4787–4794.

[50] Slattery ML, Potter J, Caan B, Edwards S, Coates A, Ma KN, Berry TD. Energy balance and colon cancer–beyond physical activity. *Cancer Res* 1997; 57: 75–80.

[51] Will JC, Galuska DA, Vinicor F, Calle EE. Colorectal cancer: another complication of diabetes mellitus? *Am J Epidemiol* 1998; 147: 816–825.

[52] Tavani A, Braga C, La Vecchia C, Conti E, Filiberti R, Montella M, Amadori, D, Russo A, Franceschi S. Physical activity and risk of cancers of the colon and rectum: an Italian case-control study. *Br J Cancer* 1999; 79: 1912–1916.

[53] Tang R, Wang JY, Lo SK, Hsieh LL. Physical activity, water intake and risk of colorectal cancer in Taiwan: a hospital-based case-control study. *Int J Cancer* 1999; 82: 484–489, 1999.

[54] Levi F, Pasche C, Lucchini F, Tavani A, La Vecchia C. Occupational and leisure-time activity and the risk of colorectal cancer. *Eur J Cancer Prev* 1999; 8: 487-493.

[55] Steindorf K, Tobiasz-Adamczyk B, Popiela T, Jedrychowski W, Penar A, Matyja A, Wahrendorf J. Combined risk assessment of physical activity and dietary habits on the development of colorectal cancer. A hospital-based case-control study in Poland. *Eur J Cancer Prev* 2000; 9: 309–316.

[56] Colbert LH, Hartman TI, Nalila N, et al. Physical activity in relation to cancer of the colon and rectum in a cohort of male smokers. *Cancer Epidemiol Biomarkers Prev* 2002; 10: 265-268.

[57] Slattery ML, Edwards S, Curtin K, Ma K, Edwards R, Holoubkov R, Schaffer D. Physical activity and colorectal cancer. *Am J Epidemiol* 2003; 158: 214-224.

[58] Wei EK, Giovannucci E, Wu K, Rosner B, Fuchs ChS, Willett WC, Colditz GA. Comparison of risk factors for colon and rectal cancer. *Int J Cancer* 2003; 108: 433-442.

[59] Slattery KL, Jacobs DR. Assessment of ability to recall physical activity of several years ago. *Ann Epidemiol* 1995; 5: 292-296.

[60] Slattery ML, Edwards SL, Ma KN, Friedman GD, Potter JD. Physical activity and colon cancer: a public health perspective. *Ann Epidemiol* 1997; 7: 137-145.

[61] Dapoigny M, Sarna SK. Effects of physical exercise on colonic motor activity. *Am J Physiol Gastroint Liver Physiol* 1991; 260: 646-652.

[62] Rao SC, Beaty J, Chamberlain M, Lambert PG, Gisolfi C. Effects of acute graded exercise on human colonic motility Am. J. Physiol. Gastrointest. *Liver Physiol* 1999; 276: 1221-1226.

[63] Dukas L, Willett WC, Giovannucci EL. Association between physical activity, fiber intake, and other lifestyle variables and constipation in a study of women. *Am J Gastroentorol* 2003; 98: 1790-1796.

[64] Krotkiewski M, Bjorntorp P, Sjostrom L, Smith U. Impact of obesity on metabolism in men and women. Importance of regional adipose tissue distribution. *J Clin Investig* 1983.72: 1150–1162.

[65] Wood PD. Impact of experimental manipulation of energy intake and expenditure on body composition. *Crit Rev Food Sci Nutr* 1993; 33*:* 369–373.

[66] Shephard RJ, Shek PN. Associations between physical activity and susceptibility to cancer. Possible mechanisms. *Sports Med* 1998; 26*:* 293–315.

In: Focus on Colorectal Cancer Research
Editor: Julia D. Martinez, pp. 41-64
ISBN #1-59454-101-9

Chapter III

ROLE OF PHYTOCHEMICALS IN COLON CARCINOGENESIS

Mary E. S. Zander, Suresh R. Volate and Michael J. Wargovich*
Division of Basic Research
South Carolina Cancer Center
Columbia, SC 29203

ABSTRACT

Epidemiological studies show that populations that rely on a plant-based diet have lower risks for common forms of cancer, suggesting that a strong relationship exists between diet and cancer. Phytochemicals, which are nonnutritive constituents of plants possessing health-protective effects, may provide protection specifically against colorectal cancer (CRC). While diet is very complex, research has identified certain foods and herbs that have some great potential to prevent CRC. Several possible mechanisms of action may explain the cancer preventive aspects of plant-based foods. Specifically, antioxidants from green tea, isothiocyanates from cruciferous vegetables, isoflavones in soy, and flavonoids such as those found in onions and turmeric, have potential anti-cancer effects. This chapter will also examine the potential cancer preventive effects of herbal supplements including garlic, ginseng, and ginger. The evidence for these food products and herbals in terms of their phytochemical components as well as the proposed mechanisms of their anti-tumor activities will be discussed.

Key Words: Phytochemicals, botanicals, anti-inflammatory, carcinogen metabolism

---

* Address for Correspondence: South Carolina Cancer Center; 14 Richland Medical Park Dr., Suite 500; Columbia, S.C. 29203

INTRODUCTION

Over the last 30 years, considerable evidence in both experimental models and human studies has amassed to validate the notion that a plant-based diet is protective for colon cancer. Several decades ago, it was noted that populations across the world characterized by a more plant-based diet were less likely to develop colon cancer when compared to those living in the U.S. and other western societies. Though strong relationships have been found supporting a diet rich in plant foods when examining vastly different cultures, controversy still exists in this area based on the lack of evidence for a plant based diet when looking at populations within a single country, within regions of countries, within sub-groups of people within a country, and at the level of the individual. Thus, though epidemiological studies regarding plant foods and cancer protection are difficult at best to interpret, experimental research using *in vitro* approaches and *in vivo* models for colon cancer has substantiated that plant-based diets contain elements that have cancer preventive effects. In addition, supplement use has been steadily increasing for several decades, and current estimates project that 1 in 3 people in the U.S. currently use some form of dietary supplements. This use can often be to add to or replace plant-based choices in the diet of an individual. The intent of this review is to highlight plant-foods with bioactive phytochemicals that inhibit the carcinogenic process. We also take a closer look at some of the more popular dietary supplements and their potential to impact colon cancer.

HOW PHYTOCHEMICALS PREVENT COLON CANCER: MECHANISMS

The Antioxidant Pathway

Oxidative damage to DNA contributes to a variety of diseases including cancer, [1] and antioxidant depletion in circulation is a characteristic finding in malignant transformation. [2] Reactive oxygen species (ROS) are generated endogenously and by chemical carcinogens. These ROS can act as second messengers to stimulate cells to activate transcription factors regulated by the intracellular redox state and promote the development of inflammation, which can lead to cancer. Many chemical carcinogens exert their mutagenic effects by covalently binding to and modifying electron-rich sources in the cells such as DNA, RNA, lipids and proteins. If modifications are not repaired and apoptosis is not initiated, mutagenesis and cancer could occur. The ability of various food components and herbals to protect against oxidative damage is thus one manner in which they can aid in the prevention of cancer development

Carcinogen Activation and Detoxification Mechanisms

Phase I and phase II enzymes represent activation and detoxification pathways, respectively, for environmental and chemical carcinogens. The mechanism of action of many herbals includes their ability to decrease phase I and/or increase phase II enzyme activity.

Phase I enzymes, including certain cytochrome P450 enzymes, aid in the activation of compounds to become DNA-reactive species, thus contributing to carcinogenesis. Therefore, the reduction of these enzymes aids in chemoprevention. [3] The induction of phase II detoxification enzymes aids in the elimination of carcinogens or their conversion to less reactive metabolites; this then decreases the mutagenesis of DNA and prevents the initiation of carcinogenesis. [3, 4]

Anti-Inflammatory Mechanisms

An important manner in which herbals aid in cancer prevention is through anti-inflammatory mechanisms. The use of traditional NSAIDs (non-steroidal anti-inflammatory drugs) such as aspirin or ibuprofen has proven to be effective in reducing the incidence of several cancers, most notably colon cancer. [5] NSAIDs are proposed to work by modulating prostaglandin synthesis via inhibition of cyclooxygenase (COX) enzymes. A potential problem with using NSAIDs is that there are numerous side effects associated with their habitual use. Thus, safe and effective natural herbals or food components with strong anti-inflammatory activities could greatly help reduce cancer rates without the adverse side effects commonly associated with habitual NSAID use.

Plant Foods and Herbals with Potential to Impact Colon Cancer

Garlic

Garlic (*Allium sativum*) has been used for seasoning foods and for medicinal purposes for thousands of years and is used in many different cultures throughout the world. [6] Today, in addition to its use in foods, garlic can be found in supplement form. In fact, garlic supplements are the fourth highest selling supplement in the United States, with $84 million in sales for 1998-1999 alone. [7] Though many people may take these supplements to aid in reducing cholesterol levels, there is great potential that garlic may also help to reduce the risk of CRC. Many studies have been performed to examine the relationship of *Allium* vegetables, particularly garlic, and the risk for gastrointestinal malignancies. Several epidemiological studies have shown decreased risks of colorectal cancer with intake of raw and/or cooked garlic. [8] *In vivo* work with garlic and garlic components has corroborated this decreased risk of CRC with their consumption. [9-12]

It is well believed that the components within garlic responsible for its chemopreventive effects are the organosulfur compounds. These compounds present in garlic represent some of the more efficient phase I/II modulators. Phase I and phase II enzymes represent activation and detoxification pathways, respectively, for environmental and chemical carcinogens.

DAS, which has been shown to inhibit chemically induced cancers of the colon and esophagus, is a potent inhibitor of cytochrome P450 2E1 (CYP2E1). CYP2E1 is involved in the metabolic activation of several carcinogens, including dimethylhydrazine and several nitrosamines. [13] DADS, also an inhibitor of experimentally-induced cancers in various animal models, [14] significantly increased several phase II enzymes, including glutathione S-transferase (GST), quinone reductase (QR), and UDP-glucuronosyltransferase (UGT), in the liver of male SPF Wistar rats. Physiologically relevant levels of DADS fed to rats have also been found to increase activities of GST and QR. [15] These enzymes catalyze the detoxification of carcinogens through reduction, hydrolysis, or conjugation with endogenous compounds, thereby blocking the ability of these carcinogens to bind to DNA. [16]

In addition to its ability to work through the phaseI/II enzyme system, garlic has shown the potential to affect the cell cycle pathway. Garlic extracts and components have been found to inhibit the proliferation of colon carcinoma and adenocarcinoma cells, and it has been demonstrated that they promote cell cycle arrest. [17-19] In addition, the compounds have been shown to induce programmed cell death, or apoptosis, in these cell lines by increasing the activity of caspase-3 as well as jun kinase. [19]

Finally, garlic has demonstrated its ability to prevent CRC through its antioxidant activities. Garlic has been reported to modulate lipid peroxidation levels and enhance the status of antioxidants. [20, 21] Aged garlic extract (AGE) is an antioxidant rich extract derived from prolonged extraction of fresh garlic at room temperature. AGE consists of water-soluble S-allylcysteine (SAC) and S-allylmercaptocysteine (SAMC), and lipid-soluble DAS, DADS, triallyl sulfide and diallyl polysulfides. AGE increases cellular glutathione in a variety of cells. As a substrate for the antioxidant enzyme glutathione peroxidase, glutathione protects cells from the damaging effects of peroxides formed in metabolism and through other ROS reactions. Decreased glutathione levels are associated with cell damage and may increase the risk of cancer development. [22]

Ginger

The spice ginger (*Zingiber officinale*) has been used in cooking as well as in medicines for thousands of years. It belongs to the Zingiberaceae family, and extracts of ginger are rich in gingerols and shogaols. These individual properties have exhibited antioxidant activities which have been shown to decrease the risk of colon cancer. [23] In addition to this generalized potential for ginger's ability to reduce risk for CRC, some research directly examining this possibility has been performed. In one such study, it has been found that a sesquiterpene zerumbone isolated from ginger had several effects on colon cancer cells *in vitro*. First, it was found to significantly inhibit the growth of the colon cells, whereas normal, non-cancerous, colon cells were either not affected or affected to a much lesser extent. In addition, this compound induced apoptosis in the cells, with 60 to 100% of treated cells being apoptotic after 48 hours of treatment. Finally, it was determined that treatment with the ginger compound dramatically and selectively decreased COX-2 levels. [24] Another study done with a supercritical fluid extraction of ginger also showed that the ginger compound inhibited CRC cell proliferation *in vitro*. In addition, this study verified the antioxidant properties of ginger. [23] All of the results from these studies indicate that ginger may show great potential as an effective CRC chemopreventive agent; furthermore, because it shows selective inhibitory effects on colon cancer cells versus normal cells, future work may lead to the possibility of using ginger or ginger extracts to treat or help treat CRC.

Ginseng

An herbal supplement which has been one of the top three most consumed supplements in the United States for many years is ginseng. [7] There are several forms of ginseng available, including Asian ginseng (*Panax ginseng*) or American ginseng (*Panax quinquefolius*), as well as fresh, white, or red ginseng. White ginseng is fresh ginseng that has been peeled and dried, and red ginseng is fresh ginseng that has been peeled, steamed and dried. [25] What is believed to be the pharmacologically active constituents in ginseng are a series of saponin glycosides collectively known as the ginsenosides. Many individual ginsenosides have been identified, and the presence and/or amount of a particular ginsenoside is dependent on the particular species as well as how the ginseng was prepared. [26]

All of the above forms of ginseng are used frequently, and have also been shown to have many beneficial characteristics. Though several epidemiological studies have been done which have shown that ginseng prevents several forms of cancer, [27] its colorectal chemopreventive properties have not yet been fully demonstrated. The *in vivo* data that is currently available indicates that further work needs to be done in order to determine the potential efficacy of ginseng preventing CRC. For instance, one study performed in a rat model showed that red ginseng is effective in preventing the pre-neoplastic lesions aberrant crypt foci (ACF), while white ginseng is not. In addition, this study indicated that red ginseng is more effective at preventing CRC before the cancerous process ever begins, and is less effective at correcting damage that has already occurred. [28] This study contradicts the findings of another study performed in rats, which showed that white ginseng but not red ginseng decreased intestinal tumor formation. Finally, a small case-control study was done in Korea which demonstrated that there was a decreased risk of CRC with habitual ginseng intake. [29] Thus, ginseng has shown strong promise as a chemopreventive agent for CRC, though studies are conflicted as to what form is effective or the most effective.

Several potential mechanisms for the chemopreventive effects of ginseng have been examined, and these include anti-inflammatory and anti-oxidant properties. It has been demonstrated that ginseng lowers the production of tumor necrosis factor-alpha (TNF-α), which is an inflammatory cytokine. [30] Furthermore, Surh *et al.* found that all of the ginsenosides tested inhibited the effects of nuclear factor kappa B (NF-κB), which stimulates cytokines in the inflammatory pathway including COX. They also found that multiple ginsenosides inhibited several of the transcription factors in the mitogen activated protein kinase (MAPK) pathway, including p38 MAPK, and ERK. The MAPK pathway is among the most extensively studied signaling cascades involved in inflammatory responses; it is believed that this pathway leads to COX-2 induction. [31] Finally, they determined that one ginsenoside in particular, Rg_3, suppressed COX-2 expression. [32] Several other groups also support the idea that ginseng suppresses COX. [33]

The anti-oxidant properties that have been demonstrated in ginseng include protection against fatty acid peroxidation and free radical-induced injury, as well as induction of the expression of superoxide dismutase [27, 30] Ginseng has been shown to attenuate lipid peroxidation, [30, 32] and suppress cytochrome P450 IIE1 (CYP2E1). [30] Furthermore, at least one study has found that this herbal's antioxidant activities are dose dependant. [30] In addition, certain ginseng fractions have been shown to scavenge reactive oxygen intermediates, including both superoxide and hydroxyl. [30, 32, 34] In addition, it increased glutathione content [35] and stimulated nitric oxide production. [27, 35] Finally, in a comparison of a large number of medicinal plants, ginseng showed some of the highest antioxidant activities of over 40 herbs tested. [36-40]

Isothiocyanates

It has been shown that the risk for CRC is decreased with a diet high in fruits and vegetables. One group of vegetables that has shown the most chemopreventive effects for CRC are the cruciferous vegetables, and specifically those in the Brassica genus, such as cabbage, broccoli, watercress, cauliflower, kale and Brussels sprouts. [4, 41, 42] The compounds within this group of vegetables believed to have the strongest chemopreventive effects are the isothiocyanates (ITCs); these compounds are thought to be responsible for the induction of the phase II detoxification enzymes, GST and QR, thereby increasing carcinogen excretion and detoxification, and decreasing interactions between the carcinogen and DNA. [3, 4, 43-45] *In vivo* as well as *in vitro* work has been done to confirm the chemopreventive effects as well as mechanisms involved. One such *in vivo* study demonstrated that ITCs decreased the number of ACFs in the azoxymethane (AOM)-induced rat colon cancer model in both the initiation and post-initiation protocols. [42] In addition, another rat study determined that the chemopreventive effects of the ITCs could be achieved at physiologically relevant levels. [43]

One of the specific manners in which ITCs may induce the phase II enzymes, and specifically QR, is by interacting with the binding sites of the promoter region of QR. [4] Though the exact manner that QR is induced is not precisely known, strong evidence exists suggesting that the addition of ITCs to colon cancer cells initially depletes the cells of glutathione, because ITCs conjugate with glutathione for their eventual elimination. This change in the glutathione pool then induces the activation of c-Jun N-terminal kinase (JNK), or the stress activated protein kinase, which is then followed by the induction of AP-1 binding, which is consequently followed by the induction of NF-κB binding, leading to an induction in the expression of QR. [4]

Besides the increase in phase II enzymes, several other mechanisms have been demonstrated that may account for the role of ITCs in decreased risk for CRC. One additional manner they have shown additional benefit is by increasing levels of apoptosis selectively in cancerous cells, while at the same time protecting undamaged DNA from genotoxic agents. [41, 45] In addition, butyrate, a bacterial by-product produced from high fiber foods (including the cruciferous vegetables), enhanced the effects of apoptosis induction, [3] indicating that consumption of the whole vegetable and not the isolated ITCs may hold the most benefit for chemoprevention. It appears that the induction of apoptosis is through a bax dependent pathway, and that the increased levels of bax induce the release of cytochrome-c, thus inducing apoptosis. [45] Other potential mechanisms of ITCs include increasing the levels of cyclins A and B1, thereby inducing cell cycle arrest in the G2/M phase. [45] A final potential mechanism that has been determined with ITC treatment on colon cancer cells *in vitro* is the increase in the acetylation of histones; this mechanism was shown to occur at concentrations that also inhibited cell proliferation, indicating that this mechanism may occur in human cells with physiologically relevant levels of ITCs. [46]

Olive Oil

Many epidemiological studies have been performed to determine if increased consumption of olive oil is associated with a concomitant decrease in CRC. The reason that these studies began to be thoroughly investigated includes the fact that many European countries in the Mediterranean area have a lower incidence of CRC (along with other cancers) relative to other Western countries. A large number of epidemiological studies have been performed in order to determine why this difference occurs. A very strong correlation that has been found in a majority of these studies is the increased consumption of olive oil. [47-51]

There are several components of olive oil that may account for its ability to decrease CRC. These include squalene, α-tocopherol, hydroxytyrosol, lignans, and various polyphenolic compounds. [47, 52, 53] These components contribute to the anti-oxidant activities in olive oil, which is one of the manners it appears to be an effective chemopreventive agent for colon cancer. [47, 51, 52] This activity has been demonstrated by its ability to scavenge free radicals and ROS. [47, 52] (This is also why olive oil rarely spoils). [47,51]

Additionally, several other chemopreventive activities have been described in studies examining olive oil. One such study using the AOM rat model showed that a high olive oil diet could significantly decrease levels of prostaglandin E2 in both the liver and the colon, indicating that it may possess anti-inflammatory properties. Furthermore, the diet significantly suppressed ornithine decarboxylase (ODC) and tyrosine-specific protein kinase (TPK) activities, which play important roles in tumor promotion. [54] Hydroxytyrosol, an antioxidant isolated from virgin olive oil, has shown to inhibit cellular proliferation in the human colon cancer cell line, HT-29; in that same study, hydroxytyrosol was found to induce cell cycle arrest as well as apoptosis. [53]

Finally, the individual component of olive oil that is believed to have the most significant effect on the prevention of CRC is squalene, which makes up 0.2% to 0.7% of the total content of olive oil. Besides its ability to act as an anti-oxidant, squalene has been shown to prevent the formation of ACF by 46% in the chemically induced AOM rat model. [55] Conversely, squalene was unable to decrease the intestinal tumor burden of the APC Min mouse model. [50] The reason that this apparent discrepancy is thought to be seen is because a mutation in the ras oncoprotein is found in the AOM rat model, while it is not found in the APC Min mouse model. Furthermore, squalene is hypothesized to inhibit the farnesylation of the ras oncoprotein. It does so indirectly by inhibiting HMGCoA reductase activity, thereby decreasing the levels of farnesyl pyrophosphate normally available as a source for the farnesylation of certain cellular signaling proteins including Ras p21. [50]

Onions

Onions (*Allium cepa*) are used as an ingredient in many dishes and are accepted by almost all traditions and cultures. The use of onions is associated with a significantly reduced risk of developing cardiovascular disease [56] and various types of cancer. [57-59] Onions, like garlic, are a member of the *Allium* family and both are rich in sulfur-containing compounds that are responsible for their pungent odors. Garlic contains predominantly allyl cysteine sulfoxides, while onions contain mainly propyl and propenyl cysteine sulfoxides. [60] These sulfur-containing compounds are the flavor precursors that generate the characteristic odor and taste of onion and are thought to be responsible for some of its health-promoting benefits. In addition to these compounds, onions contain a number of flavonoids, the most abundant of which is quercetin. Both *in vitro* and *in vivo* studies suggest this compound protects against cancer development and that this effect may exist in the intestinal tract due to the direct exposure of this compound to the intestinal epithelia.

One of the most widely used animal models for evaluating the chemopreventive activity of quercetin and its glucosides has been the AOM induced ACF model. Using this model in mice, Deschner *et al* have shown that dietary quercetin and its glucoside significantly reduced the number and multiplicity of ACFs. [61, 62] Similar studies conducted on rats showed that the decrease in the ACFs was accompanied by the reduction in crypt cell proliferation, especially in the distal portion of the large intestine. [63, 64] Furthermore, a recent study conducted on Balb-c mice reports that daily oral administration of 0.8 mg/mL and 1.6 mg/ml quercetin reduced the size of implanted human colon-25 tumors by 50%. [65]

In order to understand the molecular basis underlying the ability of quercetin to inhibit cell growth, *in vitro* studies have been conducted. Studies conducted on human colon cancer cells (COLO 320) and adenocarcinoma cells (HT-29 cells) revealed that quercetin causes a concentration dependent inhibition of cell growth by inducing cell-cycle arrest at the G1/S boundary. [66, 67] Likewise, the induction of apoptosis by quercetin has been reported in several tumor cell lines. Quercetin caused morphological changes in the cells, and agarose gel electrophoresis showed the characteristic ladder-type fragmentation of DNA. [68] Also, the synthesis of heat shock protein (HSP) 70 was inhibited by quercetin and was associated with enhancement of the quercetin-induced apoptosis. [68, 69] HSPs form a complex with mutant p53, which allows tumor cells to bypass normal mechanisms of cell cycle arrest. [70, 71] While these effects have been observed *in vivo* in certain animal models, no definitive mechanism(s) has been reported for quercetin.

Another well-known action of quercetin is its potent antioxidant activity. Oxygen-derived free radicals, such as superoxides (O_2^-), hydroxyl ($^{\cdot}OH$) and hydrogen peroxide (H_2O_2), along with metal ions such as iron ions (Fe^{2+}) appear to be important progenitors in the etiology of colorectal cancer. [72-74] The consequences of iron or free radical exposure have been shown to be associated with changes in crypt cell proliferation in rat large intestine [75] and with an alteration of colonic absorptive functions. [76] A large number of *in vitro* studies suggest that the chemopreventive capacities of quercetin and its glucosides may be due to their metal chelating ability and radical scavenging activity. *In vitro* studies conducted on human intestinal cells revealed that quercetin aglycone, at physiological concentrations, protects against hydrogen peroxide and iron-induced lipid peroxidation [77, 78] and also reduces DNA damage evoked by nickel chloride. [79] Furthermore, Plumb *et al.* demonstrated that the quercetin aglycone along with the glucosides were effective at preventing iron/ascorbate-induced lipid peroxidation of phosphatidyl choline. [80] This ability of quercetin to reduce lipid peroxidation plays a crucial role in reducing damage generated by ROS and metal ions in the colon and therefore may be contributing to its ability to reduce the risk for colon cancer.

In addition to being a powerful antioxidant, accumulating evidence also suggests that quercetin may act by inhibiting arachidonic acid (AA) metabolism. AA is known to be important in the carcinogenic processes. Many studies have shown that colon tumors produce greater amounts of prostaglandins, particularly prostaglandin E_2 (PGE_2), than the normal tissue from which they were derived. PGE_2 is overproduced in tumors as a result of the activation of inducible COX-2, an enzyme that converts arachidonic acid to prostaglandins. Selective COX-2 inhibitors have effectively attenuated the symptoms of inflammation and reduce the rate of cancer occurrence. Therefore, there is a great interest in studying the effects and usefulness of drugs on COX-2. Although numerous *in vivo* and *in vitro* studies conducted on the cells of the immune system implicate quercetin to be an effective anti-inflammatory agent, studies of this compound on colon cells are limited. Moore *et al* showed that quercetin at a concentration of 1μM was very effective at inhibiting rat and rabbit renal prostaglandin synthesis. [81] Furthermore, an *in vitro* study conducted on human colon cancer cells revealed quercetin to be the most potent suppressor of COX-2 transcription compared to other flavonoids. [82]

Soy

Populations in Asian countries have greatly reduced risk of many diseases, including CRC, which are common in Western countries. There are many aspects of the lifestyle and diet which may account for this great discrepancy between these two cultures, but one aspect which has received much attention is soy. Soy foods are eaten at a much higher rate in Asian cultures than in Western societies: the typical Asian diet is 7 to 25 times higher in soy based foods than is the typical American diet. [83]

There are many properties of soy that have been studied to determine what accounts for its ability to decrease colon cancer. These include phytochemicals, including the phytoestrogens genistein, daidzein and glycitein; phytic acid; flavonoids; isoflavones; soy proteins; and lignans. [83-87] Several of these components have been shown to decrease the risk of CRC in various models.

One such study examined the effects of a soy-based diet on AOM-induced colon tumors in rats. The results indicated that lifetime colon tumor incidence was 76% lower than the casein-based control diet; ACF and invasive adenocarcinomas also were decreased with the soy diet. [83] Another study showed that diets containing either soybean curd refuse or soy protein digest decreased tumor incidence in the AOM rat model. [88] A similar study, also in the rat AOM model, showed that diets high in genistein, soy flakes, or soy flour (both with significant levels of soy phytochemicals including genistein) significantly decreased ACFs in the rat colons. [89] Because the genistein diet had the most significant effects, this particular phytochemical may be one of the more important components of soy in preventing CRC.

Genistein, which accounts for about 50% of the isoflavones in soybeans, [87] has been found to have inhibitory effects on tyrosine kinases, which are involved in growth factor signaling pathways, suggesting that it may have cancer inhibitory properties. [86, 87, 90] In addition, genistein has been found to effect several cytochrome P450 enzymes; specifically, it has shown to increase CYP2B1 and decrease CYP24 in mouse colons. It has previously been shown that such effects could increase the synthesis and availability of 1,25-D3 in the colon, which has been shown to aid in CRC chemoprevention. [86]

Conversely, a study done with rats indicated that soy protein, but not isolated soy isoflavones, were responsible for the potential chemopreventive effects of soy foods. This study determined that the 20% soy protein diet (containing about 0.03% isoflavones) decreased polyamine levels in both the large and small intestines of the animals, whereas the 0.1% isoflavone diet did not. Decreased polyamine levels are indicative of decreased levels of cellular proliferation. [91] Other studies also found that isoflavones did not protect against CRC formation. [92] In addition, it has been suggested that the combination of components within soy are more effective than any of the single components, and that they have synergistic effects. [87]

Though the exact components of soy that protect against CRC may not yet be clarified, it has been demonstrated that soy does indeed protect against this disease. Besides the potential mechanisms already discussed in detail above, there are several other ways in which soy demonstrated chemopreventive properties. These include antioxidant activities, inducing apoptosis, inhibiting angiogenesis or the formation of new blood vessels, induction of detoxification enzymes and inhibition of carcinogen activation, inhibiting NF-κB, and down regulating transforming growth factor beta (TGF-β). [83, 87, 93, 94] Continued examination of the exact components of soy and the particular pathways through which it works to prevent colon cancer are warranted.

Tea

Tea is produced from the leaves of the plant *Camellia sinensis* and is one of the most widely consumed beverages worldwide. There are three major forms of tea (black tea, green tea and oolong tea) and each differs in the way they are processed. Black tea is processed by crushing tea leaves and allowing them to ferment, whereas green tea is unfermented dried leaves of the tea plant. Oolong tea is manufactured similar to black tea but is only allowed to ferment partially. [95] The majority of tea produced and consumed is black tea (78%) followed by green (20%) and oolong teas (2%). [95] Black tea is favored in the United States, England and other Western countries, whereas green tea is consumed primarily in China, Japan, India, and a few countries in North Africa and the Middle East. Oolong tea consumption is confined to southeastern China, Taiwan and Japan. [95, 96] While many tea drinkers find the beverage soothing, folk medicine has long valued it as a remedy for sore throats and unsettled stomachs. Recent studies have shown that the catechins and theaflavins found in tea may reduce the risk of far more serious illnesses, including atherosclerosis and various types of cancers.

Many of the beneficial effects of tea have been attributed to the polyphenols known as catechins. It has been estimated that 2.5 g of green tea leaves brewed in nine ounces of water for 3 minutes will contain 620 mg to 880 mg of water-extractable solids, with catechins making up 30–42% of the dry weight. [95] These include (—)-epicatechin (EC), (—)-epicatechin-3-gallate (ECG), (—)-epigallocatechin (EGC) and (—)-epigallocatechin-3-gallate (EGCG), with EGCG being the most abundant catechin, followed by EGC. In black tea, due to the fermentation process, the total catechin content is reduced; black tea contains approximately 20-30% of the total catechin content of green tea as well as products such as theaflavins (theaflavin, theaflavin-3- gallate, theaflavin-3'-gallate, and theaflavin-3,3'-digallate) and thearubigens. [97] The bioavailability and pharmacokinetic parameters of the tea catechins have been studied extensively in humans and rats and have been reviewed in detail by Yang *et.al.* [95, 97] After oral administrations, the pharmacokinetic profile of tea indicates that the highest tissue concentrations of the tea polyphenols are found in the organs of the digestive system and it is therefore believed that the ingested tea is more likely to protect those organs. [98-100]

The relationship between tea consumption and cancer incidence has been a complex issue. In recent years, although many studies have demonstrated chemopreventive effects of different types of tea extracts against colon tumorigenesis in rats or mice induced by AOM, 1,2-dimethylhydrazine (DMH), 2-amino-1-methyl-6-phenylimidazo [4,5-b] pyridine (PhiP) or 2-amino-3-methylimidazo [4,5-f] quinoline (IQ), [101-105] some have shown that tea has no effect. [49, 106] In studies that showed the inhibitory effects of tea, the concentration of tea polyphenols and the preparation of tea were crucial in the effectiveness of tea against colon tumorigenesis. For example, Metz *et al* reported that reconstituted green tea extracts administered daily in drinking water at a concentration of 0.02% weight/volume (w/v) were protective against colon carcinogenesis when administered after the last AOM injection. [101] At higher concentrations (0.2% w/v), Xu *et al* reported that both black and green tea extracts administered in drinking water offered protection against PhiP and IQ-induced colon cancer in the initiation and the post-initiation phases. [107] However, when similar concentrations of tea extracts were administered in a dried polyphenol powder with food, black tea but not green tea extracts provided protection against colon cancer. [103] Finally, it should also be noted that the caffeine found in tea might play a role in its effectiveness against cancer. Lou *et. al.,* reported that decaffeinated tea was less effective at inhibiting tumor formation than regular tea, and adding caffeine back to the decaffeinated tea restored biological activity. [108]

The mechanisms responsible for the anticancer actions of tea are not well understood but are being intensively investigated. Tea polyphenols display a remarkable spectrum of biochemical activities that might be able to influence processes that are dysregulated during cancer development. These include scavenging ROS, [98, 109-112, 112, 113] inhibiting enzymes in the arachidonic acid pathway (COX and LOX), [101, 114, 115] suppressing cell growth by influencing proteins that control cell cycle progression, [116-118] and inducing apoptosis. [117, 119, 120] However, because the biochemical activities are dependent on the individual polyphenolic structures, the potency of the catechins and the theaflavins vary from one biochemical activity to another. For example, although both green and black tea polyphenols have been shown to scavenge ROS, it appears that green tea is more effective. [112, 113, 116, 121] Similarly, green tea is much stronger at inhibiting LOX, [114 whereas black tea is more potent at inhibiting COX. [122] Although the mechanisms responsible for the anti-cancer actions of tea are not well understood, a number of studies suggest that the galloyl moiety on EGCG and the gallate structure on theaflavins play an important role in the growth inhibition of tumor cell lines. [116, 123]

Epidemiological studies have so far not given clear answers concerning the chemopreventive effects of tea consumption on CRC. For instance, a cohort study conducted in Saitama, Japan, has shown that women consuming more than 10 cups of green tea daily are likely to have a lower risk for various types of cancer including colon cancer. [124] On the other hand, a hospital-based case-control study conducted in Nagoya, Japan, observed that high intake of green tea (7 cups or more per day) decreased the risk for stomach cancer but had no effect on colon cancer. [125] Like the studies conducted on green tea, results from studies on black tea have also been mixed. Two population-based cohort studies, one conducted in the U.S. and the other in Sweden, found no association between black tea consumption and colon cancer. [126, 127] However, a recent cohort study conducted in the US found an inverse association between colon cancer risk and habitual tea consumption. [128] These inconsistent results may be due to a number of confounding factors including diet, smoking status, age, and alcohol consumption. Additionally, most prior studies have not distinguished hot tea from iced tea consumption, and polyphenol content can vary between these beverages. [129] Human clinical trials, although inconclusive, also indicated some positive link between the drinking of green tea and the decrease of cancer incidence. [98]

Turmeric

Turmeric (*Curcuma longa Linn*), a member of the ginger (*Zingiberaceae*) family, is native to Asia and has a long history of use in the flavoring and coloring of food. In the Indian subcontinent and Southeast Asia, turmeric has traditionally been used in Ayurvedic medicine as a treatment for inflammation, skin wounds, and tumors. [130] The root, or rhizome, has a tough brown skin and bright orange-yellow flesh and can grow up to 2 feet in length. The ground turmeric root contains a mixture of 3 related compounds (curcumin, demethoxycurcumin and bisdemethoxycurcumin) which are collectively known as curcuminoids. Curcumin (diferuloylmethane) is the most prominent of these compounds and therefore is perceived to have antitumorigenic properities. [131, 132]

Curcumin is a promising herbal colon cancer chemopreventative, and thus has generated a lot of interest in the scientific community. Phase I clinical trials indicate curcumin is apparently safe in doses up to 8 g/day [133] and studies conducted on humans showed that the bioavailability of curcumin in the digestive tract seems to be higher than elsewhere in the body (plasma, blood or urine), indicating that curcumin is a good candidate for chemoprevention of colon cancer. Indeed, *in vivo* studies (chemical and genetic rodent models) and *in vitro* studies in human colon cancer cells lines suggest that dietary curcumin has the ability to interfere with colon carcinogenesis. Curcumin (0.2% w/v) in diet inhibited the development of AOM-induced colonic adenocarcinomas in rats irrespective of whether the compound was administered during the initiation, postiniatiaion [134] or promotion/progression stages of the disease. [135] At the same dietary levels (0.2%), curcumin caused a 30% reduction in adenomas in the colons of Min mice. [136] Likewise, *in vitro* studies conducted on human colon cancer cell lines (HT-29, HCT-116, Lovo and HCT-

15) revealed that treatment with varying concentrations (2.5 – 75 μM) of curcumin led to a time and dose dependent decrease in cell proliferation. [137-140]

Curcumin has been widely used for the treatment of inflammatory disorders for centuries. Therefore, it has been suggested that one manner by which curcumin may inhibit colon carcinogenesis is its ability to interfere with AA metabolism. Rao *et al* reported that the inhibition of colon adenocarcinomas by curcumin correlated with the reduction in COX and LOX metabolites in the colonic mucosa and tumors. [141] The ability of curcumin to selectively inhibit COX-2 and decrease cell proliferation was also observed in an *in vitro* study conducted on HT-29 cells; however, this study suggested that the growth inhibitory effects of curcumin are not correlated with the inhibition of COX-2 expression. [139] Other possible mechanisms by which curcumin exerts its antiproliferative effects could be through inhibition of the cell cycle and/or induction of apoptosis. [137-139, 141-145] It has been demonstrated that curcumin inhibits proliferation by arresting the cell cycle at the G2/M phase by decreasing the expression of cyclins D and B, and induces apoptosis via both receptor- and mitochondria-mediated pathways in various cell lines. [141, 143] Additionally, curcumin has been shown to suppress DNA damage [146, 147] and upregulate carcinogen detoxification enzymes, such as GSTs. [148, 149]

Table 1: Mechanisms of Plant Foods and Herbals

Food or Herbal	Antioxidant	Phase I/II Enzymes	Anti-Inflammatory
Garlic	x	x	
Ginger	x		x
Ginseng	x		x
Isothiocyanates		x	
Olive Oil	x		x
Onions	x		x
Soy	x	x	
Tea	x		x
Turmeric	x		x

SUMMARY

Unlike the diets of high-risk areas of the world for colon cancer, such as North America, the diets of low-risk populations are often said to be more plant-based and rich in phytochemical compounds that influence risk for many cancers, including colon cancer. Based on current evidence, phytochemicals in the cancer preventive diet can modulate cancer risk through general antioxidant chemistry, modification of biotransformation pathways at the metabolic level, and suppression of chronic, sub-acute inflammation that seems to pervade and underscore many of the most common cancers afflicting countries without substantial reliance on plant foods in the daily diet.

While the evidence reviewed here is substantial for phytochemicals and protection against cancer at the molecular, cellular, and animal model levels, evidence bolstered in many cases by epidemiological evidence, gaps still remain in our understanding of whether prospective *adoption* of prudent, plant-based diets will imply a future health benefit. In the few studies to date that have examined dietary change on intermediate markers of cancer, no protective effect for a more generally plant-based diet has been found. It can be argued that these short-term studies cannot reflect the biological effects of cultures ingrained with plant foods in their diets over whole lifetimes, or perhaps there is much more to be learned about which foods truly harbor the phytochemical elements most likely to protect against human cancers, how they act singly, or, more importantly, in concert to avert risk for cancer.

REFERENCES

[1] Sharma RA, Ireson CR, Verschoyle RD, Hill KA, Williams ML, Leuratti C, Manson MM, Marnett LJ, Steward WP, Gescher A. Effects of dietary curcumin on glutathione S-transferase and malondialdehyde-DNA adducts in rat liver and colon mucosa: relationship with drug levels. *Clin Cancer Res* 2001 May;7(5):1452-8.

[2] Dreher D, Junod AF. Role of oxygen free radicals in cancer development. *Eur J Cancer* 1996 Jan;32A(1):30-8.

[3] Kirlin WG, Cai J, DeLong MJ, Patten EJ, Jones DP. Dietary compounds that induce cancer preventive phase 2 enzymes activate apoptosis at comparable doses in HT29 colon carcinoma cells. *J Nutr* 1999 Oct;129(10):1827-35.

[4] Patten EJ, DeLong MJ. Temporal effects of the detoxification enzyme inducer, benzyl isothiocyanate: activation of c-Jun N-terminal kinase prior to the transcription factors AP-1 and NFkappaB. *Biochem Biophys Res Commun* 1999 Apr;257(1):149-55.

[5] Tosetti F, Ferrari N, De Flora S, Albini A. Angioprevention': angiogenesis is a common and key target for cancer chemopreventive agents. *FASEB J* 2002 Jan;16(1):2-14.

[6] Lee BM, Park KK. Beneficial and adverse effects of chemopreventive agents. *Mutat Res* 2003 Feb;523-524:265-78.

[7] Blumenthal, Goldberg, Brinckmann. *Herbal Medicine: Expanded Commission E Monographs.* CD-ROM. 2002. Integrative Medicine Communications, Inc. Ref Type: Electronic Citation

[8] Fleischauer AT, Arab L. Garlic and cancer: a critical review of the epidemiologic literature. *J Nutr* 2001 Mar;131(3s):1032S-40S.

[9] Cheng JY, Meng CL, Tzeng CC, Lin JC. Optimal dose of garlic to inhibit dimethylhydrazine-induced colon cancer. *World J Surg* 1995 Jul;19(4):621-5.

[10] Wargovich MJ. DAS, a flavor component of garlic (Allium sativum), inhibits dimethylhydrazine-induced colon cancer. *Carcinogenesis* 1987 Mar;8(3):487-9.

[11] Wargovich MJ, Woods C, Eng VW, Stephens LC, Gray K. Chemoprevention of N-nitrosomethylbenzylamine-induced esophageal cancer in rats by the naturally occurring thioether, DAS. *Cancer Res* 1988 Dec;48(23):6872-5.

[12] Sumiyoshi H, Wargovich MJ. Chemoprevention of 1,2-dimethylhydrazine-induced colon cancer in mice by naturally occurring organosulfur compounds. *Cancer Res* 1990 Aug;50(16):5084-7.

[13] Brady JF, Li DC, Ishizaki H, Yang CS. Effect of DAS on rat liver microsomal nitrosamine metabolism and other monooxygenase activities. *Cancer Res* 1988 Nov;48(21):5937-40.

[14] Wargovich MJ. Experimental evidence for cancer preventive elements in foods. *Cancer Lett* 1997 Mar;114(1-2):11-7.

[15] Munday R, Munday CM. Low doses of DADS, a compound derived from garlic, increase tissue activities of quinone reductase and glutathione transferase in the gastrointestinal tract of the rat. *Nutr Cancer* 1999;34(1):42-8.

[16] Guyonnet D, Siess MH, Le Bon AM, Suschetet M. Modulation of phase II enzymes by organosulfur compounds from allium vegetables in rat tissues. *Toxicol Appl Pharmacol* 1999 Jan;154(1):50-8.

[17] Frantz DJ, Hughes BG, Nelson DR, Murray BK, Christensen MJ. Cell cycle arrest and differential gene expression in HT-29 cells exposed to an aqueous garlic extract. *Nutr Cancer* 2000;38(2):255-64.

[18] Ritland SR, Leighton JA, Hirsch RE, Morrow JD, Weaver AL, Gendler SJ. Evaluation of 5-aminosalicylic acid (5-ASA) for cancer chemoprevention: lack of efficacy against nascent adenomatous polyps in the Apc(Min) mouse. *Clin Cancer Res* 1999 Apr;5(4):855-63.

[19] Shirin H, Pinto JT, Kawabata Y, Soh JW, Delohery T, Moss SF, Murty V, Rivlin RS, Holt PR, Weinstein IB. Antiproliferative effects of S-allylmercaptocysteine on colon cancer cells when tested alone or in combination with sulindac sulfide. *Cancer Res* 2001 Jan;61(2):725-31.

[20] Balasenthil S, Arivazhagan S, Nagini S. Garlic enhances circulatory antioxidants during 7, 12-dimethylbenz [a]anthracene-induced hamster buccal pouch carcinogenesis. *J Ethnopharmacol* 2000 Oct;72(3):429-33.

[21] Balasenthil S, Arivazhagan S, Ramachandran CR, Nagini S. Effects of garlic on 7,12-Dimethylbenz [a]anthracene-induced hamster buccal pouch carcinogenesis. *Cancer Detect Prev* 1999;23(6):534-8.

[22] Borek C. Antioxidant health effects of aged garlic extract. *J Nutr* 2001 Mar;131(3s):1010S-5S.

[23] Leal PF, Braga ME, Sato DN, Carvalho JE, Marques MO, Meireles MA. Functional properties of spice extracts obtained via supercritical fluid extraction. *J Agric Food Chem* 2003 Apr;51(9):2520-5.

[24] Murakami A, Takahashi D, Kinoshita T, Koshimizu K, Kim HW, Yoshihiro A, Nakamura Y, Jiwajinda S, Terao J, Ohigashi H. Zerumbone, a Southeast Asian ginger sesquiterpene, markedly suppresses free radical generation, proinflammatory protein production, and cancer cell proliferation accompanied by apoptosis: the alpha,beta-unsaturated carbonyl group is a prerequisite. *Carcinogenesis* 2002 May;23(5):795-802.

[25] Yun TK, Choi SY. Non-organ specific cancer prevention of ginseng: a prospective study in Korea. *Int J Epidemiol* 1998 Jun;27(3):359-64.

[26] Shibata S. Chemistry and cancer preventing activities of ginseng saponins and some related triterpenoid compounds. *J Korean Med Sci* 2001 Dec;16 Suppl:S28-S37.

[27] Shin HR, Kim JY, Yun TK, Morgan G, Vainio H. The cancer-preventive potential of Panax ginseng: a review of human and experimental evidence. *Cancer Causes Control* 2000 Jul;11(6):565-76.

[28] Fukushima S, Wanibuchi H, Li W. Inhibition by ginseng of colon carcinogenesis in rats. *J Korean Med Sci* 2001 Dec;16 Suppl:S75-S80.

[29] Kakizoe T. Asian studies of cancer chemoprevention: latest clinical results. *Eur J Cancer* 2000 Jun;36(10):1303-9.

[30] Keum YS, Park KK, Lee JM, Chun KS, Park JH, Lee SK, Kwon H, Surh YJ. Antioxidant and anti-tumor promoting activities of the methanol extract of heat-processed ginseng. *Cancer Lett* 2000 Mar;150(1):41-8.

[31] Surh YJ, Chun KS, Cha HH, Han SS, Keum YS, Park KK, Lee SS. Molecular mechanisms underlying chemopreventive activities of anti- inflammatory phytochemicals: down-regulation of COX-2 and iNOS through suppression of NF-kappa B activation. *Mutat Res* 2001 Sep;480-481:243-68.

[32] Surh YJ, Na HK, Lee JY, Keum YS. Molecular mechanisms underlying anti-tumor promoting activities of heat- processed Panax ginseng C.A. Meyer. *J Korean Med Sci* 2001 Dec;16 Suppl:S38-S41.

[33] Ang-Lee MK, Moss J, Yuan CS. Herbal medicines and perioperative care. *JAMA* 2001 Jul;286(2):208-16.

[34] Kitts DD, Wijewickreme AN, Hu C. Antioxidant properties of a North American ginseng extract. *Mol Cell Biochem* 2000 Jan;203(1-2):1-10.

[35] Bucci LR. Selected herbals and human exercise performance. *Am J Clin Nutr* 2000 Aug;72(2 Suppl):624S-36S.

[36] Mantle D, Eddeb F, Pickering AT. Comparison of relative antioxidant activities of British medicinal plant species in vitro. *J Ethnopharmacol* 2000 Sep;72(1-2):47-51.

[37] Borchers AT, Keen CL, Stern JS, Gershwin ME. Inflammation and Native American medicine: the role of botanicals. *Am J Clin Nutr* 2000 Aug;72(2):339-47.

[38] Kimura Y, Okuda H, Arichi S. Effects of various ginseng saponins on 5-hydroxytryptamine release and aggregation in human platelets. *J Pharm Pharmacol* 1988 Dec;40(12):838-43.

[39] Park HJ, Lee JH, Song YB, Park KH. Effects of dietary supplementation of lipophilic fraction from Panax ginseng on cGMP and cAMP in rat platelets and on blood coagulation. *Biol Pharm Bull* 1996 Nov;19(11):1434-9.

[40] Teng CM, Kuo SC, Ko FN, Lee JC, Lee LG, Chen SC, Huang TF. Antiplatelet actions of panaxynol and ginsenosides isolated from ginseng. *Biochim Biophys Acta* 1989 Mar;990(3):315-20.

[41] Bonnesen C, Eggleston IM, Hayes JD. Dietary indoles and isothiocyanates that are generated from cruciferous vegetables can both stimulate apoptosis and confer protection against DNA damage in human colon cell lines. *Cancer Res* 2001 Aug;61(16):6120-30.

[42] Chung FL, Conaway CC, Rao CV, Reddy BS. Chemoprevention of colonic aberrant crypt foci in Fischer rats by sulforaphane and phenethyl isothiocyanate. *Carcinogenesis* 2000 Dec;21(12):2287-91.

[43] Munday R, Munday CM. Selective induction of phase II enzymes in the urinary bladder of rats by allyl isothiocyanate, a compound derived from Brassica vegetables. *Nutr Cancer* 2002;44(1):52-9.

[44] Hecht SS. Chemoprevention by isothiocyanates. *J Cell Biochem Suppl* 1995;22:195-209.

[45] Gamet-Payrastre L, Li P, Lumeau S, Cassar G, Dupont MA, Chevolleau S, Gasc N, Tulliez J, Terce F. Sulforaphane, a naturally occurring isothiocyanate, induces cell cycle arrest and apoptosis in HT29 human colon cancer cells. *Cancer Res* 2000 Mar;60(5):1426-33.

[46] Lea MA, Rasheed M, Randolph VM, Khan F, Shareef A, desBordes C. Induction of histone acetylation and inhibition of growth of mouse erythroleukemia cells by S-allylmercaptocysteine. *Nutr Cancer* 2002;43(1):90-102.

[47] Smith TJ. Squalene: potential chemopreventive agent. *Expert Opin Investig Drugs* 2000 Aug;9(8):1841-8.

[48] Stoneham M, Goldacre M, Seagroatt V, Gill L. Olive oil, diet and colorectal cancer: an ecological study and a hypothesis. *J Epidemiol Community Health* 2000 Oct;54(10):756-60.

[49] Weisburger JH, Rivenson A, Aliaga C, Reinhardt J, Kelloff GJ, Boone CW, Steele VE, Balentine DA, Pittman B, Zang E. Effect of tea extracts, polyphenols, and epigallocatechin gallate on azoxymethane-induced colon cancer. *Proc Soc Exp Biol* Med 1998 Jan;217(1):104-8.

[50] Newmark HL. Squalene, olive oil, and cancer risk. Review and hypothesis. *Ann N Y Acad Sci* 1999;889:193-203.

[51] Braga C, La Vecchia C, Franceschi S, Negri E, Parpinel M, Decarli A, Giacosa A, Trichopoulos D. Olive oil, other seasoning fats, and the risk of colorectal carcinoma. *Cancer* 1998 Feb;82(3):448-53.

[52] Bartsch H, Nair J, Owen RW. Exocyclic DNA adducts as oxidative stress markers in colon carcinogenesis: potential role of lipid peroxidation, dietary fat and antioxidants. *Biol Chem* 2002 Jun;383(6):915-21.

[53] Fabiani R, De Bartolomeo A, Rosignoli P, Servili M, Montedoro GF, Morozzi G. Cancer chemoprevention by hydroxytyrosol isolated from virgin olive oil through G1 cell cycle arrest and apoptosis. *Eur J Cancer Prev* 2002 Aug;11(4):351-8.

[54] Rao CV, Reddy BS. Modulating effect of amount and types of dietary fat on ornithine decarboxylase, tyrosine protein kinase and prostaglandins production during colon carcinogenesis in male F344 rats. *Carcinogenesis* 1993 Jul;14(7):1327-33.

[55] Rao CV, Newmark HL, Reddy BS. Chemopreventive effect of squalene on colon cancer. *Carcinogenesis* 1998 Feb;19(2):287-90.

[56] Kris-Etherton PM, Hecker KD, Bonanome A, Coval SM, Binkoski AE, Hilpert KF, Griel AE, Etherton TD. Bioactive compounds in foods: their role in the prevention of cardiovascular disease and cancer. *Am J Med* 2002 Dec;113 Suppl 9B:71S-88S.

[57] Hsing AW, Chokkalingam AP, Gao YT, Madigan MP, Deng J, Gridley G, Fraumeni JF, Jr. Allium vegetables and risk of prostate cancer: a population-based study. *J Natl Cancer Inst* 2002 Nov;94(21):1648-51.

[58] Ali M, Thomson M, Afzal M. Garlic and onions: their effect on eicosanoid metabolism and its clinical relevance. *Prostaglandins Leukot Essent Fatty Acids* 2000 Feb;62(2):55-73.

[59] Challier B, Perarnau JM, Viel JF. Garlic, onion and cereal fibre as protective factors for breast cancer: a French case-control study. *Eur J Epidemiol* 1998 Dec;14(8):737-47.

[60] Fenwick GR, Hanley AB. The genus Allium. Part 2. *Crit Rev Food Sci Nutr* 1985;22(4):273-377.

[61] Deschner EE, Ruperto JF, Wong GY, Newmark HL. The effect of dietary quercetin and rutin on AOM-induced acute colonic epithelial abnormalities in mice fed a high-fat diet. *Nutr Cancer* 1993;20(3):199-204.

[62] Deschner EE, Ruperto J, Wong G, Newmark HL. Quercetin and rutin as inhibitors of azoxymethanol-induced colonic neoplasia. *Carcinogenesis* 1991 Jul;12(7):1193-6.

[63] Matsukawa Y, Nishino H, Okuyama Y, Matsui T, Matsumoto T, Matsumura S, Shimizu Y, Sowa Y, Sakai T. Effects of quercetin and/or restraint stress on formation of aberrant crypt foci induced by azoxymethane in rat colons. *Oncology* 1997 Mar;54(2):118-21.

[64] Tanaka T, Kawabata K, Honjo S, Kohno H, Murakami M, Shimada R, Matsunaga K, Yamada Y, Shimizu M. Inhibition of azoxymethane-induced aberrant crypt foci in rats by natural compounds, caffeine, quercetin and morin. *Oncol Rep* 1999 Nov;6(6):1333-40.

[65] Hayashi A, Gillen AC, Lott JR. Effects of daily oral administration of quercetin chalcone and modified citrus pectin on implanted colon-25 tumor growth in Balb-c mice. *Altern Med Rev* 2000 Dec;5(6):546-52.

[66] Agullo G, Gamet L, Besson C, Demigne C, Remesy C. Quercetin exerts a preferential cytotoxic effect on active dividing colon carcinoma HT29 and Caco-2 cells. *Cancer Lett* 1994 Nov;87(1):55-63.

[67] Hosokawa N, Hosokawa Y, Sakai T, Yoshida M, Marui N, Nishino H, Kawai K, Aoike A. Inhibitory effect of quercetin on the synthesis of a possibly cell-cycle-related 17-kDa protein, in human colon cancer cells. *Int J Cancer* 1990 Jun;45(6):1119-24.

[68] Wei YQ, Zhao X, Kariya Y, Fukata H, Teshigawara K, Uchida A. Induction of apoptosis by quercetin: involvement of heat shock protein. *Cancer Res* 1994 Sep;54(18):4952-7.

[69] Hosokawa N, Hirayoshi K, Nakai A, Hosokawa Y, Marui N, Yoshida M, Sakai T, Nishino H, Aoike A, Kawai K, . Flavonoids inhibit the expression of heat shock proteins. *Cell Struct Funct* 1990 Dec;15(6):393-401.

[70] Pawlikowska-Pawlega B, Jakubowicz-Gil J, Rzymowska J, Gawron A. The effect of quercetin on apoptosis and necrosis induction in human colon adenocarcinoma cell line LS180. *Folia Histochem Cytobiol* 2001;39(2):217-8.

[71] Creagh EM, Sheehan D, Cotter TG. Heat shock proteins--modulators of apoptosis in tumour cells. *Leukemia* 2000 Jul;14(7):1161-73.

[72] Keshavarzian A, Zapeda D, List T, Mobarhan S. High levels of reactive oxygen metabolites in colon cancer tissue: analysis by chemiluminescence probe. *Nutr Cancer* 1992;17(3):243-9.

[73] Keshavarzian A, Olyaee M, Sontag S, Mobarhan S. Increased levels of luminol-enhanced chemiluminescence by rectal mucosa of patients with colonic neoplasia: a possible marker for colonic neoplasia. *Nutr Cancer* 1993;19(2):201-6.

[74] Morel I, Lescoat G, Cogrel P, Sergent O, Pasdeloup N, Brissot P, Cillard P, Cillard J. Antioxidant and iron-chelating activities of the flavonoids catechin, quercetin and diosmetin on iron-loaded rat hepatocyte cultures. *Biochem Pharmacol* 1993 Jan;45(1):13-9.

[75] Lund EK, Wharf SG, Fairweather-Tait SJ, Johnson IT. Increases in the concentrations of available iron in response to dietary iron supplementation are associated with changes in crypt cell proliferation in rat large intestine. *J Nutr* 1998 Feb;128(2):175-9.

[76] Bhaskar L, Balasubramanian KA. Luminal exposure of oxidants alter colonic absorptive function. *Life Sci* 1996;58(23):2115-23.

[77] Peng IW, Kuo SM. Flavonoid structure affects the inhibition of lipid peroxidation in Caco-2 intestinal cells at physiological concentrations. *J Nutr* 2003 Jul;133(7):2184-7.

[78] Glei M, Latunde-Dada GO, Klinder A, Becker TW, Hermann U, Voigt K, Pool-Zobel BL. Iron-overload induces oxidative DNA damage in the human colon carcinoma cell line HT29 clone 19A. *Mutat Res* 2002 Aug;519(1-2):151-61.

[79] Blasiak J, Arabski M, Pertynski T, Malecka-Panas E, Wozniak K, Drzewoski J. DNA damage in human colonic mucosa cells evoked by nickel and protective action of quercetin - involvement of free radicals? *Cell Biol Toxicol* 2002;18(4):279-88.

[80] Plumb GW, Price KR, Williamson G. Antioxidant properties of flavonol glycosides from green beans. *Redox Rep* 1999;4(3):123-7.

[81] Moore PK, Griffiths RJ, Lofts FJ. The effect of some flavone drugs on the conversion of prostacyclin to 6-oxoprostaglandin E1. *Biochem Pharmacol* 1983 Sep;32(18):2813-7.

[82] Mutoh M, Takahashi M, Fukuda K, Komatsu H, Enya T, Matsushima-Hibiya Y, Mutoh H, Sugimura T, Wakabayashi K. Suppression by flavonoids of COX-2 promoter-dependent transcriptional activity in colon cancer cells: structure-activity relationship. *Jpn J Cancer Res* 2000 Jul;91(7):686-91.

[83] Hakkak R, Korourian S, Ronis MJ, Johnston JM, Badger TM. Soy protein isolate consumption protects against azoxymethane-induced colon tumors in male rats. *Cancer Lett* 2001 May;166(1):27-32.

[84] Rosenberg Zand RS, Jenkins DJ, Diamandis EP. Flavonoids and steroid hormone-dependent cancers. *J Chromatogr B Analyt Technol Biomed Life Sci* 2002 Sep;777(1-2):219-32.

[85] McCarty MF. Vegan proteins may reduce risk of cancer, obesity, and cardiovascular disease by promoting increased glucagon activity. *Med Hypotheses* 1999 Dec;53(6):459-85.

[86] Kallay E, Adlercreutz H, Farhan H, Lechner D, Bajna E, Gerdenitsch W, Campbell M, Cross HS. Phytoestrogens regulate vitamin D metabolism in the mouse colon:

relevance for colon tumor prevention and therapy. *J Nutr* 2002 Nov;132(11 Suppl):3490S-3S.
[87] [Anonymous]. *Physicians' Desk Reference for Nutritional Supplements.* First ed. Montvale: Thomson PDR; 2003. 428 p.
[88] Azuma N, Suda H, Iwasaki H, Kanamoto R, Iwami K. Soybean curd refuse alleviates experimental tumorigenesis in rat colon. *Biosci Biotechnol Biochem* 1999 Dec;63(12):2256-8.
[89] Thiagarajan DG, Bennink MR, Bourquin LD, Kavas FA. Prevention of precancerous colonic lesions in rats by soy flakes, soy flour, genistein, and calcium. *Am J Clin Nutr* 1998 Dec;68(6 Suppl):1394S-9S.
[90] Messina MJ, Persky V, Setchell KD, Barnes S. Soy intake and cancer risk: a review of the in vitro and in vivo data. *Nutr Cancer* 1994;21(2):113-31.
[91] Wang W, Higuchi CM. Dietary soy protein is associated with reduced intestinal mucosal polyamine concentration in male Wistar rats. *J Nutr* 2000 Jul;130(7):1815-20.
[92] Davies MJ, Bowey EA, Adlercreutz H, Rowland IR, Rumsby PC. Effects of soy or rye supplementation of high-fat diets on colon tumour development in azoxymethane-treated rats. *Carcinogenesis* 1999 Jun;20(6):927-31.
[93] Fox CH, Eberl M. Phytic acid (IP6), novel broad spectrum anti-neoplastic agent: a systematic review. *Complement Ther Med* 2002 Dec;10(4):229-34.
[94] Appelt LC, Reicks MM. Soy induces phase II enzymes but does not inhibit dimethylbenz [a]anthracene-induced carcinogenesis in female rats. *J Nutr* 1999 Oct;129(10):1820-6.
[95] Yang CS, Maliakal P, Meng X. Inhibition of carcinogenesis by tea. *Annu Rev Pharmacol Toxicol* 2002;42:25-54.
[96] Trevisanato SI, Kim YI. Tea and health. *Nutr Rev* 2000 Jan;58(1):1-10.
[97] Lambert JD, Yang CS. Cancer chemopreventive activity and bioavailability of tea and tea polyphenols. *Mutat Res* 2003 Feb;523-524:201-8.
[98] Bushman JL. Green tea and cancer in humans: a review of the literature. *Nutr Cancer* 1998;31(3):151-9.
[99] Chen L, Lee MJ, Li H, Yang CS. Absorption, distribution, elimination of tea polyphenols in rats. *Drug Metab Dispos* 1997 Sep;25(9):1045-50.
[100] Kim S, Lee MJ, Hong J, Li C, Smith TJ, Yang GY, Seril DN, Yang CS. Plasma and tissue levels of tea catechins in rats and mice during chronic consumption of green tea polyphenols. *Nutr Cancer* 2000;37(1):41-8.
[101] Metz N, Lobstein A, Schneider Y, Gosse F, Schleiffer R, Anton R, Raul F. Suppression of azoxymethane-induced preneoplastic lesions and inhibition of COX-2 activity in the colonic mucosa of rats drinking a crude green tea extract. *Nutr Cancer* 2000;38(1):60-4.
[102] Lodovici M, Casalini C, De Filippo C, Copeland E, Xu X, Clifford M, Dolara P. Inhibition of 1,2-dimethylhydrazine-induced oxidative DNA damage in rat colon mucosa by black tea complex polyphenols. *Food Chem Toxicol* 2000 Dec;38(12):1085-8.
[103] Caderni G, De Filippo C, Luceri C, Salvadori M, Giannini A, Biggeri A, Remy S, Cheynier V, Dolara P. Effects of black tea, green tea and wine extracts on intestinal

carcinogenesis induced by azoxymethane in F344 rats. *Carcinogenesis* 2000 Nov;21(11):1965-9.

[104] Jia X, Han C. [Biomarkers in the studies on chemoprevention of colorectal cancer]. *Wei Sheng Yan Jiu* 2000 Mar;29(2):109-11.

[105] Luceri C, Caderni G, Sanna A, Dolara P. Red wine and black tea polyphenols modulate the expression of cycloxygenase-2, inducible nitric oxide synthase and glutathione-related enzymes in azoxymethane-induced f344 rat colon tumors. *J Nutr* 2002 Jun;132(6):1376-9.

[106] Weisburger JH, Rivenson A, Reinhardt J, Aliaga C, Braley J, Pittman B, Zang E. Effect of black tea on azoxymethane-induced colon cancer. *Carcinogenesis* 1998 Jan;19(1):229-32.

[107] Xu M, Dashwood RH. Chemoprevention studies of heterocyclic amine-induced colon carcinogenesis. *Cancer Lett* 1999 Sep;143(2):179-83.

[108] Lou YR, Lu YP, Xie JG, Huang MT, Conney AH. Effects of oral administration of tea, decaffeinated tea, and caffeine on the formation and growth of tumors in high-risk SKH-1 mice previously treated with ultraviolet B light. *Nutr Cancer* 1999;33(2):146-53.

[109] Kondo K, Kurihara M, Miyata N, Suzuki T, Toyoda M. Mechanistic studies of catechins as antioxidants against radical oxidation. *Arch Biochem Biophys* 1999 Feb;362(1):79-86.

[110] Le Marchand L. Cancer preventive effects of flavonoids--a review. *Biomed Pharmacother* 2002 Aug;56(6):296-301.

[111] Katiyar SK. Skin photoprotection by green tea: antioxidant and immunomodulatory effects. *Curr Drug Targets Immune Endocr Metabol Disord* 2003 Sep;3(3):234-42.

[112] Katiyar SK, Bergamo BM, Vyalil PK, Elmets CA. Green tea polyphenols: DNA photodamage and photoimmunology. *J Photochem Photobiol B* 2001 Dec;65(2-3):109-14.

[113] Katiyar SK, Elmets CA. Green tea polyphenolic antioxidants and skin photoprotection (Review). *Int J Oncol* 2001 Jun;18(6):1307-13.

[114] Hong J, Lu H, Meng X, Ryu JH, Hara Y, Yang CS. Stability, cellular uptake, biotransformation, and efflux of tea polyphenol (-)-epigallocatechin-3-gallate in HT-29 human colon adenocarcinoma cells. *Cancer Res* 2002 Dec;62(24):7241-6.

[115] Morand C, Manach C, Crespy V, Remesy C. Quercetin 3-O-beta-glucoside is better absorbed than other quercetin forms and is not present in rat plasma. *Free Radic Res* 2000 Nov;33(5):667-76.

[116] Salucci M, Stivala LA, Maiani G, Bugianesi R, Vannini V. Flavonoids uptake and their effect on cell cycle of human colon adenocarcinoma cells (Caco2). *Br J Cancer* 2002 May;86(10):1645-51.

[117] Ohishi T, Kishimoto Y, Miura N, Shiota G, Kohri T, Hara Y, Hasegawa J, Isemura M. Synergistic effects of (-)-epigallocatechin gallate with sulindac against colon carcinogenesis of rats treated with azoxymethane. *Cancer Lett* 2002 Mar;177(1):49-56.

[118] Jia X, Han C. Effects of green tea on colonic aberrant crypt foci and proliferative indexes in rats. *Nutr Cancer* 2001;39(2):239-43.

[119] Chen C, Shen G, Hebbar V, Hu R, Owuor ED, Kong AN. Epigallocatechin-3-gallate-induced stress signals in HT-29 human colon adenocarcinoma cells. *Carcinogenesis* 2003 Aug;24(8):1369-78.

[120] Chen ZP, Schell JB, Ho CT, Chen KY. Green tea epigallocatechin gallate shows a pronounced growth inhibitory effect on cancerous cells but not on their normal counterparts. *Cancer Lett* 1998 Jul;129(2):173-9.

[121] Paquay JB, Haenen GR, Stender G, Wiseman SA, Tijburg LB, Bast A. Protection against nitric oxide toxicity by tea. *J Agric Food Chem* 2000 Nov;48(11):5768-72.

[122] Lu J, Ho CT, Ghai G, Chen KY. Differential effects of theaflavin monogallates on cell growth, apoptosis, and Cox-2 gene expression in cancerous versus normal cells. *Cancer Res* 2000 Nov;60(22):6465-71.

[123] Yang GY, Liao J, Li C, Chung J, Yurkow EJ, Ho CT, Yang CS. Effect of black and green tea polyphenols on c-jun phosphorylation and H(2)O(2) production in transformed and non-transformed human bronchial cell lines: possible mechanisms of cell growth inhibition and apoptosis induction. *Carcinogenesis* 2000 Nov;21(11):2035-9.

[124] Imai K, Suga K, Nakachi K. Cancer-preventive effects of drinking green tea among a Japanese population. *Prev Med* 1997 Nov;26(6):769-75.

[125] Inoue M, Tajima K, Hirose K, Hamajima N, Takezaki T, Kuroishi T, Tominaga S. Tea and coffee consumption and the risk of digestive tract cancers: data from a comparative case-referent study in Japan. *Cancer Causes Control* 1998 Mar;9(2):209-16.

[126] Terry P, Wolk A. Tea consumption and the risk of colorectal cancer in Sweden. *Nutr Cancer* 2001;39(2):176-9.

[127] Cerhan JR, Putnam SD, Bianchi GD, Parker AS, Lynch CF, Cantor KP. Tea consumption and risk of cancer of the colon and rectum. *Nutr Cancer* 2001;41(1-2):33-40.

[128] Su LJ, Arab L. Tea consumption and the reduced risk of colon cancer -- results from a national prospective cohort study. *Public Health Nutr* 2002 Jun;5(3):419-25.

[129] Hakim IA, Hartz V, Harris RB, Balentine D, Weisgerber UM, Graver E, Whitacre R, Alberts D. Reproducibility and relative validity of a questionnaire to assess intake of black tea polyphenols in epidemiological studies. *Cancer Epidemiol Biomarkers Prev* 2001 Jun;10(6):667-78.

[130] Conney AH, Lou YR, Xie JG, Osawa T, Newmark HL, Liu Y, Chang RL, Huang MT. Some perspectives on dietary inhibition of carcinogenesis: studies with curcumin and tea. *Proc Soc Exp Biol Med* 1997 Nov;216(2):234-45.

[131] Sharma OP. Antioxidant activity of curcumin and related compounds. *Biochem Pharmacol* 1976 Aug;25(15):1811-2.

[132] Srimal RC, Dhawan BN. Pharmacology of diferuloyl methane (curcumin), a non-steroidal anti-inflammatory agent. *J Pharm Pharmacol* 1973 Jun;25(6):447-52.

[133] Cheng AL, Hsu CH, Lin JK, Hsu MM, Ho YF, Shen TS, Ko JY, Lin JT, Lin BR, Ming-Shiang W, Yu HS, Jee SH, Chen GS, Chen TM, Chen CA, Lai MK, Pu YS, Pan MH, Wang YJ, Tsai CC, Hsieh CY. Phase I clinical trial of curcumin, a chemopreventive agent, in patients with high-risk or pre-malignant lesions. *Anticancer Res* 2001 Jul;21(4B):2895-900.

[134] Rao CV, Rivenson A, Simi B, Reddy BS. Chemoprevention of colon cancer by dietary curcumin. *Ann N Y Acad Sci* 1995 Sep;768:201-4.

[135] Kawamori T, Lubet R, Steele VE, Kelloff GJ, Kaskey RB, Rao CV, Reddy BS. Chemopreventive effect of curcumin, a naturally occurring anti-inflammatory agent, during the promotion/progression stages of colon cancer. *Cancer Res* 1999 Feb;59(3):597-601.

[136] Perkins S, Verschoyle RD, Hill K, Parveen I, Threadgill MD, Sharma RA, Williams ML, Steward WP, Gescher AJ. Chemopreventive efficacy and pharmacokinetics of curcumin in the min/+ mouse, a model of familial adenomatous polyposis. *Cancer Epidemiol Biomarkers Prev* 2002 Jun;11(6):535-40.

[137] Hanif R, Qiao L, Shiff SJ, Rigas B. Curcumin, a natural plant phenolic food additive, inhibits cell proliferation and induces cell cycle changes in colon adenocarcinoma cell lines by a prostaglandin-independent pathway. *J Lab Clin Med* 1997 Dec;130(6):576-84.

[138] Moragoda L, Jaszewski R, Majumdar AP. Curcumin induced modulation of cell cycle and apoptosis in gastric and colon cancer cells. *Anticancer Res* 2001 Mar;21(2A):873-8.

[139] Goel A, Boland CR, Chauhan DP. Specific inhibition of COX-2 expression by dietary curcumin in HT-29 human colon cancer cells. *Cancer Lett* 2001 Oct;172(2):111-8.

[140] Chen H, Zhang ZS, Zhang YL, Zhou DY. Curcumin inhibits cell proliferation by interfering with the cell cycle and inducing apoptosis in colon carcinoma cells. *Anticancer Res* 1999 Sep;19(5A):3675-80.

[141] Rao CV, Rivenson A, Simi B, Reddy BS. Chemoprevention of colon carcinogenesis by dietary curcumin, a naturally occurring plant phenolic compound. *Cancer Res* 1995 Jan;55(2):259-66.

[142] Chen H, Zhang ZS, Zhang YL, Zhou DY. Curcumin inhibits cell proliferation by interfering with the cell cycle and inducing apoptosis in colon carcinoma cells. *Anticancer Res* 1999 Sep;19(5A):3675-80.

[143] Khar A, Ali AM, Pardhasaradhi BV, Varalakshmi CH, Anjum R, Kumari AL. Induction of stress response renders human tumor cell lines resistant to curcumin-mediated apoptosis: role of reactive oxygen intermediates. *Cell Stress Chaperones* 2001 Oct;6(4):368-76.

[144] Rashmi R, Santhosh Kumar TR, Karunagaran D. Human colon cancer cells differ in their sensitivity to curcumin-induced apoptosis and heat shock protects them by inhibiting the release of apoptosis-inducing factor and caspases. *FEBS Lett* 2003 Mar;538(1-3):19-24.

[145] Samaha HS, Kelloff GJ, Steele V, Rao CV, Reddy BS. Modulation of apoptosis by sulindac, curcumin, phenylethyl-3-methylcaffeate, and 6-phenylhexyl isothiocyanate: apoptotic index as a biomarker in colon cancer chemoprevention and promotion. *Cancer Res* 1997 Apr;57(7):1301-5.

[146] Shalini VK, Srinivas L. Lipid peroxide induced DNA damage: protection by turmeric (Curcuma longa). *Mol Cell Biochem* 1987 Sep;77(1):3-10.

[147] Subramanian M, Sreejayan, Rao MN, Devasagayam TP, Singh BB. Diminution of singlet oxygen-induced DNA damage by curcumin and related antioxidants. *Mutat Res* 1994 Dec;311(2):249-55.

[148] Piper JT, Singhal SS, Salameh MS, Torman RT, Awasthi YC, Awasthi S. Mechanisms of anticarcinogenic properties of curcumin: the effect of curcumin on glutathione linked detoxification enzymes in rat liver. *Int J Biochem Cell Biol* 1998 Apr;30(4):445-56.

[149] Susan M, Rao MN. Induction of glutathione S-transferase activity by curcumin in mice. *Arzneimittelforschung* 1992 Jul;42(7):962-4.

In: Focus on Colorectal Cancer Research
Editor: Julia D. Martinez, pp. 65-96

ISBN #1-59454-101-9

Chapter IV

COLORECTAL CANCER AND THE GROWTH HORMONE/INSULIN-LIKE GROWTH FACTOR-I AXIS

Stephen A. Bustin*
Centre for Academic Surgery
Paul J. Jenkins
Department of Endocrinology

ABSTRACT

Colorectal cancer risk is determined by a combination of environmental factors and genetic predisposition. Recent evidence suggests that dietary and related factors such as physical activity and body size may influence colorectal cancer risk through their effects on the serum concentration of insulin-like growth factor-I (IGF-I) and insulin-like growth factor binding protein (IGFBP)-3, two members of the growth hormone (GH)/IGF-I axis. The GH/IGF-I axis is involved in both human development as well as the maintenance of normal function and homeostasis in most cells of the body. In addition to their classical role as endocrine hormones, its members regulate a wide range of biological functions such as cell proliferation, differentiation and apoptosis through paracrine and autocrine mechanisms. This is particularly evident in its critical role as a regulator of rapidly renewing epithelial cell populations such as those found in the colon. Here its appropriate expression is responsible for the ordered migration of differentiating cells from the bottom towards the top of the colonic crypt and their eventual demise through apoptosis. During cancer development this complex network regulating tissue homeostasis breaks down, with inappropriate expression of the GH/IGF-I axis making an important contribution. The increased understanding of the molecular mechanisms and

* Address for Correspondence: Centre for Academic Surgery, Barts and the London Queen Mary's School of Medicine and Dentistry London E1 1BB, Tel: +44-020-7377-7000 Ext 2431, Fax: ++44-020-7377-7283, Email: s.a.bustin@qmul.ac.uk

signalling pathways regulated by the GH/IGF-I axis has started to provide significant insights into the aetiology, prevention and therapy for this cancer.

Keywords: proliferation; differentiation; mitogen; apoptosis; signal transduction; hybrid receptors; growth hormone; IGF-I; colorectal cancer

INTRODUCTION

The risk of developing colorectal cancer is determined by a combination of genetic factors and environmental effects, in particular diet and lifestyle. Rates of colorectal cancer vary by as much as 10-fold between low-incidence areas, generally in the third world, to much higher rates in the developed world, paralleling changes in diet and lifestyle [1]. Furthermore, migrants from low-risk areas to developed countries experience rapid increases in colorectal cancer risk within the same generation. This is clear evidence that non-hereditary factors play a major aetiological role in colorectal cancer.

Two uncertainties remain: first, what precisely are the dietary and lifestyle factors that contribute to the increased risk and second, what is the mechanism by which they effect that risk? In contrast to long-held views, most recent data suggest at best a weak link between dietary fibre [2;3], fat and meat intake [4;5] and risk of adenomas and colorectal cancer. On the other hand, it is now clear that low levels of physical activity and greater adiposity increase risks and folic acid, calcium supplements and adequate vitamin D levels may act as protective agents [6;7].

A link between these factors and the development of cancers is provided by endogenous hormones and growth factors. Dietary and other factors stimulate their secretion from distant organs, e.g. the liver (endocrine), from nearby (paracrine) and adjacent (juxtacrine) cells or from the cell itself (autocrine). They may bind to specific membrane-bound receptors and initiate a signal transduction cascade, or they may enter the nucleus directly and bind to specific target sequences on the cell's DNA. In either event, cells alter their pattern of gene expression and respond to the external stimulus by modifying their behaviour in an appropriate manner (Figure 1). Consequently, growth factors and their respective receptors are central to the regulation of normal cell proliferation, differentiation and apoptosis. Subtle changes in cellular location, e.g. whether it is at the bottom or at the top of the colonic crypt, will result in that cell being exposed to different combinations and concentrations of growth factors and result in the expression of a different repertoire of genes. Clearly, the complex structure of the colon requires very tight regulation of the expression of any growth factors in order to maintain the homeostastic balance between cellular proliferation, differentiation and apoptosis. Therefore, it is not surprising that aberrant expression of hormones and growth factors also has a key role in tumour promotion and growth.

One important group of growth factors is the growth hormone (GH)/ insulin-like growth factor-I (IGF-I) axis, which plays an important role in the regulation of normal human growth and development [8]. Its inappropriate expression appears to contribute to the growth, maintenance and progression of the most common cancers, including cancers of the breast, lung and colon [9]. Conversely, the reduction of serum IGF-I levels as occurs with caloric intake restriction leads to a significant reduction in the frequency of intestinal cancers [10].

Recent epidemiological and experimental studies have associated the increased colorectal cancer risk of dietary factors with their effects on the bioavailability of members of the GH/IGF-I axis, in particular IGF-I and its predominant binding protein insulin-like growth factor binding protein (IGFBP)-3. However, it is also becoming clear that there are extensive interactions between the IGF-I, epidermal growth factor (EGF), oestrogen and insulin signal transduction pathways which provide further potential mechanisms through which dietary and other factors, *e.g.* bile acids, sodium butyrate, folate and vitamin D, may modulate the risk of colorectal cancer.

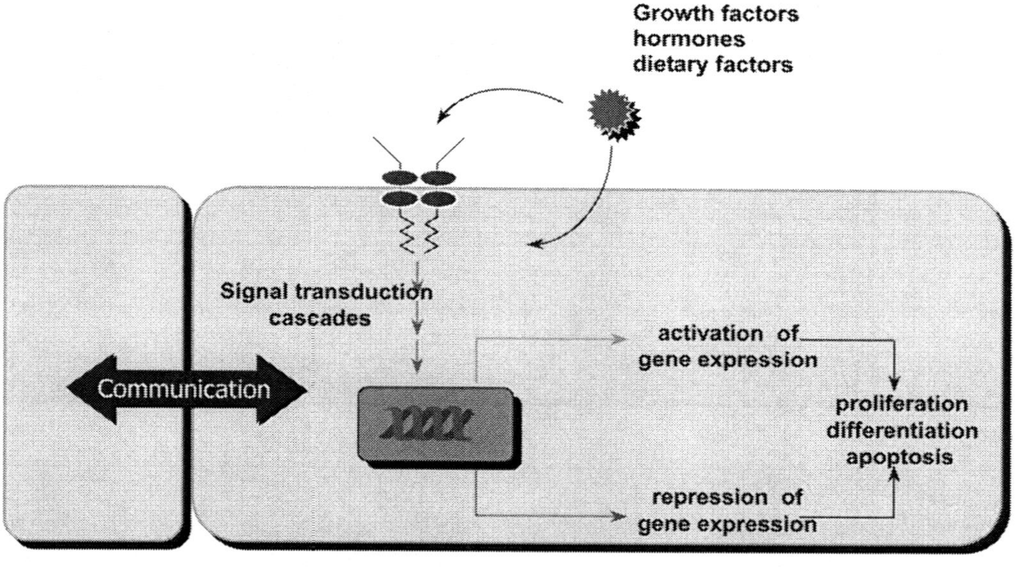

Figure 1. Regulation of cell behaviour. External stimuli, whether endocrine, paracrine, juxtacrine or autocrine, trigger signal transduction cascades that result in a cell altering its expression profile to adjust to an altered environmental condition or location. Some factors can bind directly to specific sites on promoters and activate or repress gene expression.

Colorectal Cancer

Most colorectal cancers arise sporadically, with inherited cancer syndromes accounting for about 5% of all cases. Alterations in cellular behaviour in response to environmental changes are reversible, once that change is reversed. However, over the course of several decades, genetic and epigenetic changes accumulate within a cell and these can modify its behavioural responses. Most important are those changes that result in alterations within key signalling pathways and that give the cells some growth and survival advantage. Eventually, this leads to the pathologic transformation, first to an adenomatous polyp and ultimately an invasive cancer [11]. Two distinct pathways of tumorigenesis exist in sporadic colorectal cancer. The chromosomal instability (CIN) phenotype, which accounts for 85% of sporadic colorectal cancers, is characterized by gross chromosomal lesions. The microsatellite instability pathway (MIN), which is characterized by widespread microsatellite instability due to aberrant DNA mismatch repair machinery, accounts for 15% of all sporadic colorectal cancers [12].

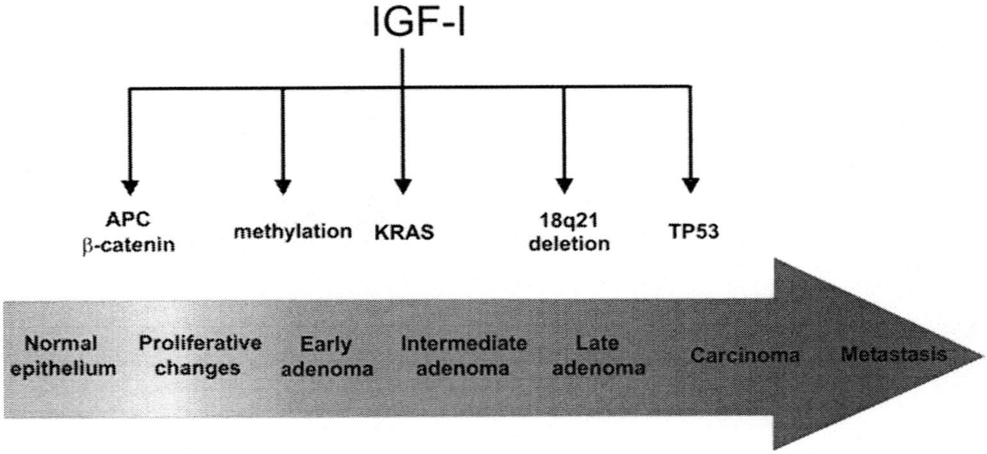

Figure 2. IGF-I and colorectal cancer development. The stepwise progression from normal colonic epithelium to an invasive carcinoma is shown, together with the main alteration underlying these changes. IGF-I directly affects every step of this progression. Its effects on methylation [196] and p53 expression [197;198] have not yet been demonstrated in the colon.

The concept of colorectal carcinogenesis as a multistep process is well established, and a series of mutations have been identified that result in a colorectal cancer-specific genetic pathway (Figure 2) [13]. In CIN cancers at least four sequential alterations in a number of oncogenes and tumour suppressor genes have to occur to permit a colorectal cancer to develop. Inactivating mutations of the adenomatous polyposis coli (APC) tumour suppressor gene on chromosome 5q21 are one of the earliest events in colorectal tumorigenesis and are found in 60-80% of sporadic colorectal cancers [14]. APC is a multifunctional protein that contains several amino acid domains that mediate its interactions with numerous other proteins [15], many of which are influential in mediating the effects of the GH/IGF-I axis. APC's key functions include (i) regulation of the steady state levels of β-catenin and its degradation by the ubiquitin-proteasome pathway, (ii) maintenance of apoptosis, (iii) cell-cycle progression and (iv) maintenance of chromosomal stability. Activating mutations of the K-ras protooncogene, which are found in up to 50% of sporadic colorectal tumours, are another early event and have been reported in histologically normal colonic mucosa [16]. K-RAS is involved in signal transduction from numerous growth factor receptors, including the GH and IGF-I receptors and overexpression can affect both cell adhesion and the cell cycle [17]. Loss of heterozygosity on 18q is a later event, and results in the inactivation of two tumour-suppressor genes, SMAD2 and SMAD4 of the transforming growth factor beta (TGFβ) pathway [18]. Mutations in the tumour-suppressor gene p53 on chromosome 17p appears to be a late event in the adenoma to carcinoma sequence, and are found in up to 70% of sporadic colorectal cancers [19]. Numerous other genetic events accompany neoplastic progression and are indicated by allelic loss on most chromosomes [20;21].

A different pathway is followed by colorectal tumours that display microsatellite instability, found in most cancers from patients with hereditary non-polyposis colorectal cancer (HNPCC) and approximately 15% of sporadic colorectal cancers. This instability is caused by mutations in (HNPCC) or epigenetic silencing of (sporadic cancers) DNA mismatch repair genes [22]. Their gene products control the repair of DNA base pair mismatches and ensure faithful DNA polymerisation during replication. DNA polymerases are apt to be especially error-prone in areas of DNA containing nucleotide repeat sequences and inappropriate insertion of nucleotides or slippage of the polymerase at these sites results in insertions or deletions consisting of multiples of the nucleotide repeat sequence. These are normally repaired by the DNA mismatch repair enzymes, but in their absence can become fixed during the next cycle of replication and generate alleles of different sizes. Consequently, MIN tumours have an increased mutation rate ("mutator phenotype"), with genes carrying microsatellite and other repeat sequences becoming targets for insertion/deletion type mutations. Several colorectal cancer-associated genes with such targets within their coding sequences have been identified, *e.g.* type II TGFβ receptor [23], insulin-like growth-factor II receptor [24], Bcl-2-associated X protein (BAX) [25]and the E2F4 cell cycle regulator [26]. Importantly, all of these genes are linked by their regulation through GH/IGF-I signalling (see below).

THE GH/IGF-I AXIS

Growth Hormone Releasing Hormone and Somatostatin

Classical endocrine regulation of the GH/IGF1 axis is orchestrated by the differential effects of growth hormone releasing hormone (GHRH) and somatostatin (SS) (Figure 3). These are secreted from the hypothalamus, bind to their respective receptors in the pituitary and effect pituitary GH release. Both the GHRH receptor (GHRH-R) and SS receptor (SSR) are G-protein-coupled seven-transmembrane proteins (7-TM), but whereas there is only a single GHRH-R, there are at least six molecular subtypes of SSR [27]. SS [28] and several subtypes of SSR are expressed in the human colon [29;30] and in the rat their levels increase after fasting [31]. SS works as an inhibitory peptide for inflammation [32] and can inhibit the growth of human colorectal cancer cell lines *in vitro* [33], but the molecular mechanisms underlying these effects remain unknown. Expression of the GHRH-R has been reported in one colorectal cancer cell line and GHRH-R antagonists inhibit cell growth *in vivo* and *in vitro* [34], but it is remains unclear whether GHRH is expressed in the human colon *in vivo* [35].

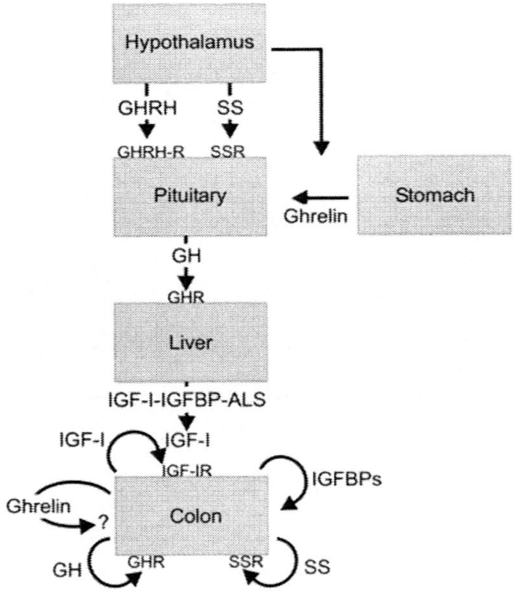

Figure 3. The growth hormone(GH)/insulin-like growth factor-I (IGF-I) axis. The secretion of GH from the pituitary is regulated through a complex neuroendocrine control system that comprises two stimulatory regulators, GH-releasing hormone (GHRH) and ghrelin, and inhibitory somatostatin (SS). GHRH and ghrelin binding to their respective receptors (GHRHR and GHSR) in the pituitary stimulates GH release which enters the circulation and binds to its receptor, principally located in the liver. This activates the expression and release of IGF-I. IGF-I is bound by IGF binding proteins (IGFBPs), especially IGFBP-3, and the acid labile subunit (ALS). Expression of all three components is regulated by the binding of GH to GHR and hence affected by the GH status of the individual. In addition, important autocrine/paracrine functions of GH are mediated through locally expressed GHR, IGF-I and IGF-IR.

Ghrelin

The recent identification of a second signalling pathway regulating GH release from the pituitary is a further indication that the regulation of GH release is still not fully understood. This pathway results in GH release that is distinct from its regulation by hypothalamic GHRH, and involves small synthetic molecules called growth-hormone secretagogues (GHSs) [36]. They act through the GH secretagogue receptor (GHS-R), which is related to the motilin receptor [37], although several observations suggest the presence of additional receptors. An endogenous ligand, ghrelin, was identified recently and shown to effect pituitary GH release in humans [38;39]. Its role in the human colon is unclear as conflicting reports concerning the gastrointestinal distribution and function of the GHS-R have emerged: whilst ghrelin mRNA has been detected in the colon [40], it is still unclear whether [41], or not [42] GHS-R is expressed. Expression may be difficult to detect, as it has recently been shown that expression of the GHS-R is confined to neuronal cell bodies and fibres, entero-endocrine and mast cells, whereas it is absent from epithelial cells [43].

GH and GHR

GH is a peptide hormone synthesised and secreted mainly by the anterior pituitary gland. Its biological effects are mediated by its interaction with a specific growth hormone receptor (GHR). This is a transmembrane glycoprotein member of the cytokine receptor superfamily and it is expressed in most tissue types [44]. Transcription of the GH gene in the pituitary is regulated by a tissue-specific transcriptional activator protein, PIT-1. However, the contextual details of GH gene regulation are still not well understood [45] and PIT-1 by itself does not activate the GH gene. The GHR gene is transcribed as a primary mRNA that can undergo alternative processing to produce several related mRNAs, including membrane bound GHR itself, the circulating GH binding protein, and a truncated GHR comprising the extracellular part of the GHR that inhibits normal cellular responses to GH [46]. Transcription is initiated from multiple promoters which, in conjunction with alternative splicing, allows for exquisite regulation of gene expression [47].

Most biological effects of GH appear to be indirect and are mediated by its interaction with its hepatic receptor, which stimulates expression and the release of IGF-I peptide from the liver. A GH-like activity was first detected in the colon in 1981 [48], but there have been no further reports about whether GH is transcribed in the colon, or how its expression might be regulated.

We have used a real-time RT-PCR assay to investigate the expression of GH mRNA in a consecutive series of 40 paired normal and malignant human colon biopsies. GH mRNA was detected in all samples, with little variation in mRNA levels between individuals. Steady-state mRNA levels were low, with a median of about $1 x 10^6$copy numbers/μg RNA, which equates to approximately 1 copy per cell, probably an indication that GH expression is not universal, but is confined to a subpopulation of cells. There was no significant difference between normal ($7.8 x 10^5$ copies/μg RNA) and tumour ($1.6 x 10^6$ copies/μg RNA) samples, or between samples taken from the proximal or distal colon (Figure 4).

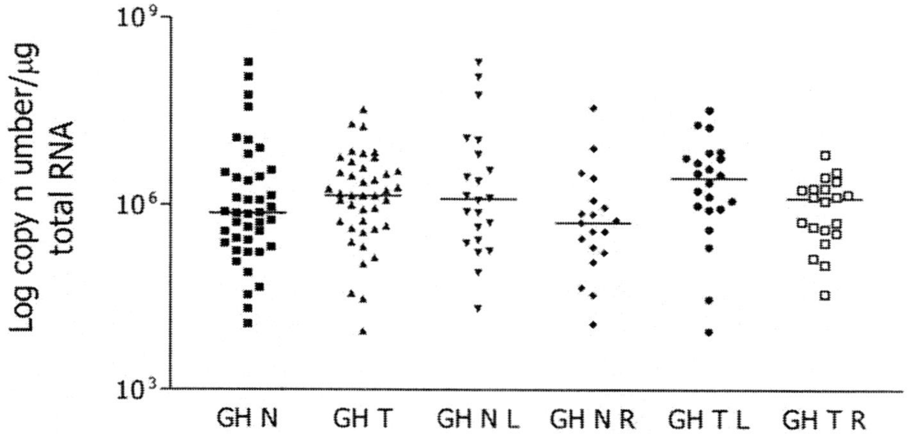

Figure 4. Quantification of GH mRNA levels in the human colon. GH mRNA is universally expressed, but there is no evidence for differential expression between normal and tumour tissue or between the left and the right side of the colon. (N is normal, T is tumour, R is right and L is left side).

Highest GHR mRNA levels in the colon are observed in the proliferating and differentiating zones of the colonic crypt [49] and expression is mainly intracellular, probably a result of endoplasmic reticulum and Golgi localisation [50]. However, nothing is known about the function in the colon of the numerous regulatory elements directing GHR transcription, about the mechanisms directing splicing, the role of its truncated isoform (GHRtr) or its cleavage to GH binding protein. Many downstream components of the GHR signal transduction pathway are similar to, and may complement those involved in IGF-I signalling [44]. In particular, signalling molecules such as SHC and insulin receptor substrates 1 and 2 are activated, resulting in the activation of enzymes such as mitogen-activated protein kinased (MAPK), protein kinase C (PKC) and phosphatidylinositol 3'-kinase.

IGF-I and IGF1R

The functions of IGF-I as a mitogen [51] and anti-apoptotic survival factor [52;53] are well documented, as are its role in protein synthesis, glucose metabolism and in innate as well as acquired immunity [54]. However, it has become clear that in addition to its endocrine function, IGF-I can act in an autocrine/paracrine manner [55;56] and recent evidence suggests another function within the colon: IGF-I may have an important role in controlling the timing of the maturation process of the epithelial cells migrating along the crypt. Although the initial effects of IGF-I are mitogenic, it subsequently stimulates intestinal cell differentiation and induces growth arrest of colon cancer cells. The initial stimulation is due to AKT1 phosphorylation of forkhead-1. This results in the inactivation of forkhead-1 so that it no longer can activate the expression of the cdk inhibitor p27(kip1). However, this effect is short-lived and following a limited number of cell divisions, forkhead1 becomes dephosphorylated and p27(kip1) is upregulated, with resulting growth arrest [57]. This growth inhibition by IGF-I can be blocked by concurrent addition of IGFBP-3.

The single copy IGF-I gene consists of six exons and is transcribed from two promoters located 5' to exons 1 and 2, respectively [58]. As with the GHR, alternative RNA splicing and differential polyadenylation results in considerable heterogeneity in mature IGF-I transcripts, not all of which are expressed in the colon [59]. Most reports, although not all [60], are able to detect the presence of IGF-I mRNA in normal colon [61;62], and we have recently used a real-time RT-PCR assay to show its expression in 60% of normal and 54% of tumour biopsies [63].

In addition to GH, genetic predisposition plays an important role in determining circulating IGF-I levels [64], although the relative importance of genetic and environmental factors in intra- and inter-individual variation in IGF-I-signalling levels remains to be determined. Although low serum IGF-I levels are associated with a polymorphic CA microsatellite within the IGF-I gene [65], its relevance to colorectal cancer risk is uncertain [66].

IGF-I exerts its effects predominantly via the type I insulin-like growth factor receptor (IGF-IR), which also serves as a receptor for IGF-II. However, since regulation of IGF-II is GH-independent, its actions will not be discussed in this review. The IGF-IR, together with the insulin receptor (IR) with which it shares 70% homology, comprises the type II receptor tyrosine kinase (RTK) family [67].

IGF-IR mRNA contains an internal ribosome entry site (IRES) that may allow the cell to synthesise sufficient amount of IGF-IR to initiate anti-apoptotic pathways when normal protein synthesis is inhibited [68]. The receptor is synthesised as a single peptide that is cleaved to a 350 kDa heterotetrameric, disulphide linked, transmembrane glycoprotein. It consists of two extracellular 135 kDa α subunits, which bind IGF-I, and two intracellular 90 kDa β subunits, which have intrinsic tyrosine-specific protein kinase activity. Binding of ligands to IGF-IR results in the autophosphorylation of several tyrosines within the β subunits in an intramolecular trans-reaction [67]. This enhances its tyrosine kinase activity and provides docking sites for various SH2 and phosphotyrosine-binding (PTB) domain-containing proteins that mediate the signalling cascades originating from the IGF-IR. The specific signalling pathways engaged depend on the number of activated IGF-IRs, availability of intracellular signal transducers, the action of negative regulators, and is influenced by extracellular modulators such as the IGF binding proteins (IGFBPs) [69]. IGF-IR is expressed in most normal colon epithelia [70], colorectal carcinomas [71] and colorectal cell lines [72;73]. Most reports, although not all [74;75], agree that IGF-IR levels are upregulated in colorectal cancers compared with adjacent non-malignant colon [60;76;77]. Certainly, blocking of signalling through the IGF-IR blocks IGF-I-induced activation of Akt-1, suppresses tumorigenicity *in vitro* and *in vivo* and up-regulates apoptosis [78]. Furthermore, it inhibits growth and abrogates expression of VEGF [79]. This agrees with our finding that local expression of IGF-I is significantly correlated with angiogenesis in colorectal cancers [80].

Expression from the IGF-IR promoter is downregulated by the WT1 Wilms' tumour suppressor protein [81] and by wild-type 53, in contrast to mutant p53 which stimulates its activity without binding to its promoter [82]. Physical interaction of p53 and WT1 [83] stabilises p53 and inhibits its ability to induce apoptosis [84]. Conversely, the transcriptional activity of WT1 protein depends on the cellular status of p53 and in the presence of mutant p53 WT1 cannot suppress IGF-IR activity [85]. The importance of the interaction of these two proteins is illustrated by the finding that in breast cancers WT1 and mutant p53 are co-expressed in more aggressive, oestrogen receptor-negative cancers [86]. A recent report suggests universal upregulation of non-mutated WT1 in colorectal cancers [87], although a previous report did not concur [88]. Therefore, the upregulation of IGF-1R in colorectal cancers could be a consequence of a possible sequestration of WT1 by mutant p53.

IGFBPs

Most of the seven, possibly more, IGF binding proteins (IGFBPs) [89] are expressed in the colon [90]. They are members of a group of structurally related proteins that bind IGF-I competitively and significantly extend its half life [91]. Indeed, more than 90% of circulating IGF-I is complexed with IGFBPs, principally IGFBP-3 which is also up-regulated by GH [91]. This binding can result in growth-inhibitory as well as growth-promoting effects [92]. IGFBP-1, -2 and –4 can cross endothelial barriers and may transport IGF-I from the circulation to colonic tissue. IGFBP-3 and –5 can form alternative ternary complexes with

IGF-I and an acid-labile subunit (ALS), thus modulating the bioavailability of free IGF-I and retain it in the circulation [93]. It is not known whether the colon expresses ALS, but one could speculate that differential heterotrimerisation of locally produced IGF-I and ALS with IGFBP-3 and IGFBP-5 might be involved in regulating local IGF-I bioactivity. In addition to sequestration, IGFBP-3 can also prevent IGF-I-induced signalling by interacting competitively with the IGF-IR [94]. High IGF-I exposure results in the down regulation of IGF-IR; hence the binding of IGF-I to IGFBPs may protect it from down regulation by providing a reservoir of IGF-I that is presented to the IGF-IR in a controlled fashion [95]. These opposing effects of the IGFBPs probably play a role in regulating the actions of IGF-I on the turnover of rapidly proliferating colon cells.

In addition, IGFBPs can also bind to ECM components, cell surface binding sites, cytoplasmic proteins and nuclear receptors and these interactions result in IGF-I-independent actions of IGFBPs on cells. Polymorphisms within the IGFBP3 gene may result in subtle changes to IGFBP-3 protein function [96].

From a colorectal cancer point of view, the most relevant effects are those affecting cell behaviour associated with unregulated growth. For example, there is some suggestion that various forms of IGFBPs might play a modulatory role in the maintenance of a functional polarity in differentiated colon epithelial cells [97]. One important IGF-I-independent action of IGFBP-3 involves apoptosis, with several cell cycle regulators implicated. IGFBP-3-specific cell surface association receptors that have been detected in several tissue-types [98] and one is the retinoid X receptor-α, which is required for the actions of multiple natural ligands including thyroid hormone, vitamin D, and retinoic acid. Binding results in IGFBP-3 translocation to the nucleus and regulates the transcription of genes involved in the modulation of cell proliferation and apoptosis [99]. The aformentioned link between pathways regulated by the tumour suppressor p53 and IGF-I may arise through direct regulation of IGF- 1 receptor levels, [82] or by modulation of IGF-I via transactivation of the IGFBP-3 gene [100], which specifically enhances the response of colorectal cells to DNA damage [101]. The level of IGFBP-3 protein expression in colonic epithelial cells correlates with the p53 status of the cells, with wild type p53 cells secreting higher levels of IGFBP3 protein than mutant p53 cell lines. Sodium butyrate (NaB), which induces apoptosis in colorectal cancer cells, upregulates IGFBP-3 mRNA and protein in both wild type and mutant p53 expressing cell lines. This suggests that IGFBP-3 may act as a positive regulator of NaB-induced apoptosis in colonic epithelial cells [102]. Interestingly, and in contrast to the reduced serum levels reported in colorectal cancer patients, elevated local IGFBP-3 levels have been reported in colon cancers, compared with adjacent normal tissue, and IGFBP-3 appears to mediate TGFβ-induced proliferation of metastatic colon carcinoma cell lines [103]. Together this suggests that there may be a selective advantage for colon cancers with elevated IGFBP-3 levels *in vivo* because their IGFBP-3 could bind and inactivate high serum IGF-I levels, allowing the cancers to continue to proliferate.

IGFBP activity is also regulated by IGFBP proteases and phosphorylation, which affect the relative affinities of IGFBPs, IGFs and IGF-1R. Proteolytic cleavage of the IGFBPs results in a rapid, irreversible modification of their structure and function [104], whereas their phosphorylation transiently affects their affinity for IGF-I [105]. Autocrine regulation of IGFBPs by colorectal cancer cells is suggested by the finding that IGFBP-2, but not IGFBP-3 and –4, is selectively degraded by extracts prepared from normal colon and from cancer tissue [62] and may be implicated in colon cancer metastases and prognosis [106].

A ROLE FOR THE GH/IGF-I AXIS IN COLORECTAL TUMOURIGENESIS

A role for the GH/IGF-I axis in colorectal cancer pathogenesis is suggested by several prospective health screens. These indicate that individuals with higher IGF-I and lower IGFBP-3 serum levels within the normal range have an increased colorectal cancer risk [107-112]. One study finds an increased colon, but not rectal cancer risk [113]. These findings are supported by studies carried out in patients with acromegaly, who by definition have high levels of serum GH and IGF-I, and whose colonic epithelium is characterised by increased proliferation which is proportional to serum IGF-I levels [114]. These patients are at an increased risk of colorectal cancer [115-118] and their tumours are larger, more dysplastic and are often synchronous. There is also a suggestion that not only do adenomas occur more frequently in acromegaly but they behave more aggressively with an increased tendency for malignant progression. Importantly, a prospective study involving a second colonoscopic evaluation at intervals after the original screening examination when all visible polyps had been removed revealed new adenomas in a significant number of acromegalic patients and their occurrence was significantly related to both serum growth hormone and IGF-1 levels [119]. We have also recently shown that the increased colonic epithelial proliferation in acromegaly is accompanied by significantly reduced apoptosis and a disordered pattern of the bcl-2 family of apoptotic proteins (unpublished observation).

However, not all studies show this association between serum IGF-I levels and sporadic cancer risk [120;121], and one study reports increased levels of IGFBP-3 (and IGFBP-2) in patients with colorectal cancer [122]. Certainly, causality has not yet been established and elevated serum IGF-I levels in cancer patients may simply be a surrogate measure of some other process [123]. For example, it remains to be explained why serum levels of IGFBP3 and IGF-I, which are normally both regulated by GH and strongly and directly correlated, become decoupled so that despite increased GH and IGF-I levels, IGFBP-3 serum levels are negatively correlated with colorectal cancer risk.

The circulating levels of several members of the GH/IGF-I axis vary in response to nutritional status and in response to changes in energy metabolism. In the energy-restricted state, which is strongly protective against colorectal cancer, circulating levels of IGF-I, IGFBP-3, and insulin are decreased, whereas levels of IGFBPs-1 and -2 are increased [124]. Overeating and obesity, on the other hand, lead to hyperinsulinaemia and decreased levels of IGFBPs-1 and -2 but have little effect on IGF-I and IGFBP-3 levels. A recent report suggests that energy intake is positively related to plasma IGF-I levels, but only in certain sub-populations [125].

The regulation of the GH/IGF-I axis in the colon remains largely unexplored, both in terms of the regulation of GH and IGF-I expression itself, but also with respect to the role of the various IGFBPs and proteases, as well as the intracellular signalling pathways involved in transducing its numerous effects. This is important, since cellular responses to various stimuli are usually cell-type specific and pathways activated in one tissue-type may not be the ones relevant for colorectal tumour development. It is not even clear what cells within the colon express which GH/IGF-I axis proteins.

The colonic epithelium is arranged in crypts with actively dividing stem cells located towards the base, and differentiating daughter cells moving up the crypt towards the lumenal surface to undergo apoptosis (Figure 5). The steady state of cell growth of normal colonic epithelium is maintained by a dynamic balance between the different actions being performed by the cells and the extent of the various functional compartments along the crypt axis is maintained within precise boundaries by multiple homeostatic signals. Epithelial cells are separated from the connective tissue, comprising fibroblasts, myofibroblasts, endothelial and neuroendocrine cells, by a basement membrane composed of extracellular matrix (ECM). The ECM provides an intricate and organised meshwork of numerous growth factors that are secreted and act locally to regulate gene expression [126]. This cellular make-up of the colon would predict an important regulatory role for the GH/IGF-I axis and it is not surprising that IGF-I exerts paracrine actions to regulate crypt cell proliferation [127] as well as colonic restitution [128] through reorganisation of integrin receptors and modulation of E-cadherin/catenin complex function.

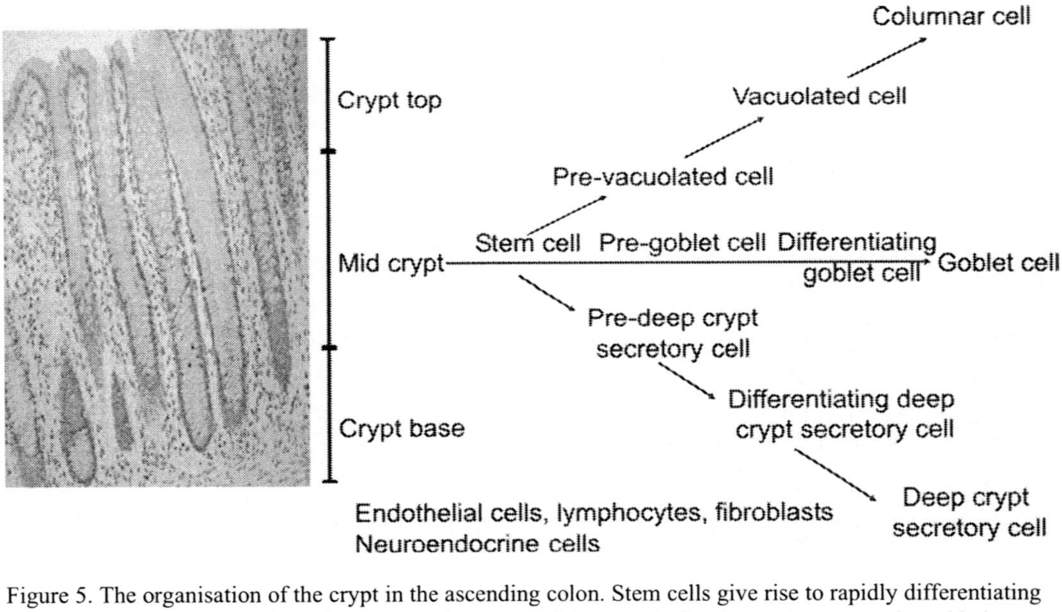

Figure 5. The organisation of the crypt in the ascending colon. Stem cells give rise to rapidly differentiating specialised epithelial cells that migrate towards the top of the crypt before becoming apoptotic and being sloughed off into the lumen. The connective tissue beneath the epithelial cells contains endothelial cells, lymphocytes, fibroblasts, myofibroblasts and neuroendocrine cells.

Downstream Effects of IGF-IR Activation

Mutational analyses of the IGF-IR show that the different functions are mediated by distinct domains within the cytoplasmic parts of the receptor. Ligand binding results in activation of the tyrosine kinase domains within the β-subunit and creates high affinity binding sites for signalling proteins, with the insulin receptor substrate-1 (IRS-1) being the major substrate of the IGF-IR, along with IRS-2, Shc, Crk, Grb-2 and Grb-10 [8]. Phosphorylated IRS-1 employs its src-homology domains to recruit other SH-domain proteins, and the result is the intracytoplasmic assembly of a complex consisting of a variety of proteins that are responsible for stimulating diverse downstream signal transduction pathways. The two main signaling pathways involve the p21 ras/mitogen-activated protein (MAP) kinase and the phosphatidyl inositol-3 kinase (PI-3K) pathways (Figure 6). Activation of Ras and the MAP kinase pathway is initiated by Grb-2 binding to IRS-1, SOS binding to this complex via SH3 domains, followed by Ras and Raf activation and downstream MAP kinases. In addition, the IGF-IR can bind directly to Crk and Shc which can activate the Grb-2/SOS complex. This results in the activation of early response genes such as c-fos and c-jun, and thus in cell cycle progression [129]. Alternatively, or complementary, interaction of the phosphotyrosines of IRS-1with the p85 subunit of the phosphatidylinositol-3 kinase (PI-3K) [130] couples IGF-IR signalling to the S6 kinase cascade [131]. PI-3k associates with membranes where its p110 catalytic subunit phosphorylates phosphoinositides. These, in turn, trigger the phosphorylation of protein kinase B (PKB/Akt), which phosphorylates Bad, an apoptosis-inducing member of the Bcl-2 family of proteins [132]. Bad becomes sequestered by 14-3-3 proteins and becomes unable to bind and inactivate anti-apoptotic Bcl-2 and Bcl-x_L and suppresses c-Myc-induced apoptosis. Therefore, activation of this pathway frequently results in anti-apoptotic signalling. However, pathways are cell type dependent and a strict separation of pathways is not possible since anti-apoptotic effects of IGF-1 can be effected through either pathway [133], and they can interact with and may even be able to replace each other [134]. This is illustrated by the anti-apoptotic protein, mirk, whose expression is downregulated by the IGF-I-induced ERKs in colon cancer cells [135]. One important element in this crosstalk may be Ras, which appears to have a dual function, since it is also an upstream effector of PI(3)K [136]. Furthermore, novel signalling pathways are constantly being identified, e.g. an IGF-IR-mediated survival signalling pathway that is independent of PI(3)K and PKB/Akt activity [137] and there is some suggestion that tumour cells can employ different pathways from those described in non-transformed cells [138]. Finally, polymorphisms in IRS-1 [139] and in the p85α-subunit of PI3-kinase [140] interfere with insulin-, and may well also do so with IGF-I-stimulated signalling.

Choice of signalling pathway is also stimulus dependent: IGF-I can protect colon cancer cells from TNF-α -induced apoptosis by potentiating the MAPK and NFκB signalling pathways induced by TNF-α itself [53], even in the absence of cell adhesion-mediated signaling [141].

Another important effect of IGF-IR signalling concerns its role in colon epithelial restitution, which is crucial to the maintenance of a continuous physical and functional barrier that protects the colon from the external milieu. Local IGF-I and IGFBP-4 levels are significantly increased following surgical resection, with IGFBP3 being down regulated [142]. Colorectal cancer cell lines expressing high levels of the IGF-IR have a higher migratory capability and higher levels of activated c-Src compared with cells expressing low levels of IGF-IR [143]. IGF-I promotes the migration of human colon tumour cells by reorganising the integrins at the leading edge of the migration cells and modulating the function of theE-cadherin/β-catenin complex [128]. Again IGF-I stimulated colonic migration proceeds though the activation of multiple signalling pathways including PI-3k, PKCγ and δ, and MAPK, although the detailed contributions by individual members of the different pathways are contradictory.

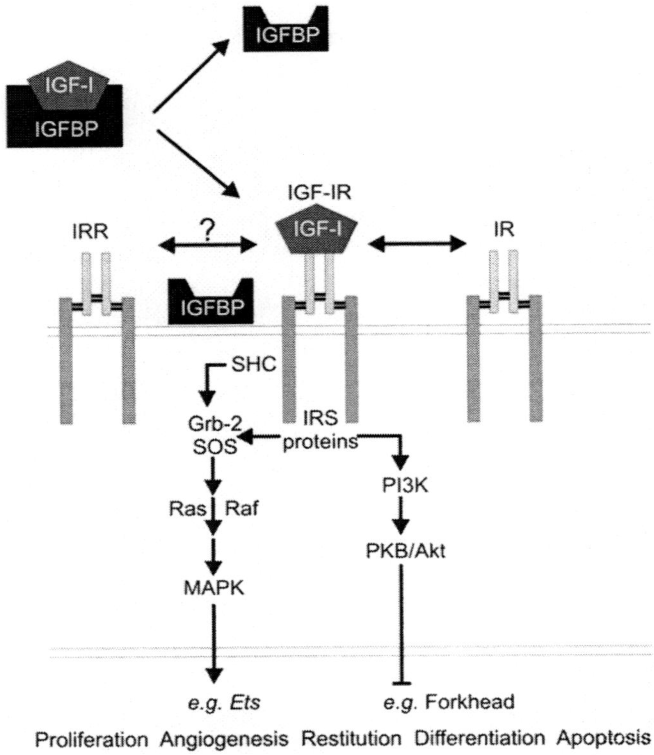

Figure 6. IGF-IR signalling. Insulin receptor (IR) and IGF-IR are structurally homologous and the complexity of IGF-I signalling is increased by the formation of hybrid receptors that result from the dimerisation of IGF-IR and IR hemireceptors. The IGF-IR consists of two extracellular α subunits, which bind IGF-I and two intracellular β subunits, which have intrinsic tyrosine-specific protein kinase activity. Proteolysis of IGFBPs leads to the release of IGF-I from its complex with IGFBPs and ALS (not shown) and cell-associated IGFBPs may have an additive or inhibitory effect. Binding of IGF-I to IGF-IR results in the autophosphorylation on tyrosine residues and provides docking sites for various proteins that mediate the signalling cascades originating from the IGF-IR. The specific signalling pathways engaged depend on the number of activated IGF-IRs, their interaction with other receptors (IR and IRR), availability of intracellular signal transducers, the action of negative regulators, and is influenced by extracellular modulators such as the IGFBPs. The insulin receptor substrate-1 (IRS-1) is the major substrate of the IGF-IR and activation of the mitogen-activated protein (MAP) kinase pathway is initiated by GRB2 binding to IRS-1, SOS binding to this complex via SH3 domains, followed by activation of Ras and Raf and of downstream MAP kinases. In addition, IRS-1 can associate with PI-3 kinase, thus triggering the phosphorylation of the serine kinase PKB/Akt. Similarly, the coupling of Shc with the IRS homologues Gab-1 or Gab-2 can activate the PI3 kinase pathway. Two examples of transcription factors affected by IGF-I are shown. The proto-oncogene, ets-1, is a transcription factor known to control the expression of a number of genes involved in extracellular matrix remodelling and has been postulated to play a role in colorectal cell migration and tumour invasion. It is activated by IGF-I [199] and a family member, PEA3, is upregulated by wnt1 signalling and is a potent activator of COX-2 transcription [200]. IGF-I down regulates the activity of Forkhead1 via the PI3K/Akt kinase pathway, leading to inhibition of this apoptotic transcription factor [57].

SIGNALLING SPECIFICITY

There is increasing evidence that the various signal transduction pathways interact with one another to generate complex networks with properties that the individual pathways lack. The IGF-IR appears to be at a convergence point in the control of cell growth and a functional IGF-I/IGF-IR autocrine loop is required for the mitogenic effects of a variety of growth factors, e.g. EGF [144]. Therefore, it is interesting that GH can phosphorylate ERbB-2 and inhibit EGF-induced mitogenic signalling in fibroblasts [145], whereas IGF-IR can phosphorylate and activate the EGF-R family member. In the colon, ErbB-2 expression may be associated with the early stages of tumour development. In addition, IGF-IR and ErbB-2 receptor can form heteromeric complexes, a process that is induced in breast cancer cells by IGF-I itself.

IGF-IR and IR have different capacities to activate specific cellular responses despite their high degree of homology and their interaction with apparently identical immediate downstream adaptors. For example, signalling through the IGF-IR is more effective at stimulating DNA synthesis [146] whereas the IR is more tightly coupled to the stimulation of glycogen synthesis and to the p44mapk pathway [147]. This raises important questions concerning the mechanisms by which IGF-I elicits its effects and how IGF-IR and IR initiated intracellular signalling differs [148]. Several proteins interacting preferentially with IGF-IR or IR have been identified [149;150] and this results in more efficient phosphorylation of PI-3K isoforms and of IRS-1 by the IR [151] and, more effective Shc phosphorylation, association of Shc with Grb-2 and activation of MAP kinase by the IGF-IR [152]. Furthermore, hybrid receptors that contain one each of the IR and IGF-IR α and β subunits have been identified [153-155]. Both hormone binding and signaling properties of the hybrid receptor appear to be different from that of either the IR or IGF-IR [156] and they appear to play a major role in mediating the IGF-I signal response in breast cancer [157]. The insulin receptor-related receptor (IRR) is another receptor with extensive sequence similarity with the IGF-IR [158] and, as it can associate with the IR [159], it may well also do so with the IGF-IR. On its own IRR does not bind IGF-I [160], but since IGF-I can bind efficiently to either IGF-IRα subunit, a hybrid IGF-IR/IRR molecule could be expected to bind IGF-I and display altered signalling specificity.

Clearly, hybrid receptors expand the possible repertoire of cellular responses to IGF-I stimulation and pathology in one receptor could affect both the hybrid and other receptor, or perhaps be partially compensated for by a hybrid receptor. It is likely that such hybrids also exist in colonic epithelium and could again indicate possible cooperation with IGF-IR in mitogenic signal transduction, facilitating the development and maintenance of the malignant phenotype.

The question of how cells distinguish between IGF-I and IGF-II binding to the IGF-IR also remains unanswered. It is likely that the interaction of IGF-I and IGF-II with their binding proteins direct their overall biological activities. Clearly, *in vivo* IGF-IR may be activated by different ligands and this activation occurs contemporaneously with signalling from multiple receptors. This results in the activation of similar signalling networks involving multiple interacting components, many of which are, in addition, promiscuous intermediates for multiple hormone, growth factor and cytokine receptors. It remains to be understood how such signalling is integrated and is able to confer specificity [161;162]. The ultimate impact on cell function depends on the patterns of interaction within these networks, their kinetics and sub cellular compartmentalisation.

In addition, IGF-I mRNA levels are regulated by oestrogen, which has a protective effect against colon cancer [163]. The extent of crosstalk between IGF-I and oestrogens in colorectal cancer remains unclear, but the effects of oestrogen in the colon are mediated through the oestrogen receptor (ER)-β and results in the inhibition of transcription from AP-1 containing promoters. The IGF-I promoter contains an AP-1 site and, interestingly, expression of ER-β is downregulated during malignant transformation of the colon [164].

TARGETS OF THE GH/IGF-I AXIS

Wnt

During embryonic development Wnt signalling is involved with patterning in the gut and each of the Wnt signalling components shows a characteristic and region-specific pattern of expression along the anterior-posterior axis of the digestive tube. In adult tissue, the Wnt signalling pathway regulates cell proliferation and its proper regulation is critical for a highly proliferative tissue such as the colonic epithelium where the epithelial cells proliferate from the bottom of the crypt at a rate that perfectly balances the death of cells that have reached the top [165]. Deregulation of this pathway, either through the inactivation of the adenomatous polyposis coli (APC) tumour suppressor gene or an activation mutation of β-catenin, is the first, virtually obligatory step, on the pathway leading to colorectal neoplasia [166]. IGF-I signalling results in the inactivation of glycogen synthase kinase (GSK-3β), a key negative regulator of the pathway, which mediates the downregulation of cytoplasmic β-catenin via the ubiquitin-proteasome pathway [167]. It also leads to the rapid phosphorylation of β-catenin, its dissociation from E-cadherin, nuclear accumulation and significantly increased transcription from Tcf-4 responsive promoters [168]. IGF-I-dependent stimulation of the β-catenin pathway also involves activation of the Ras signalling pathway [169]. Hence, IGF-I regulates the two events that are required for modulation of the ß-catenin/TCF-mediated transcription: the loss of E-cadherin function and the activation of the Wnt-signalling cascade. This suggests that IGF-I acts early in the adenoma-carcinoma progression sequence. However, a late function is not excluded as another function of IGF-I is the promotion of colonic cell migration through reorganisation of integrin receptors and through modulation of E-cadherin/catenins complex function [128]. Several cancer-associated genes are regulated by Tcf-4, including c-jun [170], cyclin D1 [171], matrilysin [172], eEF4E [173] and for at least one, c-myc [174], there is perfect correlation with nuclear β-catenin expression [175].

TGFβ

The observed increase in TGFβ mRNA levels in response to IGF-I signalling [176]is, at first sight, slightly paradoxical, since TGFβ signalling has a key role in counteracting the effects of mitogenic growth factors and results in inhibition of cell proliferation and promotion of apoptosis [177]. Hence reduced responsiveness to the inhibitory effects of TGFβ plays an important event in the loss of growth control in colorectal tumorigenesis [178]. Nevertheless, most colorectal cancers express high levels of TGFβ *in vitro* [179] and *in vivo* [180], and this correlates with disease progression [181] and metastasis [182]. The answer may lie in the finding that TGFβ receptor expression is downregulated in most MSI+ [23], and possibly also most other colorectal carcinomas [180], although there is some contradictory evidence [183]. TGFβ signalling in the absence of type II receptor expression results in the induction of cyclo-oxygenase-2 (Cox-2) [184], which is overexpressed in many colorectal cancers [185]. High levels of Cox-2 make colon epithelial cells more invasive [177] and upregulate angiogenic factors [186].

Angiogenesis

Tumour growth above a certain size depends on the recruitment of a new vasculature and tumours express a number of autocrine and paracrine factors that activate or otherwise facilitate this process. Vascular endothelial growth factor (VEGF) is the main pro-angiogenesis factor responsible for neo-vascularisation of colorectal tumours and signalling through the IGF-IR [187] increases its expression at the level of transcription and mRNA stability [188] as well as at the protein level in several colorectal cancer cell lines [189]. A recent report shows that it effects this through the MAPK pathway activating hypoxia-inducible factor-1 [190]. The biological relevance of this is revealed by the finding that the increase in VEGF levels is accompanied by an increase in microvessel density [63], which suggests that neovascularisation promoted by IGF-I-induced expression of VEGF in colorectal carcinoma cells may be another mechanism through which it encourages tumour growth.

Apoptosis

Tumour cells are believed to contain a block in differentiation that renders them more susceptible than normal cells to the induction of apoptosis. Therefore, mutations that inhibit apoptosis and promote survival through pathways such as those mediated by the IGF-IR are actively selected in tumour cells. Expression of the anti-apoptotic Bcl-xL protein c is elevated in colorectal tumourigenesis [191] and is up regulated by IGF-I [192]. It can either homodimerise and inhibit apoptosis or it can heterodimerise with Bad and cause apoptosis. IGF-I prevents heterodimerisation by activating Akt, which phosphorylates Bad and can no longer bind Bcl-x_L [193]. In addition, IGF-I activated-Akt phosphorylates pro-caspase-9, which then cannot bind to cytochrome c/Apaf-1 to undergo proteolytic cleavage to caspase-9. It also binds to caspase-9 itself, rendering it unable to cleave caspase-3 and prevents progression of the caspase cascade to apoptosis. [194]

Clinical Benefits

This review has discussed the considerable evidence in support of an important role for the GH/IGF-I axis in the development and growth of colorectal cancer. Further knowledge of the mechanisms regulating this influence and the downstream signalling pathways by which these components exert their effects may have important clinical applications. For instance, confirmation of the link between the prospective development of colon cancer and circulating IGF-I levels may allow the identification of individuals at increased risk to be identified. Next, more vigilant screening procedures could be put in place and manoeuvres taken to reduce IGF-I levels. This concerns in particular patients with acromegaly, amongst whom high IGF-I levels correlate with the development of new adenomas and in whom colonoscopic screening intervals are influenced by serum IGF-I levels [119].

Confirmation of this link also raises long-term safety issues regarding the increasing use of recombinant human growth hormone, not only in patients with pituitary growth hormone deficiency but also to adults (especially elderly) with normal growth hormone secretion, as a supposed tonic and 'elixir of youth'.

Therapeutic implications lie not only in possible chemoprevention but also in chemotherapy. Manipulation of the GH/IGF-I axis may be important in preventing the development of colon cancer, especially if colon-specific strategies can be devised. The effects of IGF-I in angiogenesis are also exciting considerable interest, particularly following the recent development of a specific GH receptor antagonist. Preliminary studies have suggested a marked inhibition of metastasis of colonic tumours in animals when this antagonist 'Pegvisomant' is combined with more standard cytotoxic drugs [195].

Conclusion

In vivo, signalling pathways initiated by IGF-IR activation in the colon are extremely complex: several ligands bind to the IGF-IR, which itself can heterodimerise with at least two other receptors, but perhaps most importantly, activation occurs contemporaneously with signalling from numerous other hormone and cytokine receptors. Therefore, signals are transduced along networks that involve multiple interacting components, many of which are shared and are intermediates for numerous hormone, growth factor and cytokine receptors. The pattern of the interactions within these networks, their kinetics and their subcellular compartmentalisation result in alterations to cellular behaviour that increase the risk of deregulated colon cell growth and, ultimately, permits the growth of neoplastic cells that are more likely to develop into carcinomas in the presence of high IGF-I levels. The contribution of the GH/IGF-I axis to the increased colorectal cancer risk and the contribution of this axis to the key regulatory signalling pathways remains a challenge for the future.

Acknowledgement

The authors' work is supported by grants from the Bowel and Cancer Research, the Joint Research Board and Cancer Research Committee of St Bartholomew's Hospital.

REFERENCES

[1] Koyama Y, Kotake K: Overview of colorectal cancer in Japan: report from the Registry of the Japanese Society for Cancer of the Colon and Rectum. *Dis.Colon Rectum* 1997;40:S2-S9.

[2] Terry P, Giovannucci E, Michels KB, Bergkvist L, Hansen H, Holmberg L, Wolk A: Fruit, vegetables, dietary fiber, and risk of colorectal cancer. *J Natl.Cancer Inst.* 2001;93:525-533.

[3] Fuchs CS, Giovannucci EL, Colditz GA, Hunter DJ, Stampfer MJ, Rosner B, Speizer FE, Willett WC: Dietary fiber and the risk of colorectal cancer and adenoma in women. *N.Engl.J Med.* 1999;340:169-176.

[4] Jarvinen R, Knekt P, Hakulinen T, Rissanen H, Heliovaara M: Dietary fat, cholesterol and colorectal cancer in a prospective study. *Br.J Cancer* 2001;85:357-361.

[5] Flood A, Velie EM, Sinha R, Chaterjee N, Lacey JV, Jr., Schairer C, Schatzkin A: Meat, fat, and their subtypes as risk factors for colorectal cancer in a prospective cohort of women. *Am.J Epidemiol.* 2003;158:59-68.

[6] Giovannucci E: Diet, body weight, and colorectal cancer: a summary of the epidemiologic evidence. *J Womens Health (Larchmt.)* 2003;12:173-182.

[7] Lamprecht SA, Lipkin M: Chemoprevention of colon cancer by calcium, vitamin D and folate: molecular mechanisms. *Nat.Rev.Cancer* 2003;3:601-614.

[8] Baserga R, Hongo A, Rubini M, Prisco M, Valentinis B: The IGF-I receptor in cell growth, transformation and apoptosis. *Biochim.Biophys.Acta* 1997;1332:F105-F126.

[9] Khandwala HM, McCutcheon IE, Flyvbjerg A, Friend KE: The effects of insulin-like growth factors on tumorigenesis and neoplastic growth. *Endocr.Rev.* 2000;21:215-244.

[10] Mai V, Colbert LH, Berrigan D, Perkins SN, Pfeiffer R, Lavigne JA, Lanza E, Haines DC, Schatzkin A, Hursting SD: Calorie restriction and diet composition modulate spontaneous intestinal tumorigenesis in Apc(Min) mice through different mechanisms. *Cancer Res.* 2003;63:1752-1755.

[11] Breivik J, Gaudernack G: Carcinogenesis and natural selection: a new perspective to the genetics and epigenetics of colorectal cancer. *Adv.Cancer Res.* 1999;76:187-212.

[12] Lindblom A: Different mechanisms in the tumorigenesis of proximal and distal colon cancers. *Curr.Opin.Oncol.* 2001;13:63-69.

[13] Fearon ER, Vogelstein B: A genetic model for colorectal tumorigenesis. *Cell* 1990;61:759-767.

[14] Cottrell S, Bicknell D, Kaklamanis L, Bodmer WF: Molecular analysis of APC mutations in familial adenomatous polyposis and sporadic colon carcinomas. *Lancet* 1992;340:626-630.

[15] Polakis P: The adenomatous polyposis coli (APC) tumor suppressor. *Biochim.Biophys.Acta* 1997;1332:F127-F147.

[16] Minamoto T, Yamashita N, Ochiai A, Mai M, Sugimura T, Ronai Z, Esumi, H.: Mutant K-ras in apparently normal mucosa of colorectal cancer patients. Its potential as a biomarker of colorectal tumorigenesis. *Cancer* 1995;75:1520-1526.

[17] Yang JJ, Kang JS, Krauss RS: Ras signals to the cell cycle machinery via multiple pathways to induce anchorage-independent growth. *Mol Cell Biol.* 1998;18:2586-2595.

[18] Thiagalingam S, Lengauer C, Leach FS, Schutte M, Hahn SA, Overhauser J, Willson JK, Markowitz S, Hamilton SR, Kern SE, Kinzler KW, Vogelstein B: Evaluation of candidate tumour suppressor genes on chromosome 18 in colorectal cancers. *Nat.Genet.* 1996;13:343-346.

[19] Cawkwell L, Lewis FA, Quirke P: Frequency of allele loss of DCC, p53, RBI, WT1, NF1, NM23 and APC/MCC in colorectal cancer assayed by fluorescent multiplex polymerase chain reaction. *Br.J Cancer* 1994;70:813-818.

[20] Ilyas M, Straub J, Tomlinson IP, Bodmer WF: Genetic pathways in colorectal and other cancers. *Eur.J Cancer* 1999;35:1986-2002.

[21] Robbins DH, Itzkowitz SH: The molecular and genetic basis of colon cancer. *Med.Clin.North Am.* 2002;86:1467-1495.

[22] Jacob S, Praz F: DNA mismatch repair defects: role in colorectal carcinogenesis. *Biochimie* 2002;84:27-47.

[23] Markowitz S, Wang J, Myeroff L, Parsons R, Sun L, Lutterbaugh J, Fan RS, Zborowska E, Kinzler KW, Vogelstein B: Inactivation of the type II TGF-beta receptor in colon cancer cells with microsatellite instability. *Science* 1995;268:1336-1338.

[24] Souza RF, Appel R, Yin J, Wang S, Smolinski KN, Abraham JM, Zou TT, Shi YQ, Lei J, Cottrell J, Cymes K, Biden K, Simms L, Leggett B, Lynch PM, Frazier M, Powell SM, Harpaz N, Sugimura H, Young J, Meltzer SJ: Microsatellite instability in the insulin-like growth factor II receptor gene in gastrointestinal tumours. *Nat.Genet.* 1996;14:255-257.

[25] Rampino N, Yamamoto H, Ionov Y, Li Y, Sawai H, Reed JC, Perucho M: Somatic frameshift mutations in the BAX gene in colon cancers of the microsatellite mutator phenotype. *Science* 1997;275:967-969.

[26] Souza RF, Yin J, Smolinski KN, Zou TT, Wang S, Shi YQ, Rhyu MG, Cottrell J, Abraham JM, Biden K, Simms L, Leggett B, Bova GS, Frank T, Powell SM, Sugimura H, Young J, Harpaz N, Shimizu K, Matsubara N, Meltzer SJ: Frequent mutation of the E2F-4 cell cycle gene in primary human gastrointestinal tumors. *Cancer Res.* 1997;57:2350-2353.

[27] Muller EE, Locatelli V, Cocchi D: Neuroendocrine control of growth hormone secretion. *Physiol Rev.* 1999;79:511-607.

[28] Chayvialle JA, Paulin C, Dubois PM, Descos F, Dubois MP: Ontogeny of somatostatin in the human gastro-intestinal tract, endocrine pancreas and hypothalamus. *Acta Endocrinol (Copenh)* 1980;94:1-10.

[29] Radulovic SS, Milovanovic SR, Cai RZ, Schally AV: The binding of bombesin and somatostatin and their analogs to human colon cancers. *Proc.Soc.Exp.Biol.Med.* 1992;200:394-401.

[30] Hope N, Butt G, Ross I, Warhurst G, Arn M, Grigor M, Lubcke R, Barbezat GO: Somatostatin enhances cAMP-dependent short-circuit current in human colon via somatostatin receptor subtype-2. *Dig.Dis.Sci.* 2001;46:2499-2503.

[31] Kido T, Sumii K, Kawano M, Sumii M, Yoshihara M, Chayama K: Food deprivation enhances somatostatin and somatostatin receptor subtype expression in rat colon. *Regul.Pept.* 2003;114:167-173.

[32] Watanabe T, Kubota Y, Sawada T, Muto T: Distribution and quantification of somatostatin in inflammatory disease. *Dis.Colon Rectum* 1992;35:488-494.

[33] Smith JP, Solomon TE: Effects of gastrin, proglumide, and somatostatin on growth of human colon cancer. *Gastroenterology* 1988;95:1541-1548.

[34] Szepeshazi K, Schally AV, Groot K, Armatis P, Halmos G, Herbert F, Szende B, Varga JL, Zarandi M: Antagonists of growth hormone-releasing hormone (GH-RH) inhibit IGF-II production and growth of HT-29 human colon cancers. *Br.J.Cancer* 2000;82:1724-1731.

[35] Shibasaki T, Kiyosawa Y, Masuda A, Nakahara M, Imaki T, Wakabayashi I, Demura H, Shizume K, Ling N: Distribution of growth hormone-releasing hormone-like immunoreactivity in human tissue extracts. *J Clin.Endocrinol.Metab* 1984;59:263-268.

[36] Dieguez C, Casanueva FF: Ghrelin: a step forward in the understanding of somatotroph cell function and growth regulation. *Eur.J.Endocrinol.* 2000;142:413-417.

[37] Feighner SD, Tan CP, McKee KK, Palyha OC, Hreniuk DL, Pong SS, Austin CP, Figueroa D, MacNeil D, Cascieri MA, Nargund R, Bakshi R, Abramovitz M, Stocco R, Kargman S, O'Neill G, Van Der Ploeg LH, Evans J, Patchett AA, Smith RG, Howard AD: Receptor for motilin identified in the human gastrointestinal system. *Science* 1999;284:2184-2188.

[38] Takaya K, Ariyasu H, Kanamoto N, Iwakura H, Yoshimoto A, Harada M, Mori K, Komatsu Y, Usui T, Shimatsu A, Ogawa Y, Hosoda K, Akamizu T, Kojima M, Kangawa K, Nakao K: Ghrelin Strongly Stimulates Growth Hormone Release in Humans. *J.Clin.Endocrinol.Metab* 2000;85:4908-4911.

[39] Peino R, Baldelli R, Rodriguez-Garcia J, Rodriguez-Segade S, Kojima M, Kangawa K, Arvat E, Ghigo E, Dieguez C, Casanueva FF: Ghrelin-induced growth hormone secretion in humans. *Eur.J Endocrinol.* 2000;143:R11-R14.

[40] Gnanapavan S, Kola B, Bustin SA, Morris DG, McGee P, Fairclough P, Bhattacharya S, Carpenter R, Grossman AB, Korbonits M: The Tissue Distribution of the mRNA of Ghrelin and Subtypes of Its Receptor, GHS-R, in Humans. *J Clin Endocrinol Metab* 2002;87:2988.

[41] Date Y, Kojima M, Hosoda H, Sawaguchi A, Mondal MS, Suganuma T, Matsukura S, Kangawa K, Nakazato M: Ghrelin, a novel growth hormone-releasing acylated peptide, is synthesized in a distinct endocrine cell type in the gastrointestinal tracts of rats and humans. *Endocrinology* 2000;141:4255-4261.

[42] Papotti M, Ghe C, Cassoni P, Catapano F, Deghenghi R, Ghigo E, Muccioli G: Growth hormone secretagogue binding sites in peripheral human tissues. *J.Clin.Endocrinol.Metab* 2000;85:3803-3807.

[43] Dass NB, Munonyara M, Bassil AK, Hervieu GJ, Osbourne S, Corcoran S, Morgan M, Sanger GJ: Growth hormone secretagogue receptors in rat and human gastrointestinal tract and the effects of ghrelin. *Neuroscience* 2003;120:443-453.

[44] Thomas MJ: The molecular basis of growth hormone action. *Growth Horm.IGF.Res.* 1998;8:3-11.

[45] Tuggle CK, Trenkle A: Control of growth hormone synthesis. *Domest.Anim Endocrinol.* 1996;13:1-33.

[46] Edens A, Talamantes F: Alternative processing of growth hormone receptor transcripts. *Endocr.Rev.* 1998;19:559-582.

[47] Schwartzbauer G, Menon RK: Regulation of growth hormone receptor gene expression. *Mol.Genet.Metab* 1998;63:243-253.

[48] Kyle CV, Evans MC, Odell WD: Growth hormone-like material in normal human tissues. *J.Clin.Endocrinol.Metab* 1981;53:1138-1144.

[49] Delehaye-Zervas MC, Mertani H, Martini JF, Nihoul-Fekete C, Morel G, Postel-Vinay MC: Expression of the growth hormone receptor gene in human digestive tissue. *J Clin Endocrinol.Metab* 1994;78:1473-1480.

[50] Lincoln DT, Kaiser HE, Raju GP, Waters MJ: Growth hormone and colorectal carcinoma: localization of receptors. *In Vivo* 2000;14:41-49.

[51] Culouscou JM, Remacle-Bonnet M, Garrouste F, Marvaldi J, Pommier G: Simultaneous production of IGF-I and EGF competing growth factors by HT- 29 human colon cancer line. *Int.J.Cancer* 1987;40:646-652.

[52] Guo YS, Jin GF, Houston CW, Thompson JC, Townsend CM, Jr.: Insulin-like growth factor-I promotes multidrug resistance in MCLM colon cancer cells. *J Cell Physiol* 1998;175:141-148.

[53] Remacle-Bonnet MM, Garrouste FL, Heller S, Andre F, Marvaldi JL, Pommier GJ: Insulin-like growth factor-I protects colon cancer cells from death factor-induced apoptosis by potentiating tumor necrosis factor alpha- induced mitogen-activated protein kinase and nuclear factor kappaB signaling pathways. *Cancer Res.* 2000;60:2007-2017.

[54] Heemskerk VH, Daemen MA, Buurman WA: Insulin-like growth factor-1 (IGF-1) and growth hormone (GH) in immunity and inflammation. *Cytokine Growth Factor Rev.* 1999;10:5-14.

[55] Sjogren K, Liu JL, Blad K, Skrtic S, Vidal O, Wallenius V, LeRoith D, Tornell J, Isaksson OG, Jansson JO, Ohlsson C: Liver-derived insulin-like growth factor I (IGF-I) is the principal source of IGF-I in blood but is not required for postnatal body growth in mice. *Proc.Natl.Acad.Sci.U.S.A* 1999;96:7088-7092.

[56] Yakar S, Liu JL, Stannard B, Butler A, Accili D, Sauer B, LeRoith D: Normal growth and development in the absence of hepatic insulin-like growth factor I. *Proc.Natl.Acad.Sci.U.S.A* 1999;96:7324-7329.

[57] Ewton DZ, Kansra S, Lim S, Friedman E: Insulin-like growth factor-I has a biphasic effect on colon carcinoma cells through transient inactivation of forkhead1, initially mitogenic, then mediating growth arrest and differentiation. *Int.J Cancer* 2002;98:665-673.

[58] Rotwein P: Structure, evolution, expression and regulation of insulin-like growth factors I and II. *Growth Factors* 1991;5:3-18.

[59] Lund PK, Ulshen MH, Rountree DB, Selub SE, Buchan AM: Molecular biology of gastrointestinal peptides and growth factors: relevance to intestinal adaptation. *Digestion* 1990;46 Suppl 2:66-73.

[60] Freier S, Weiss O, Eran M, Flyvbjerg A, Dahan R, Nephesh I, Safra T, Shiloni E, Raz I: Expression of the insulin-like growth factors and their receptors in adenocarcinoma of the colon. *Gut* 1999;44:704-708.

[61] Tricoli JV, Rall LB, Karakousis CP, Herrera L, Petrelli NJ, Bell GI, Shows TB: Enhanced levels of insulin-like growth factor messenger RNA in human colon carcinomas and liposarcomas. *Cancer Res.* 1986;46:6169-6173.

[62] Michell NP, Langman MJ, Eggo MC: Insulin-like growth factors and their binding proteins in human colonocytes: preferential degradation of insulin-like growth factor binding protein 2 in colonic cancers. *Br.J Cancer* 1997;76:60-66.

[63] Bustin SA, Dorudi S, Phillips SM, Feakins RM, Jenkins PJ: Local expression of insulin-like growth factor-I affects angiogenesis in colorectal cancer. *Tumour.Biol* 2002;23:130-138.

[64] Kao PC, Matheny AP, Jr., Lang CA: Insulin-like growth factor-I comparisons in healthy twin children. *J.Clin.Endocrinol.Metab* 1994;78:310-312.

[65] Rosen CJ, Kurland ES, Vereault D, Adler RA, Rackoff PJ, Craig WY, Witte S, Rogers J, Bilezikian JP: Association between serum insulin growth factor-I (IGF-I) and a simple sequence repeat in IGF-I gene: implications for genetic studies of bone mineral density. *J.Clin.Endocrinol.Metab* 1998;83:2286-2290.

[66] Giovannucci E, Haiman CA, Platz EA, Hankinson SE, Pollak MN, Hunter DJ: Dinucleotide repeat in the insulin-like growth factor-I gene is not related to risk of colorectal adenoma. *Cancer Epidemiol.Biomarkers Prev.* 2002;11:1509-1510.

[67] LeRoith D, Werner H, Beitner-Johnson D, Roberts CT, Jr.: Molecular and cellular aspects of the insulin-like growth factor I receptor. *Endocr.Rev.* 1995;16:143-163.

[68] Giraud S, Greco A, Brink M, Diaz JJ, Delafontaine P: Translation initiation of the insulin-like growth factor I receptor mRNA is mediated by an internal ribosome entry site. *J Biol.Chem.* 2001;276:5668-5675.

[69] Baserga R: The IGF-I receptor in cancer research. Exp.Cell Res. 1999;253:1-6.

[70] Rouyer-Fessard C, Gammeltoft S, Laburthe M: Expression of two types of receptor for insulinlike growth factors in human colonic epithelium. *Gastroenterology* 1990;98:703-707.

[71] Pollak MN, Perdue JF, Margolese RG, Baer K, Richard M: Presence of somatomedin receptors on primary human breast and colon carcinomas. *Cancer Lett.* 1987;38:223-230.

[72] Guo YS, Narayan S, Yallampalli C, Singh P: Characterization of insulinlike growth factor I receptors in human colon cancer. *Gastroenterology* 1992;102:1101-1108.

[73] Lahm H, Amstad P, Wyniger J, Yilmaz A, Fischer JR, Schreyer M, Givel JC: Blockade of the insulin-like growth-factor-I receptor inhibits growth of human colorectal cancer cells: evidence of a functional IGF-II- mediated autocrine loop. *Int.J Cancer* 1994;58:452-459.

[74] Zenilman ME, Graham W: Insulin-like growth factor I receptor messenger RNA in the colon is unchanged during neoplasia. *Cancer Invest* 1997;15:1-7.

[75] Adenis A, Peyrat JP, Hecquet B, Delobelle A, Depadt G, Quandalle P, Bonneterre J, Demaille A: Type I insulin-like growth factor receptors in human colorectal cancer. *Eur J Cancer* 1995;31A:50-55.

[76] Hakam A, Yeatman TJ, Lu L, Mora L, Marcet G, Nicosia SV, Karl RC, Coppola D: Expression of insulin-like growth factor-1 receptor in human colorectal cancer. *Hum.Pathol.* 1999;30:1128-1133.

[77] Weber MM, Fottner C, Liu SB, Jung MC, Engelhardt D, Baretton GB: Overexpression of the insulin-like growth factor I receptor in human colon carcinomas. *Cancer* 2002;95:2086-2095.

[78] Adachi Y, Lee CT, Coffee K, Yamagata N, Ohm JE, Park KH, Dikov MM, Nadaf SR, Arteaga CL, Carbone DP: Effects of genetic blockade of the insulin-like growth factor receptor in human colon cancer cell lines. *Gastroenterology* 2002;123:1191-1204.

[79] Reinmuth N, Liu W, Fan F, Jung YD, Ahmad SA, Stoeltzing O, Bucana CD, Radinsky R, Ellis LM: Blockade of insulin-like growth factor I receptor function inhibits growth and angiogenesis of colon cancer. *Clin.Cancer Res.* 2002;8:3259-3269.

[80] Bustin SA, Dorudi S, Phillips SM, Feakins RM, Jenkins PJ: Local expression of insulin-like growth factor-I affects angiogenesis in colorectal cancer. *Tumour.Biol.* 2002;23:130-138.

[81] Tajinda K, Carroll J, Roberts CT, Jr.: Regulation of insulin-like growth factor I receptor promoter activity by wild-type and mutant versions of the WT1 tumor suppressor. *Endocrinology* 1999;140:4713-4724.

[82] Werner H, Karnieli E, Rauscher FJ, LeRoith D: Wild-type and mutant p53 differentially regulate transcription of the insulin-like growth factor I receptor gene. *Proc.Natl.Acad.Sci.U.S.A* 1996;93:8318-8323.

[83] Maheswaran S, Park S, Bernard A, Morris JF, Rauscher FJ, III, Hill DE, Haber DA: Physical and functional interaction between WT1 and p53 proteins. *Proc.Natl.Acad.Sci.U.S.A* 1993;90:5100-5104.

[84] Maheswaran S, Englert C, Bennett P, Heinrich G, Haber DA: The WT1 gene product stabilizes p53 and inhibits p53-mediated apoptosis. *Genes Dev.* 1995;9:2143-2156.

[85] Idelman G, Glaser T, Roberts CT, Jr., Werner H: WT1-p53 interactions in insulin-like growth factor-I receptor gene regulation. *J Biol.Chem.* 2003;278:3474-3482.

[86] Silberstein GB, Van Horn K, Strickland P, Roberts CT, Jr., Daniel CW: Altered expression of the WT1 wilms tumor suppressor gene in human breast cancer. *Proc.Natl.Acad.Sci.U.S.A* 1997;94:8132-8137.

[87] Oji Y, Yamamoto H, Nomura M, Nakano Y, Ikeba A, Nakatsuka S, Abeno S, Kiyotoh E, Jomgeow T, Sekimoto M, Nezu R, Yoshikawa Y, Inoue Y, Hosen N, Kawakami M, Tsuboi A, Oka Y, Ogawa H, Souda S, Aozasa K, Monden M, Sugiyama H: Overexpression of the Wilms' tumor gene WT1 in colorectal adenocarcinoma. *Cancer Sci.* 2003;94:712-717.

[88] Hiltunen MO, Koistinaho J, Alhonen L, Myohanen S, Marin S, Kosma VM, Paakkonen M, Janne J: Hypermethylation of the WT1 and calcitonin gene promoter regions at chromosome 11p in human colorectal cancer. *Br.J Cancer* 1997;76:1124-1130.

[89] Collet C, Candy J: How many insulin-like growth factor binding proteins? *Mol.Cell Endocrinol.* 1998;139:1-6.

[90] Hoeflich A, Yang Y, Huber S, Rascher W, Koepf G, Blum WF, Heinz-Erian P, Kolb HJ, Kiess W: Expression of IGFBP-2, -3, and -4 mRNA during differentiation of Caco-2 colon epithelial cells. *Am.J Physiol* 1996;271:E922-E931.

[91] Jones JI, Clemmons DR: Insulin-like growth factors and their binding proteins: biological actions. *Endocr.Rev.* 1995;16:3-34.

[92] Michell NP, Dent S, Langman MJ, Eggo MC: Insulin-like growth factor binding proteins as mediators of IGF-I effects on colon cancer cell proliferation. *Growth Factors* 1997;14:269-277.

[93] Twigg SM, Baxter RC: Insulin-like growth factor (IGF)-binding protein 5 forms an alternative ternary complex with IGFs and the acid-labile subunit. *J.Biol.Chem.* 1998;273:6074-6079.

[94] Mohseni-Zadeh S, Binoux M: Insulin-like growth factor (IGF) binding protein-3 interacts with the type 1 IGF receptor, reducing the affinity of the receptor for its ligand: an alternative mechanism in the regulation of IGF action. *Endocrinology* 1997;138:5645-5648.

[95] Conover CA: Potentiation of insulin-like growth factor (IGF) action by IGF-binding protein-3: studies of underlying mechanism. *Endocrinology* 1992;130:3191-3199.

[96] Zou T, Fleisher AS, Kong D, Yin J, Souza RF, Wang S, Smolinski KN, Abraham JM, Meltzer SJ: Sequence alterations of insulin-like growth factor binding protein 3 in neoplastic and normal gastrointestinal tissues. *Cancer Res.* 1998;58:4802-4804.

[97] Remacle-Bonnet M, Garrouste F, el Atiq F, Marvaldi J, Pommier G: Cell polarity of the insulin-like growth factor system in human intestinal epithelial cells. Unique apical sorting of insulin-like growth factor binding protein-6 in differentiated human colon cancer cells. *J.Clin.Invest* 1995;96:192-200.

[98] Oh Y, Muller HL, Pham H, Rosenfeld RG: Demonstration of receptors for insulin-like growth factor binding protein-3 on Hs578T human breast cancer cells. *J.Biol.Chem.* 1993;268:26045-26048.

[99] Liu B, Lee HY, Weinzimer SA, Powell DR, Clifford JL, Kurie JM, Cohen P: Direct functional interactions between insulin-like growth factor- binding protein-3 and retinoid X receptor-alpha regulate transcriptional signaling and apoptosis. *J.Biol.Chem.* 2000;275:33607-33613.

[100] Buckbinder L, Talbott R, Velasco-Miguel S, Takenaka I, Faha B, Seizinger BR, Kley N: Induction of the growth inhibitor IGF-binding protein 3 by p53. *Nature* 1995;377:646-649.

[101] Williams AC, Collard TJ, Perks CM, Newcomb P, Moorghen M, Holly JM, Paraskeva C: Increased p53-dependent apoptosis by the insulin-like growth factor binding protein IGFBP-3 in human colonic adenoma-derived cells. *Cancer Res.* 2000;60:22-27.

[102] Collard TJ, Guy M, Butt AJ, Perks CM, Holly JM, Paraskeva C, Williams AC: Transcriptional upregulation of the insulin-like growth factor binding protein IGFBP-3 by sodium butyrate increases IGF-independent apoptosis in human colonic adenoma-derived epithelial cells. *Carcinogenesis* 2003;24:393-401.

[103] Kansra S, Ewton DZ, Wang J, Friedman E: IGFBP-3 mediates TGF beta 1 proliferative response in colon cancer cells. *Int.J.Cancer* 2000;87:373-378.

[104] Rajah R, Katz L, Nunn S, Solberg P, Beers T, Cohen P: Insulin-like growth factor binding protein (IGFBP) proteases: functional regulators of cell growth. *Prog.Growth Factor Res.* 1995;6:273-284.

[105] Jones JI, Busby WH, Wright G, Clemmons DR: Human IGFBP-1 is phosphorylated on 3 serine residues: effects of site- directed mutagenesis of the major phosphoserine. *Growth Regul.* 1993;3:37-40.

[106] Mishra L, Bass B, Ooi BS, Sidawy A, Korman L: Role of insulin-like growth factor-I (IGF-I) receptor, IGF-I, and IGF binding protein-2 in human colorectal cancers. *Growth Horm.IGF.Res.* 1997;8:473-479.

[107] Ma J, Pollak MN, Giovannucci E, Chan JM, Tao Y, Hennekens CH, Stampfer MJ: Prospective study of colorectal cancer risk in men and plasma levels of insulin-like growth factor (IGF)-I and IGF-binding protein-3. *J Natl.Cancer Inst.* 1999;91:620-625.

[108] Manousos O, Souglakos J, Bosetti C, Tzonou A, Chatzidakis V, Trichopoulos D, Adami HO, Mantzoros C: IGF-I and IGF-II in relation to colorectal cancer. *Int.J.Cancer* 1999;83:15-17.

[109] Giovannucci E, Pollak M, Platz EA, Willett WC, Stampfer MJ, Majeed N, Colditz GA, Speizer FE, Hankinson SE: Insulin-like growth factor I (IGF-I), IGF-binding protein-3 and the risk of colorectal adenoma and cancer in the Nurses' Health Study. *Growth Horm.IGF.Res.* 2000;10 Suppl A:S30-S31.

[110] Ma J, Pollak M, Giovannucci E, Chan JM, Tao Y, Hennekens C, Stampfer MJ: A prospective study of plasma levels of insulin-like growth factor I (IGF-I) and IGF-binding protein-3, and colorectal cancer risk among men. *Growth Horm.IGF.Res.* 2000;10 Suppl A:S28-S29.

[111] Kaaks R, Toniolo P, Akhmedkhanov A, Lukanova A, Biessy C, Dechaud H, Rinaldi S, Zeleniuch-Jacquotte A, Shore RE, Riboli E: Serum C-peptide, insulin-like growth factor (IGF)-I, IGF-binding proteins, and colorectal cancer risk in women. *J.Natl.Cancer Inst.* 2000;92:1592-1600.

[112] Renehan AG, Painter JE, Atkin WS, Potten CS, Shalet SM, O'Dwyer ST: High-risk colorectal adenomas and serum insulin-like growth factors. *Br.J.Surg.* 2001;88:107-113.

[113] Palmqvist R, Hallmans G, Rinaldi S, Biessy C, Stenling R, Riboli E, Kaaks R: Plasma insulin-like growth factor 1, insulin-like growth factor binding protein 3, and risk of colorectal cancer: a prospective study in northern Sweden. *Gut* 2002;50:642-646.

[114] Cats A, Dullaart RP, Kleibeuker JH, Kuipers F, Sluiter WJ, Hardonk MJ, de Vries EG: Increased epithelial cell proliferation in the colon of patients with acromegaly. *Cancer Res.* 1996;56:523-526.

[115] Brunner JE, Johnson CC, Zafar S, Peterson EL, Brunner JF, Mellinger RC: Colon cancer and polyps in acromegaly: increased risk associated with family history of colon cancer. *Clin.Endocrinol.(Oxf)* 1990;32:65-71.

[116] Ron E, Gridley G, Hrubec Z, Page W, Arora S, Fraumeni JF, Jr.: Acromegaly and gastrointestinal cancer. *Cancer* 1991;68:1673-1677.

[117] Jenkins PJ, Fairclough PD, Richards T, Lowe DG, Monson J, Grossman A, Wass JA, Besser M: Acromegaly, colonic polyps and carcinoma. *Clin.Endocrinol.(Oxf)* 1997;47:17-22.

[118] Jenkins PJ, Besser M: Clinical perspective: acromegaly and cancer: a problem. *J.Clin.Endocrinol.Metab* 2001;86:2935-2941.

[119] Jenkins PJ, Frajese V, Jones AM, Camacho-Hubner C, Lowe DG, Fairclough PD, Chew SL, Grossman AB, Monson JP, Besser GM: Insulin-like growth factor I and the development of colorectal neoplasia in acromegaly. *J.Clin.Endocrinol.Metab* 2000;85:3218-3221.

[120] Glass AR, Kikendall JW, Sobin LH, Bowen PE: Serum concentrations of insulin-like growth factor 1 in colonic neoplasia. *Acta Oncol.* 1994;33:70-71.

[121] Paterson AC, Leeding KS, Bach LA, Baldwin GS, Macrae FA, Shulkes A: More about: prospective study of colorectal cancer risk in men and plasma levels of insulin-like growth factor (IGF)-I and IGF-binding protein-3. *J.Natl.Cancer Inst.* 2000;92:1947-1948.

[122] el Atiq F, Garrouste F, Remacle-Bonnet M, Sastre B, Pommier G: Alterations in serum levels of insulin-like growth factors and insulin- like growth-factor-binding proteins in patients with colorectal cancer. *Int J Cancer* 1994;57:491-497.

[123] Cohen P, Clemmons DR, Rosenfeld RG: Does the GH-IGF axis play a role in cancer pathogenesis? *Growth Horm.IGF.Res.* 2000;10:297-305.

[124] Thissen JP, Ketelslegers JM, Underwood LE: Nutritional regulation of the insulin-like growth factors. *Endocr.Rev.* 1994;15:80-101.

[125] Giovannucci E, Pollak M, Liu Y, Platz EA, Majeed N, Rimm EB, Willett WC: Nutritional predictors of insulin-like growth factor I and their relationships to cancer in men. *Cancer Epidemiol.Biomarkers Prev.* 2003;12:84-89.

[126] de Fougerolles AR, Chi-Rosso G, Bajardi A, Gotwals P, Green CD, Koteliansky VE: Global expression analysis of extracellular matrix-integrin interactions in monocytes. *Immunity.* 2000;13:749-758.

[127] Simmons JG, Pucilowska JB, Lund PK: Autocrine and paracrine actions of intestinal fibroblast-derived insulin-like growth factors. *Am.J.Physiol* 1999;276:G817-G827.

[128] Andre F, Rigot V, Thimonier J, Montixi C, Parat F, Pommier G, Marvaldi J, Luis J: Integrins and E-cadherin cooperate with IGF-I to induce migration of epithelial colonic cells. *Int.J Cancer* 1999;83:497-505.

[129] Egan SE, Weinberg RA: The pathway to signal achievement. *Nature* 1993;365:781-783.

[130] Fedi P, Pierce JH, di Fiore PP, Kraus MH: Efficient coupling with phosphatidylinositol 3-kinase, but not phospholipase C gamma or GTPase-activating protein, distinguishes ErbB-3 signaling from that of other ErbB/EGFR family members. *Mol Cell Biol.* 1994;14:492-500.

[131] Ming XF, Burgering BM, Wennstrom S, Claesson-Welsh L, Heldin CH, Bos JL, Kozma SC, Thomas G: Activation of p70/p85 S6 kinase by a pathway independent of p21ras. *Nature* 1994;371:426-429.

[132] Datta SR, Dudek H, Tao X, Masters S, Fu H, Gotoh Y, Greenberg ME: Akt phosphorylation of BAD couples survival signals to the cell- intrinsic death machinery. *Cell* 1997;91:231-241.

[133] Parrizas M, Saltiel AR, LeRoith D: Insulin-like growth factor 1 inhibits apoptosis using the phosphatidylinositol 3'-kinase and mitogen-activated protein kinase pathways. *J Biol.Chem.* 1997;272:154-161.

[134] Petley T, Graff K, Jiang W, Yang H, Florini J: Variation among cell types in the signaling pathways by which IGF-I stimulates specific cellular responses. *Horm.Metab Res.* 1999;31:70-76.

[135] Lee K, Deng X, Friedman E: Mirk protein kinase is a mitogen-activated protein kinase substrate that mediates survival of colon cancer cells. *Cancer Res.* 2000;60:3631-3637.

[136] Kauffmann-Zeh A, Rodriguez-Viciana P, Ulrich E, Gilbert C, Coffer P, Downward J, Evan G: Suppression of c-Myc-induced apoptosis by Ras signalling through PI(3)K and PKB. *Nature* 1997;385:544-548.

[137] Kulik G, Weber MJ: Akt-dependent and -independent survival signaling pathways utilized by insulin-like growth factor I. *Mol.Cell Biol.* 1998;18:6711-6718.

[138] Burtscher I, Compagni A, Lamm GM, Christofori G: An insulin-like growth factor-mediated, phosphatidylinositol 3' kinase- independent survival signaling pathway in beta tumor cells. *Cancer Res.* 1999;59:3923-3926.

[139] Almind K, Inoue G, Pedersen O, Kahn CR: A common amino acid polymorphism in insulin receptor substrate-1 causes impaired insulin signaling. Evidence from transfection studies. *J.Clin.Invest* 1996;97:2569-2575.

[140] Hansen T, Andersen CB, Echwald SM, Urhammer SA, Clausen JO, Vestergaard H, Owens D, Hansen L, Pedersen O: Identification of a common amino acid polymorphism in the p85alpha regulatory subunit of phosphatidylinositol 3-kinase: effects on glucose disappearance constant, glucose effectiveness, and the insulin sensitivity index. *Diabetes* 1997;46:494-501.

[141] Garrouste F, Remacle-Bonnet M, Fauriat C, Marvaldi J, Luis J, Pommier G: Prevention of cytokine-induced apoptosis by insulin-like growth factor-I is independent of cell adhesion molecules in HT29-D4 colon carcinoma cells-evidence for a NF-kappaB-dependent survival mechanism. *Cell Death.Differ.* 2002;9:768-779.

[142] Mantell MP, Ziegler TR, Adamson WT, Roth JA, Zhang W, Frankel W, Bain A, Chow JC, Smith RJ, Rombeau JL: Resection-induced colonic adaptation is augmented by IGF-I and associated with upregulation of colonic IGF-I mRNA. *Am.J.Physiol* 1995;269:G974-G980.

[143] Sekharam M, Nasir A, Kaiser HE, Coppola D: Insulin-like growth factor 1 receptor activates c-SRC and modifies transformation and motility of colon cancer in vitro. *Anticancer Res.* 2003;23:1517-1524.

[144] Coppola D, Ferber A, Miura M, Sell C, D'Ambrosio C, Rubin R, Baserga R: A functional insulin-like growth factor I receptor is required for the mitogenic and transforming activities of the epidermal growth factor receptor. *Mol.Cell Biol.* 1994;14:4588-4595.

[145] Kim SO, Houtman JC, Jiang J, Ruppert JM, Bertics PJ, Frank SJ: Growth hormone-induced alteration in ErbB-2 phosphorylation status in 3T3-F442A fibroblasts. *J.Biol.Chem.* 1999;274:36015-36024.

[146] Lammers R, Gray A, Schlessinger J, Ullrich A: Differential signalling potential of insulin- and IGF-1-receptor cytoplasmic domains. *EMBO J.* 1989;8:1369-1375.

[147] Tartare S, Mothe I, Kowalski-Chauvel A, Breittmayer JP, Ballotti R, Van Obberghen E: Signal transduction by a chimeric insulin-like growth factor-1 (IGF-1) receptor having the carboxyl-terminal domain of the insulin receptor. *J.Biol.Chem.* 1994;269:11449-11455.

[148] Adamo M, Roberts CT, LeRoith D: How distinct are the insulin and insulin-like growth factor I signalling systems? *Biofactors* 1992;3:151-157.

[149] Furlanetto RW, Dey BR, Lopaczynski W, Nissley SP: 14-3-3 proteins interact with the insulin-like growth factor receptor but not the insulin receptor. *Biochem.J.* 1997;327 (Pt 3):765-771.

[150] Laviola L, Giorgino F, Chow JC, Baquero JA, Hansen H, Ooi J, Zhu J, Riedel H, Smith RJ: The adapter protein Grb10 associates preferentially with the insulin receptor as compared with the IGF-I receptor in mouse fibroblasts. *J.Clin.Invest* 1997;99:830-837.

[151] Urso B, Brown RA, O'Rahilly S, Shepherd PR, Siddle K: The alpha-isoform of class II phosphoinositide 3-kinase is more effectively activated by insulin receptors than IGF receptors, and activation requires receptor NPEY motifs. *FEBS Lett.* 1999;460:423-426.

[152] Urso B, Cope DL, Kalloo-Hosein HE, Hayward AC, Whitehead JP, O'Rahilly S, Siddle K: Differences in signaling properties of the cytoplasmic domains of the insulin receptor and insulin-like growth factor receptor in 3T3-L1 adipocytes. *J.Biol.Chem.* 1999;274:30864-30873.

[153] Moxham CP, Duronio V, Jacobs S: Insulin-like growth factor I receptor beta-subunit heterogeneity. Evidence for hybrid tetramers composed of insulin-like growth factor I and insulin receptor heterodimers. *J.Biol.Chem. 1*989;264:13238-13244.

[154] Soos MA, Siddle K: Immunological relationships between receptors for insulin and insulin- like growth factor I. Evidence for structural heterogeneity of insulin- like growth factor I receptors involving hybrids with insulin receptors. *Biochem.J.* 1989;263:553-563.

[155] Belfiore A, Pandini G, Vella V, Squatrito S, Vigneri R: Insulin/IGF-I hybrid receptors play a major role in IGF-I signaling in thyroid cancer. *Biochimie* 1999;81:403-407.

[156] Moxham CP, Jacobs S: Insulin/IGF-I receptor hybrids: a mechanism for increasing receptor diversity. *J.Cell Biochem.* 1992;48:136-140.

[157] Pandini G, Vigneri R, Costantino A, Frasca F, Ippolito A, Fujita-Yamaguchi Y, Siddle K, Goldfine ID, Belfiore A: Insulin and insulin-like growth factor-I (IGF-I) receptor overexpression in breast cancers leads to insulin/IGF-I hybrid receptor overexpression: evidence for a second mechanism of IGF-I signaling. *Clin.Cancer Res.* 1999;5:1935-1944.

[158] Shier P, Watt VM: Primary structure of a putative receptor for a ligand of the insulin family. *J Biol.Chem.* 1989;264:14605-14608.

[159] Jui HY, Accili D, Taylor SI: Characterization of a hybrid receptor formed by dimerization of the insulin receptor-related receptor (IRR) with the insulin receptor (IR): coexpression of cDNAs encoding human IRR and human IR in NIH-3T3 cells. *Biochemistry* 1996;35:14326-14330.

[160] Zhang B, Roth RA: Binding properties of chimeric insulin receptors containing the cysteine-rich domain of either the insulin-like growth factor I receptor or the insulin receptor related receptor. *Biochemistry* 1991;30:5113-5117.

[161] Dey BR, Spence SL, Nissley P, Furlanetto RW: Interaction of human suppressor of cytokine signaling (SOCS)-2 with the insulin-like growth factor-I receptor. *J.Biol.Chem.* 1998;273:24095-24101.

[162] Dey BR, Furlanetto RW, Nissley P: Suppressor of cytokine signaling (SOCS)-3 protein interacts with the insulin-like growth factor-I receptor. *Biochem.Biophys.Res.Commun.* 2000;278:38-43.

[163] Newcomb PA, Storer BE: Postmenopausal hormone use and risk of large-bowel cancer. *J.Natl.Cancer Inst.* 1995;87:1067-1071.

[164] Foley EF, Jazaeri AA, Shupnik MA, Jazaeri O, Rice LW: Selective loss of estrogen receptor beta in malignant human colon. *Cancer Res.* 2000;60:245-248.

[165] Polakis P: The oncogenic activation of beta-catenin. *Curr.Opin.Genet.Dev.* 1999;9:15-21.

[166] Bienz M, Clevers H: Linking colorectal cancer to Wnt signaling. *Cell* 2000;103:311-320.

[167] Quevedo C, Alcazar A, Salinas M: Two different signal transduction pathways are implicated in the regulation of initiation factor 2B activity in insulin-like growth factor-1-stimulated neuronal cells. *J.Biol.Chem.* 2000;275:19192-19197.

[168] Playford MP, Bicknell D, Bodmer WF, Macaulay VM: Insulin-like growth factor 1 regulates the location, stability, and transcriptional activity of beta -catenin. *Proc.Natl.Acad.Sci.U.S.A* 2000;97:12103-12108.

[169] Desbois-Mouthon C, Cadoret A, Blivet-Van Eggelpoel MJ, Bertrand F, Cherqui G, Perret C, Capeau J: Insulin and IGF-1 stimulate the beta-catenin pathway through two signalling cascades involving GSK-3beta inhibition and Ras activation. *Oncogene* 2001;20:252-259.

[170] Mann B, Gelos M, Siedow A, Hanski ML, Gratchev A, Ilyas M, Bodmer WF, Moyer MP, Riecken EO, Buhr HJ, Hanski C: Target genes of beta-catenin-T cell-factor/lymphoid-enhancer-factor signaling in human colorectal carcinomas. *Proc.Natl.Acad.Sci.U.S.A* 1999;96:1603-1608.

[171] Tetsu O, McCormick F: Beta-catenin regulates expression of cyclin D1 in colon carcinoma cells. *Nature* 1999;398:422-426.

[172] Crawford HC, Fingleton BM, Rudolph-Owen LA, Goss KJ, Rubinfeld B, Polakis P, Matrisian LM: The metalloproteinase matrilysin is a target of beta-catenin transactivation in intestinal tumors. *Oncogene* 1999;18:2883-2891.

[173] Rosenwald IB, Chen JJ, Wang S, Savas L, London IM, Pullman J: Upregulation of protein synthesis initiation factor eIF-4E is an early event during colon carcinogenesis. *Oncogene* 1999;18:2507-2517.

[174] He TC, Sparks AB, Rago C, Hermeking H, Zawel L, da Costa LT, Morin PJ, Vogelstein B, Kinzler KW: Identification of c-MYC as a target of the APC pathway. *Science* 1998;281:1509-1512.

[175] Brabletz T, Herrmann K, Jung A, Faller G, Kirchner T: Expression of nuclear beta-catenin and c-myc is correlated with tumor size but not with proliferative activity of colorectal adenomas. *Am.J.Pathol.* 2000;156:865-870.

[176] Ghahary A, Shen Q, Shen YJ, Scott PG, Tredget EE: Induction of transforming growth factor beta 1 by insulin-like growth factor-1 in dermal fibroblasts. *J Cell Physiol* 1998;174:301-309.

[177] Van Laethem JL, Robberecht P: Growth factors in colorectal tumorigenesis. *Acta Gastroenterol.Belg.* 1995;58:274-279.

[178] Manning AM, Williams AC, Game SM, Paraskeva C: Differential sensitivity of human colonic adenoma and carcinoma cells to transforming growth factor beta (TGF-beta): conversion of an adenoma cell line to a tumorigenic phenotype is accompanied by a reduced response to the inhibitory effects of TGF-beta. *Oncogene* 1991;6:1471-1476.

[179] Anzano MA, Rieman D, Prichett W, Bowen-Pope DF, Greig R: Growth factor production by human colon carcinoma cell lines. *Cancer Res.* 1989;49:2898-2904.

[180] Matsushita M, Matsuzaki K, Date M, Watanabe T, Shibano K, Nakagawa T, Yanagitani S, Amoh Y, Takemoto H, Ogata N, Yamamoto C, Kubota Y, Seki T, Inokuchi H, Nishizawa M, Takada H, Sawamura T, Okamura A, Inoue K: Down-regulation of TGF-beta receptors in human colorectal cancer: implications for cancer development. *Br.J Cancer* 1999;80:194-205.

[181] Tsushima H, Kawata S, Tamura S, Ito N, Shirai Y, Kiso S, Imai Y, Shimomukai H, Nomura Y, Matsuda Y, Matsuzawa Y: High levels of transforming growth factor beta 1 in patients with colorectal cancer: association with disease progression. *Gastroenterology* 1996;110:375-382.

[182] Picon A, Gold LI, Wang J, Cohen A, Friedman E: A subset of metastatic human colon cancers expresses elevated levels of transforming growth factor beta1. *Cancer Epidemiol.Biomarkers Prev.* 1998;7:497-504.

[183] Eskinazi R, Resibois A, Svoboda M, Peny MO, Adler M, Robberecht P, Van Laethem JL: Expression of transforming growth factor beta receptors in normal human colon and sporadic adenocarcinomas. *Gastroenterology* 1998;114:1211-1220.

[184] Sheng H, Shao J, O'Mahony CA, Lamps L, Albo D, Isakson PC, Berger DH, DuBois RN, Beauchamp RD: Transformation of intestinal epithelial cells by chronic TGF-beta1 treatment results in downregulation of the type II TGF-beta receptor and induction of COX-2. *Oncogene* 1999;18:855-867.

[185] Eberhart CE, Coffey RJ, Radhika A, Giardiello FM, Ferrenbach S, DuBois RN: Up-regulation of COX-2 gene expression in human colorectal adenomas and adenocarcinomas. *Gastroenterology* 1994;107:1183-1188.

[186] Tsujii M, Kawano S, Tsuji S, Sawaoka H, Hori M, DuBois RN: COX-2 regulates angiogenesis induced by colon cancer cells. *Cell* 1998;93:705-716.

[187] Di Popolo A, Memoli A, Apicella A, Tuccillo C, di Palma A, Ricchi P, Acquaviva AM, Zarrilli R: IGF-II/IGF-I receptor pathway up-regulates COX-2 mRNA expression and PGE2 synthesis in Caco-2 human colon carcinoma cells. *Oncogene* 2000;19:5517-5524.

[188] Warren RS, Yuan H, Matli MR, Ferrara N, Donner DB: Induction of vascular endothelial growth factor by insulin-like growth factor 1 in colorectal carcinoma. *J Biol.Chem.* 1996;271:29483-29488.

[189] Akagi Y, Liu W, Zebrowski B, Xie K, Ellis LM: Regulation of vascular endothelial growth factor expression in human colon cancer by insulin-like growth factor-I. *Cancer Res.* 1998;58:4008-4014.

[190] Fukuda R, Hirota K, Fan F, Jung YD, Ellis LM, Semenza GL: Insulin-like growth factor 1 induces hypoxia-inducible factor 1-mediated vascular endothelial growth factor expression, which is dependent on MAP kinase and phosphatidylinositol 3-kinase signaling in colon cancer cells. *J Biol.Chem.* 2002;277:38205-38211.

[191] Krajewska M, Moss SF, Krajewski S, Song K, Holt PR, Reed JC: Elevated expression of Bcl-X and reduced Bak in primary colorectal adenocarcinomas. *Cancer Res.* 1996;56:2422-2427.

[192] Parrizas M, LeRoith D: Insulin-like growth factor-1 inhibition of apoptosis is associated with increased expression of the bcl-xL gene product. *Endocrinology* 1997;138:1355-1358.

[193] Zha J, Harada H, Yang E, Jockel J, Korsmeyer SJ: Serine phosphorylation of death agonist BAD in response to survival factor results in binding to 14-3-3 not BCL-X(L). *Cell* 1996;87:619-628.

[194] Cardone MH, Roy N, Stennicke HR, Salvesen GS, Franke TF, Stanbridge E, Frisch S, Reed JC: Regulation of cell death protease caspase-9 by phosphorylation. *Science* 1998;282:1318-1321.

[195] Muller AF, Janssen JA, de Herder WW, van der Lely AJ: Growth hormone receptor antagonists: potential indications. *Ned.Tijdschr.Geneeskd.* 2001;145:69-73.

[196] Mirpuri E, Garcia-Trevijano ER, Castilla-Cortazar I, Berasain C, Quiroga J, Rodriguez-Ortigosa C, Mato JM, Prieto J, Avila MA: Altered liver gene expression in CCl4-cirrhotic rats is partially normalized by insulin-like growth factor-I. *Int.J Biochem Cell Biol.* 2002;34:242-252.

[197] Chen WH, Pellegata NS, Wang PH: Coordinated effects of insulin-like growth factor I on inhibitory pathways of cell cycle progression in cultured cardiac muscle cells. *Endocrinology* 1995;136:5240-5243.

[198] Wang PH, Schaaf GJ, Chen WH, Feng J, Prins BA, Levin ER, Bahl JJ: IGF I induction of p53 requires activation of MAP kinase in cardiac muscle cells. *Biochem Biophys.Res.Commun.* 1998;245:912-917.

[199] Dunn SE, Torres JV, Oh JS, Cykert DM, Barrett JC: Up-regulation of urokinase-type plasminogen activator by insulin-like growth factor-I depends upon phosphatidylinositol-3 kinase and mitogen-activated protein kinase kinase. *Cancer Res.* 2001;61:1367-1374.

[200] Howe LR, Crawford HC, Subbaramaiah K, Hassell JA, Dannenberg AJ, Brown AM: PEA3 is up-regulated in response to Wnt1 and activates the expression of COX-2. *J Biol Chem.* 2001;276:20108-20115.

In: Focus on Colorectal Cancer Research
Editor: Julia D. Martinez, pp. 97-122

ISBN #1-59454-101-9

Chapter V

ANTITUMOUR ACTIVITY OF YOGURT

***A. de Moreno de LeBlanc*[1,2] *and G. Perdigón* [1,2,*]**

[1] Centro de Referencias para Lactobacilos (CERELA). Chacabuco 145, (4000) Tucumán. Argentina.

[2] Cátedra de Inmunología. Instituto de Microbiología. Facultad de Bioquímica, Química y Farmacia. Universidad Nacional de Tucumán, Argentina

ABSTRACT

Several studies have demonstrated that fermented milk consumption decrease the incidence of colorectal cancer. Using a chemically induced murine colon cancer model it was reported that conventional yogurt inhibits tumour development. In this model, the inflammatory immune response caused by the carcinogen (DMH) showed a great increase in IgG+ B cells, CD8+ T lymphocytes and in proinflammatory cytokines (TNFα and IFNγ). Yogurt feeding inhibited tumour development by decreasing the inflammatory immune response and increasing the number of IgA+ cells, CD4+ T lymphocytes, cytokines such as IL-10 and decreasing NO radicals. Yogurt also induced the apoptosis mechanisms. The local immune stimulation produced by yogurt feeding increased monocytes/macrophages population and the cytokines release in the nodular tissue and in the Peyer's patches suggesting that these cells could be responsible for IFNγ and TNFα production. The enhancement of IL-10 found would favour the regulation of the immune response, not only in the inhibition model of the tumour growth, but also when yogurt is given long term. The immune mechanisms involved by yogurt to decrease the inflammatory immune response caused by the carcinogen were different to those observed with an antiinflammatory drug (indomethacin). Indomethacin did not increase immune infiltrative cell activity in the large intestine and the cytokine levels were diminished. Nitric oxide synthase enzyme determinations showed that in mice fed with yogurt, the IFNγ enhancement was not related to inflammation, but to an immunomodulation. We demonstrated that the only single yogurt supplementation was unable to inhibit tumour development in the initiation stage, however it inhibited the

* To whom the correspondence should be addressed. E-mail: perdigon@cerela.org.ar, FAX: 54-381-4005600.

tumour growth (promption and progression) when it was administered cyclically after tumour induction. Cellular apoptosis increase observed could explain the importance for the TNFα levels found in the mice fed long term with yogurt. The normal microflora has an important function in the intestinal inflammatory process preceding tumour development, lactic acid bacteria present in yogurt play a role in this process since it has been shown that these bacteria and fermented milk products act on the microbial enzyme activities associated with colon carcinogenesis. This chapter will show that yogurt can inhibit the promotion and progression of chemically induced colon cancer in mice through its antiinflammatory effect, cell apoptosis and by its immunomodulating properties.

Anticarcinogenic Activity of Probiotics

Probiotics have been given credit for numerous health-promoting effects; they stimulate the immune system, possess anticarcinogenic and hypocholesterolemic properties, exert an antagonistic action against enteric pathogens and various intestinal disorders (Mital and Garg, 1995; Kato, 2000; Perdigón *et al.,* 2001) and play a role in the control of gastrointetsinal health. Their connection with animal and human cancers has been extensively reviewed (Rolfe, 2000; Hughes and Rowland, 2003). Probiotics such as lactobacilli and bifidobacteria in fermented or culture-containing dairy foods such as yogurt may play a role in reducing the risk of colon cancer (Fernandes and Shahani, 1990; Braddy *et al.,* 2000; Wolloski *et al.*, 2001). The increase of immune cells activity in the prevention of cancer by lactic acid bacteria (LAB) consumption has also been described (Kato *et al.*, 1984; Hayashi and Ohwaki, 1989).

The intake of products containing viable LAB may lower the risk of colon cancer either directly by reducing procarcinogenic substances or indirectly by reducing the level of the enzymes (β-glucuronidase, azoreductase, nitroreductase, among others) that convert procarcinogens to carcinogens in the intestine (Goldin *et al.*, 1980; Goldin and Gorbach, 1984; Fernandes and Shahani, 1990). The consumption of *L. acidophilus* in experimental animal models reduced the activity of fecal enzymes such as β-glucuronidase, azoreductase and nitroreductase (Goldin and Gorbach, 1976; 1980), this activity having been well correlated with the number of LAB in the intestine. The products of these enzymes are known to be mutagenic and carcinogenic. Goldin and Gorbach (1976) showed the relationship between diet and rat fecal bacterial enzymes implicated in colon cancer. Furthermore, the effect of the diet on various cancer types has been the subject of many reviews (Cummings and Bingham, 1998; Reddy, 1998).

A specific strain of *lactobacillus*, *Lactobacillus* GG, has been shown to reduce the incidence of tumours in carcinogen-treated laboratory rats, particularly during the early promotional stages of carcinogenesis and when animals are fed with a high fat diet (Goldin *et al.*, 1996). Likewise, *Bifidobacterium longum* inhibited cell proliferation and the development of colon tumours in laboratory rats treated with a chemical carcinogen and fed with high fat diets (Singh *et al.*, 1997, Abdelali *et al.*, 1995; Reddy and Riverson, 1993). Sreekumar and Husono (2000) showed that *L. acidophilus* reduced fecal β-glucuronidase activity and the number of bacteria in the intestinal tract of rats.

Studies in humans have also shown that *L. acidophilus* supplements decrease the activity of fecal bacterial enzymes (β-glucuronidase and nitroreductase) that may convert procarcinogens to carcinogens (Goldin *et al.*, 1980; Goldin and Gorbach, 1984). When healthy female adults in Finland supplemented their diets with yogurt containing viable *Lactobacillus* GG for four weeks, fecal bacterial enzyme activity decreased (Ling *et al.*, 1994).

Another mechanism involved in tumour supression by LAB is the modulation of the host immune response (Perdigón *et al.*, 2001).

FERMENTED MILKS AND PROBIOTICS. THEIR RELATIONSHIP WITH THE HOST IMMUNE SYSTEM

Live microbial food supplements added to improve the intestinal microbial balance, which benefically affect the host animal, are known as probiotics (Fuller, 1989). Schrezenenmeir and deVrese (2001) proposed the following definition, which confines the probiotic concept to effects produced by viable microorganisms; this concept is independent of the probiotic site of action and the route of administration: "A preparation of or a product containing viable, defined microorganisms in sufficient numbers, which alter the microflora (by implantation or colonization) in a compartment of the host and that exert beneficial health effects on this host." It is important to note that these definitions comprise not only preparations specifically designed to act as probiotics but also traditional yogurt and other fermented products with LAB which have beneficial effects on the consumer.

Lactic acid bacteria, the most commonly used microorganisms in probiotic products, exert effects on the immune system of the host (Perdigon *et al.* 2001). Feeding with LAB and yogurt stimulates the systemic immune response (macrophage function and number of immunoglobulin secreting cells) as well as the local immune response (IgA secretion into the intestine) (Perdigón *et al.*, 1999; Vintiñi *et al.*, 2000). Consequently, the consumption of fermented dairy products containing viable microorganisms such as yogurt has increased. Besides enhancing the immune response, the consumption of fermented milks and LAB has been shown to increase resistance to neoplasia and infections (Kato, 2000). Gut associated lymphoid tissue (GALT) is under constant exposure to environmental antigens, the digestive flora being its main antigenic stimulus (Cebra, 1999). Another mechanism by which LAB is thought to promote health is through the normalization of intestinal flora which has been disturbed by disease or drugs (Kato, 2000).

Immunomodulation by LAB depends on the contact of these microorganisms with the lymphoid tissue which transitorily colonize the intestinal lumen. By this mechanism most LAB have the ability to survive in the gastrointestinal tract passage that can influence their immunogenicity (Schiffrin *et al.*, 1997, Saxelin, 1996). LAB which survive the conditions of the gastrointestinal tract can adhere to the intestinal epithelial cells or M cells from Peyer's patches, stimulating the GALT and increasing the production of cytokines and antibodies (principally secretory IgA). (Perdigón *et al.*, 2002a; Perdigón *et al.*, 2001; Meydani and Ha, 2000).

Yogurt has been defined in the Codex Alimentarius as a coagulated milk product that results from the lactic acid fermentation of milk by *Lactobacillus delbrueckii* subsp. *bulgaricus* and *Streptococcus thermophilus*. In this definition, in addition to the LAB present in the yogurt, the peptides released during the fermentation process are important from the nutritional point of view. Many investigators have studied the therapeutic effects of yogurt and LAB commonly used in yogurt production against diseases such as cancer, infections and gastroinstestinal disorders. The immunomodulating and immunostimulating properties of yogurt and fermented milks have also been well documented (Matar *et al.*, 2003).

The immunomodulation effects of yogurt are in part caused by the bacteria contained in it. When viable or biologically active LAB enter the intestine, they can activate the GALT specific or nonspecific inmune responses as well as the systemic immune response (Meydani and Ha, 2000).

Perdigón *et al.* (1999) studied different LAB as well as the mechanisms involved in the mucosal immune system activation. Some LAB induced specific secretory immunity while others increased the intestinal inflammatory response. Vintiñi *et al.* (2000) demonstrated the importance of the LAB strain to be used. They studied, using BALB/c mice, the effect of different LAB (*Lactobacillus casei, L. acidophilus, L. rhamnosus, L. delbrueckii* subsp. *bulgaricus, L. plantarum, Lactococcus lactis* and *Streptococcus thermophilus*) on the intestinal mucosal response. They showed that not all LAB can be utilized as oral adjuvants and that their beneficial effects on the intestinal immune system are not limited for one bacterial genus or species. Consequently, the immunomodulating properties of LAB are strain specific.

Simulated commercial yogurt feeding of BABL/c mice induced a marked immune cell infiltration with plasm cells and lymphocytes prevalence (Perdigón *et al.*, 1994). Yogurt feeding for 7 days increased the number of IgA+ cells in the small and large intestine of mice, but IgM+ and IgG+ cells did not increase (Perdigón *et al.*, 1998). Macrophage numbers were higher in regard to non-treatment control group, but they did not show increased activity. The above observations explain why yogurt does not over stimulate the undesirable inflammatory response (Valdéz *et al.*, 1997).

In addition to LAB, yogurt possesses other non bacterial components produced during fermentation which can contribute to immunogenicity and to other properties like its antitumour activity of yogurt, which is related to its immunological modulator potential.

Peptides and free fat acids released during fermentation were shown to increase the immune response. In this way, peptidic fractions liberated during milk fermentation with a strain of *Lactobacillus helveticus* stimulated the immune system and inhibited the growth of an immuno dependent fibrosarcoma in a mice model (LeBlanc *et al.*, 2002). The peptidic profiles of milk proteins were significantly different after fermentation by LAB, suggesting that microbial proteolysis could be a potential source of bioactive peptides (Matar *et al.*, 1996). Milk fermented with *Lactobacillus helveticus* R389, a bacterium with high protease and peptidase activity, exerted an antimutagenic effect while a mutant strain, deficient in proteolytic activity, did not (Matar *et al.*, 1997). In a similary way, milk fermented with the proteolytic strain increased the number of IgA+ cells in the small intestine as well as in the bronchi of mice, but fermented milk obtained with the mutant strain did not show the same *in vivo* results (Matar *et al.*, 2001).

Fractions separated by dialysis from yogurt showed tumour inhibition in *in vivo* murine assays (Ayebo *et al.*, 1982). Certain soluble components produced by LAB during milk fermentation could be used to prevent certain malignant gastrointestinal pathologies (Biffi *et al.*, 1997). The filtrate of yogurt was reported to increase IFNγ production by natural killer cells (de Simone *et al.*, 1986).

YOGURT AND COLON CANCER. A STUDY OF THE IMMUNE POPULATIONS AND CYTOKINE PROFILES INVOLVED

In our laboratory, colon cancer inhibition by yogurt was studied in an experimental model using BALB/c mice. Animals were fed with yogurt for 10 consecutive days (the dose with the best effects of yogurt on the intestinal immune system). The colon tumour was chemically induced with dimethylhydrazine (DMH) and the animals were given yogurt cyclically again after tumour induction (for ten consecutive days followed by a one week break and then again for ten days) until the end of the experiment (six months).

Yogurt feeding inhibed tumour growth (yogurt-DMH-yogurt group) (Figure 1A). In this experimental model, a large inflammatory immune response was observed during the tumour development in the large intestine in the mice treated only with DMH (tumour control or DMH group). The inflammatory response was observed histologically by identification of the immune cells. The increase in IgG-producing B cells and CD8+ T lymphocytes (Table 1) would point to their participationin the inflammatory process. The increased number of CD8+ cells enhanced the cytotoxic immune response with an increase in the inflammatory immune response. Furthermore, the IgG+ cells determined could increase the inflammation by the cytolytic activity of IgG through the complement system. When the DMH injected mice were fed with yogurt, an increase in the number of IgA-secreting cells and CD4+ T lymphocytes (Table 1) in the lamina propria of the large intestine with a decrease in the IgG+ and CD8+ cells was observed (Perdigón *et al.*, 1998). The antitumour activity observed with yogurt feeding could be caused either by the immunomodulatory capacity of the LAB (Perdigón and Oliver, 2000) or of yogurt (Perdigón *et al.*, 1994). The increase in the number of IgA+ cells but not of IgG+ cells in the large intestine of the mice fed with yogurt could limit the inflammatory response, since IgA is considered as an important barrier in colonic neoplasia (Isaacson, 1982).

Since mice were fed with yogurt for long periods, another experimental group (yogurt group) was added in order to determine the effect of long term feeding with the fermented product. The histological studies showed that a large number of immune cells infiltrated the lamina propria of the large intestine in this group (figure 1C). However, CD4+ and CD8+ T lymphocytes did not increase in comparison with non-treatment control mice (de Moreno de LeBlanc and Perdigón, 2004) while long term yogurt feeding increased IgA-secreting cells, being remarkable in the fourth and sixth months (Table 1). All these results suggest that the antitumour activity of yogurt may be exerted by its ability to mediate the down regulation of the inflammatory response induced by the carcinogen, since it is known that inflammation is a risk factor for several types of cancer (Prescott and Fitzpatrick, 2000).

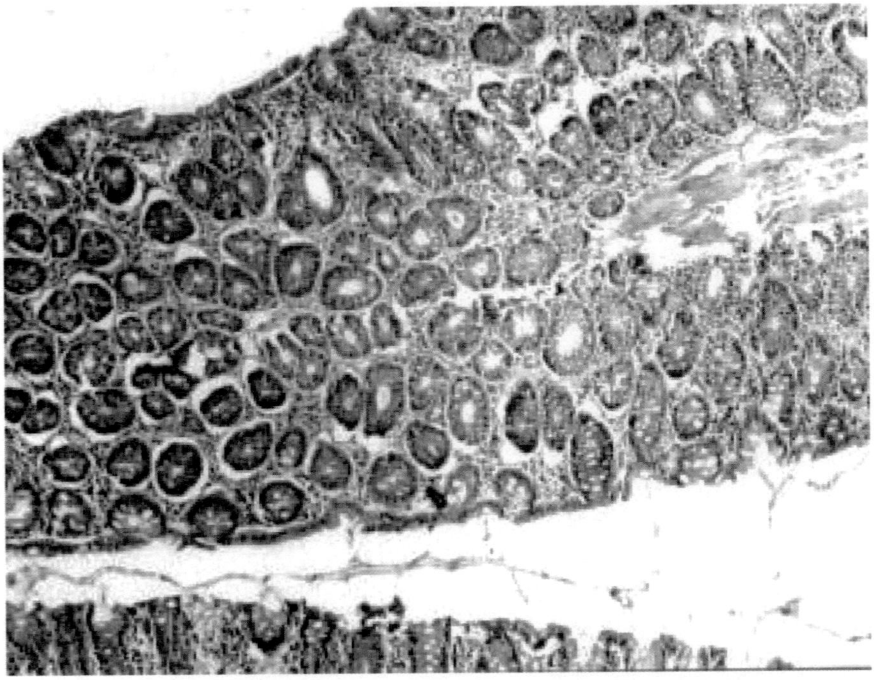

A

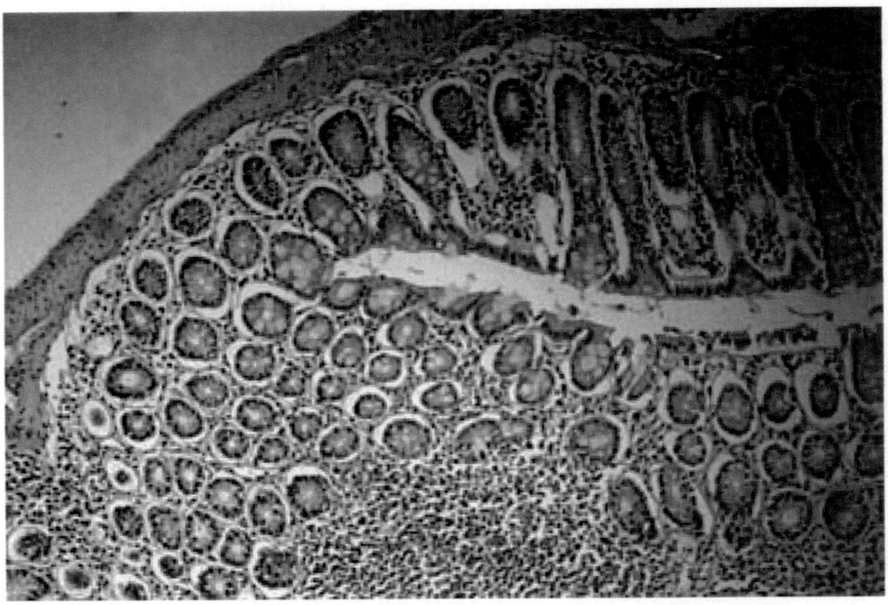

B

Figure 1. Continued on next page

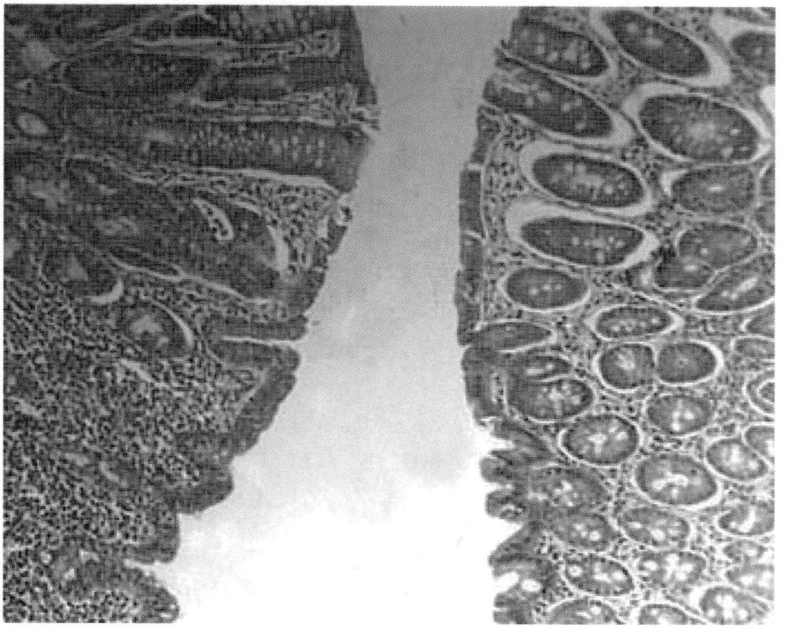

C

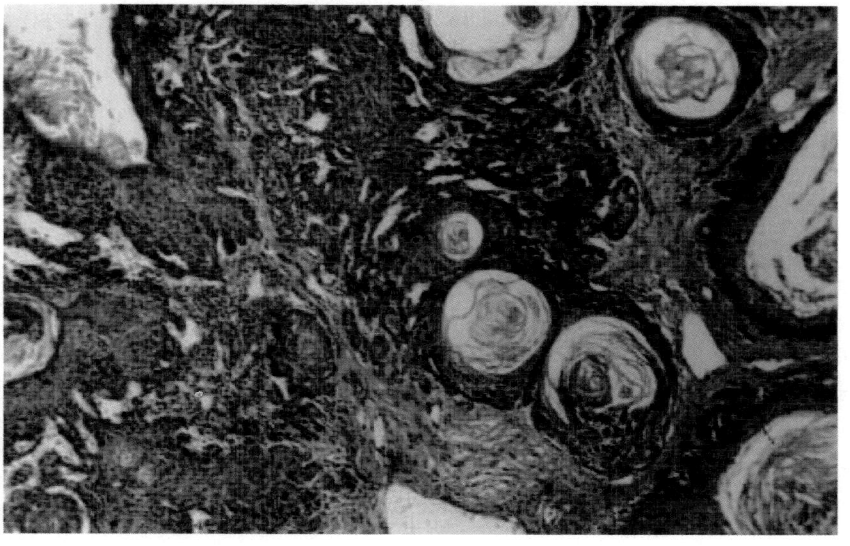

D

Figure 1. Histological study comparing the differnet experimental groups. Slices from large intetsine of mice were studied stain them with hematoxilin-eosin. Microphotographs B, C, and D were taking to compare the mice only fed with yoghrut, others treated with DMH and fed with yoghrut and the tumour control group. All the samples were obtained in the end of the study (6 months). A) Non-treatment control group (100X). B) Yogurt group. Tissue maintaine the typical structure of the large intestine but it is possible observe cell increase in the lamina propria (100X). C) Yogurt-DMH-yogurt group. The tissue organization is conserve with inportant increases in the lamina propria cells and goblet cells (100X). D) DMH group. Tumor tissue compound of fibrous tissue and queratin nucleus (100X).

Table 1. Comparative study of the cell populations, proinflammatory cytokines and iNOS enzyme

Experimental Group	Period of treatment	IgA	CD4	CD8	TNFα	IFNγ	iNOS
DMH	2 months	60*±8	20±3	50*±2	68*±4	86*±15	23*±5
	3 months	60*±8	22±3	50*±3	97*±15	162*±15	19±6
	4 months	70*±7	ND	ND	155*±22	140*±17	41*±5
	5 months	40±4	36±2	80*±4	123*±16	134*±3	22±4
	6 months	ND	ND	ND	125*±10	99*±22	25*±5
Y-DMH-Y	2 months	100*±10	40±2	30*±2	64*±8	105*±6	15*±5
	3 months	130*±8	82*±5	40*±2	78*±11	1 115*±10	1 15*±6
	4 months	100*±7	ND	ND	57*±18	121*±27	14*±4
	5 months	50±3	35*±2	10±1	130*±21	144*±9	12*±3
	6 months	ND	ND	ND	75*±10	86*±6	12*±2
Yogurt	2 months	ND	ND	ND	ND	ND	ND
	3 months	84±17	29±8	12±4	50*±7	100*±10	19*±5
	4 months	108*±12	22±4	14±4	57*±8	112*±9	11*±2
	5 months	79±10	21±2	15±6	81*±9	129*±14	14*±3
	6 months	95*±13	17±4	10±3	101*±14	86*±17	12*±2
DMH-indomethacin	2 months	76±14	41*±6	24*±5	42*±9	69*±9	24*±5
	3 months	62±12	31*±5	20*±7	20±8	40*±8	16±5
	4 months	106*±24	22±4	17±6	27±10	23±5	18±3
	5 months	125*±3	18±3	16*±3	16±7	24±6	8±2
	6 months	114*±22	32*±7	22*±5	26±7	35*±8	20*±2
Yogurt basal	10 days	84±11	19±3	10±3	29±3	25±3	8±2
Non-treatment control		65±5	20±3	11±2	17±2	21±2	10±2

Results are expressed as number of positive cell for the correspondient cellular marker, cytokine or enzyme counted in 10 fields of vision as seen at 1000X magnification using a fluorescence light microscope. * = significant differences of each group comparing with non-treatment control. $P < 0.001$. Y-DMH-Y= yogurt-DMH-yogurt; ND = Not determined.

The studies concerning the cell population in our model allowed us to suggest the possible antinflammatory role of yogurt to account for its antitumour activity. Since cytokines are the biological messengers for the regulation and modulation of the immune response, are produced by activated immune cells and are able to activate other cells during the inflammatory response, they are a pontential target for the study of the mechanisms induced by LAB or yogurt to modulate the immune response.

We studied different cytokines using immunohistochemic or immunfluorescent methods on large intestine slices from the different groups of mice treated with DMH, yogurt-DMH-yogurt or yogurt. TNFα (tumour necrosis factor), one of the selected cytokines, was initially identified as a tumoral necrosis mediator in the serum of animals treated with lipopolisacharides (LPS). It was studied due to the monocyte/macrophage prevalence in our experimental model and because these actived cells release it. TNFα has proinflammatory properties but can also mediate cellular apoptosis (Sellers and Fisher, 1999).

IFNγ was selected at first as the Th-1 lymphocyte population marker. The number of CD4+ cells reported for the mice fed with yogurt after DMH treatment could account for the decrease in the inflammatory response through cytokines release for CD4+ population (IL-4, IL-10, IFNγ). Although IFNγ is a proinflammatory cytokine, it is able to kill colonic epithelial cells (Numata *et al.*, 1991).

We observed that the proinflammatory cytokines (TNFα and IFNγ) were increased in the cells from the large intestine of tumour control mice (DMH group) and in the yogurt-DMH-yogurt group (Table 1). Yogurt feeding itself also produced high levels of these proinflammatory cytokines (Perdigón *et al.*, 2002b).

In mice injected with DMH, the nodular infiltrates in the large intestine showed an enhacement in their number and size. The cells from these nodules were important to study the effect on the immune responses of the DMH and the yogurt-DMH-yogurt groups (de Moreno de LeBlanc et al., 2004). In all the assayed periods, up to six months, yogurt feeding increased TNFα producing cells in comparison with the tumour control group. These cells comprise non-adherent (fibroblast, mast cells and some T and NK cells) as well as adherent (macrophages / monocytes) cells (Feghali and Wright, 1997). In our experimental model, adherent cells produced large amounts of TNFα than non-adherent. The number of IFNγ+ cells also increased with yogurt supplementation. This cytokine is produced mainly by cells belonging to non-adherent populations such as T cells and NK cells (Feghali and Wright, 1997). IFNγ production by other cells such as macrophages and dendritic cells, which are considered adherent cells, was reprted recently (Frucht *et al.*, 2001). In our study, in addition to non-adherent cells, we detected IFNγ (nearly 50%) in the adherent cells. All these observations show that yogurt stimulates the activity of infiltrative cells (adherent and non adherent), which increased cytokine production, necessary for tumour resolution. As previously suggested by de Moreno de LeBlanc *et al.* (2004), adherent cells play an important role in the immune responses observed in our tumour model. They would also be accompanied by activated non-adherent cells.

The above results led us to study the effect of long term yogurt feeding on the cytokine released from Peyer's patches cells in order to evaluate its effect on the intestinal immune system, since Peyer's patches are inductor sites of the mucosal immune reponse. TNFα and IFNγ significantly increased in mice fed with yogurt for ten days, after which time values remained constant. TNFα increase was due to the adherent population, whereas both adherent and non-adherent populations were responsible for IFNγ production (de Moreno de LeBlanc and Perdigón, 2004a). Yogurt only stimulated cytokine production by Peyer's patch cells at the beginning of yogurt supplementation, after which a basal cytokine level was maintained in these cells.

We analyzed other regulatory cytokines (IL-10 and IL-4) that could be involved in the immune response of the mice fed with yogurt since, unlike the DMH group, the increased proinflammatory cytokine positive cells were not related to the inflammation and tumour development observed in those animals.

IL-10 and IL-4 are rassociated with activated Th-2 lymphocytes but IL-10 can also be produced by other cell populations such as macrophages and dendritic cells.

In different experimental models, TNFα and IL-10 were demonstrated to have opposite effects (Bogdan *et al.*, 1992). The balance betweeen TNFα and IL-10 could modulate the effector function of macrophages and cellular apoptosis. Furthermore, IL-10 is important as a regulator in the intestine. Berg *et al.* (1996) demonstrated the IL-10 role in intestinal inflammation and carcinogenesis. Mice with a disruption of the IL-10 gene showed inflammatory changes in caecum, colon and rectum with a high incidence of colorectal adenocarcinomas. IL-10 also participates in the normal tolerance to indigenous bacterial flora and its lack is related to inflammation (Sydora *et al*,. 2003).

In our model, the number of IL-10+ cells increased significativelly in all the samples from the three experimetal groups (DMH, yogurt-DMH-yogurt and yoghrut) (Perdigón *et al*, 2002a). It is important to remark that yogurt feeding always produced more IL-10+ cells in the yogurt-DMH-yogurt group than in the DMH group.

IL-4 plays a significant role both in controlling cell growth and in modulating the immune response (Chang *et al.*, 2000). This cytokine has antagonist functions to IFNγ and appears to possess certain antiinflammatory properties, IL-4 can inhibit the production of several proinflammatory cytokines such as IL-1, IL-6, IL-8 and TNFα (Feghali and Wright, 1997). Patton *et al.* (2002) showed that *Schistosoma mansoni*-infected IL-4 deficient mice (IL-4 $^{-/-}$) developed a Th-1 response with excessive and prolonged production of nitric oxide (NO) associated with enhanced IFNγ production and IL-4 is also associated with immune modulation in some tumour models (Nishihori *et al.*, 2000).

The increase in IFNγ values led us to measure IL-4 production since we thought that IL-4 would modulate the production of IFNγ. We determined that, among the groups studied, IL-4 was the cytokine that presented the most remarkable differences. The number of IL-4+ cells increased at the beginning of the experiment in the yogurt-DMH-yogurt group; IL-4 probably exerts control over the inflammation, which helps in the non-development of the tumour; afterwards, the number of IL-4+ cells was similar to those obtained with the non-treatment control group (figure 2). IL-4+ cells only increased at the end of the experience (six months) in the DMH group, in which time the mice presented important lesions in the large intestine and development of the tumour. In this group it is possible that the great alterations produced in the intestine together with the high levels of cytokines such as IFNγ and TNFα increased the IL-10 levels to regulate the immune response. This could not by itself control the inflammatory response induced by the carcinogen so that the IL-4 regulatory cytokine was released. However, at this stage of tumour evolution (fourth and fifth months), tumour growth could be not reverted.

Yogurt feeding by itself did not increase IL-4+ cells, although it increased IL-10+ cells in the large intestine (figure 2). These results suggest that yogurt could modulate the immune response; it stimulates cytokine production when this is required, or induces down regulation of the immune cells to avoid exacerbation of the immune response. This effect would occur mainly through IL-10, which showed increases in the tissue during all the periods assayed.

The increase in cell number and cytokines production in mice after long term feeding with yogurt led us to study the Bcl-2 protein as a marker of cell activity and mitosis. This protein is a measure of cell survival due to its antiapoptotic activity (Sellers and Fisher, 1999). We found that the number of Bcl-2(+) cells increased in the large intestine of mice after long term yogurt feeding as well as in the samples obtained after assay for two and three months in the yogurt-DMH-yogurt group. The number of Bcl-2(+) cells did not increase in the DMH group except in the sixth month, when the animals had developed tumour (de Moreno de LeBlanc *et al.*, 2004). The increase in Bcl2(+) cells observed in the group of mice after long term yogurt feedding may be related to cell infiltration and survival caused by the fermented milk and would explain the enhancement in the number of cytokine positive cells observed in this group of animals.

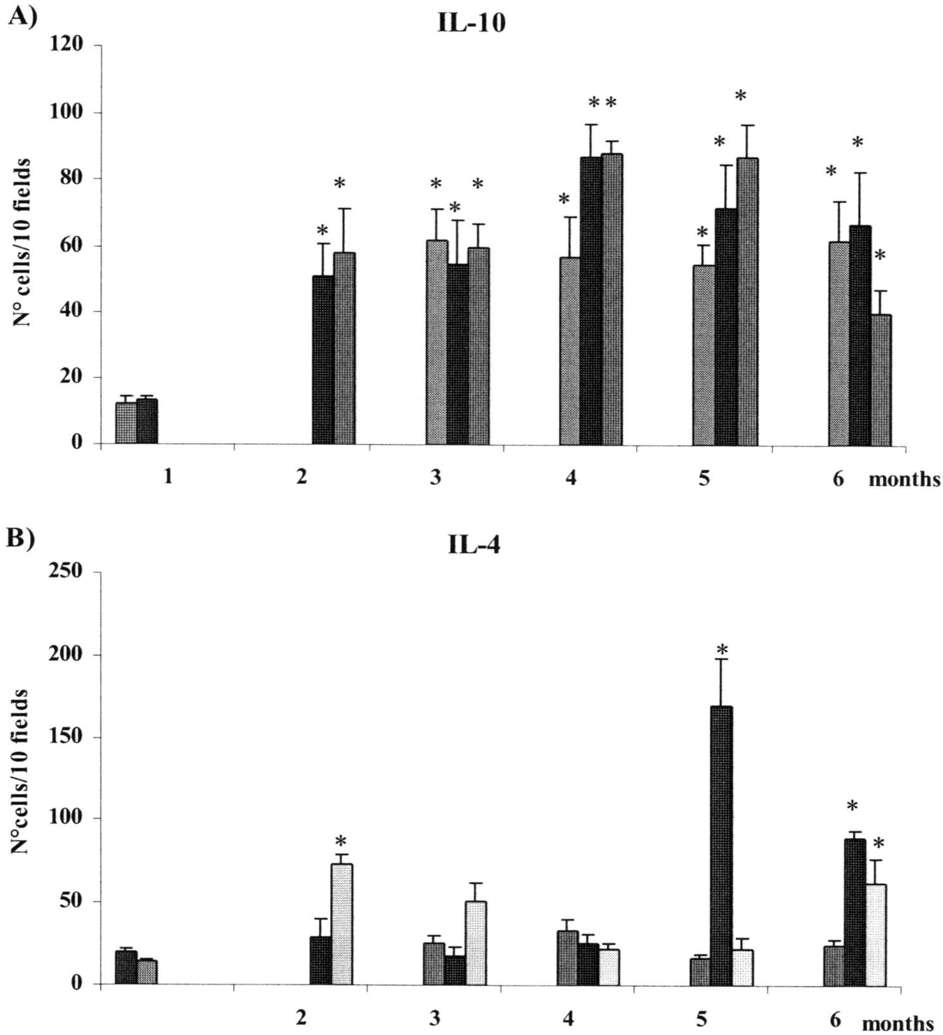

Figure 2. Comparative study of two regulatory cytokines. Cytokines were analized in large intetsine slices from different experimental groups using indirect immunofluorescent technique. Results are expresed as number of positive cells counted in ten fileds of vision at 1000X of magnification. * represent significative diference comparing with the non-treatment control using Student's Test P<0,001. Non-treatment control; Basal yogurt (10 days); Yogurt; DMH; Yogurt-DMH-Yogurt

We were able to study another role of CD4+ T lymphocytes due to their increase in the DMH group when yogurt was added to the diet. There is now evidence that CD4+ T cells which express the CD25 marker play a critical role in immune regulation through IL-10 production (Read and Powrie, 2001). There are discrepancies regarding the regulatory activity and the CD25 marker. Curotto de Lafaille and Lafaille (2002) reported that CD4+CD25- T cells are as effective as CD4+CD25+ T cells in controlling T-cell mediated diseases. We analyzed the CD25 marker of the large intestine in the treatment periods in which the number of IL-10+ cells was highest. We found that the CD25+ marker had increased in some samples (de Moreno de LeBlanc and Perdigón, 2004). The results obtained showed that the CD4+CD25+ T regulatory cells were not the only cell population responsible for the increased levels of IL10 observed in our tumour model.

In order to determine the importance of CD4+ T cells enhancement in the yogurt-DMH-yogurt group, we decided to study the T cell receptor (TCR). Infiltrative lymphocytes in certain solid tumours are characterized by the γ/δ chains presents in the TCR. These lymphocytes would produce certain molecules in the tumour site which would contribute to the antitumour immune response (perforines and cytokin es). The IFNγ released by γ/δ (+) TCR lymphocytes present in the tumour is one of the cytokines responsible for this action (Ferrarini *et al.*, 2002). In our experimental colon cancer model, as mentioned above, IFN+ cells increased in all the group assayed; thus the study of the TCR will permit to know whether these T lymphocytes play an important role in the antitumor immune response exerted by yogurt through IFNγ.

T γ/δ (+) and α/β(+) cells were studied in the different experimental groups. We did not observe any significative increases in either α/β(+) or γ/δ (+) TCR in any of the groups, so that γ/δ (+) TCR cells would not be the mainl source of the IFNγ enhancement observed.

It has been reported (Perdigon *et al.*, 2000) that *Lactobacillus delbruekii* subsp *bulgariccus* and S*treptococcus thermophilus* interact with the small intestine cells of mice but not with those of the large intestine. Yogurt preparation is a symbiotic interaction between both bacterial species where the starter culture is a strain pools of each bacterial species. Consequently, we analized in mice the interaction between yogurt starter bacteria or bacterial antigens and the intestine using a fluorescent bacterial suspension grown under conditions similar to commercial yogurt. We determined that fluorescent cells from the starter culture were able to interact with Peyer's patches and with the large intestine (figure 3). This finding allowed us to understand why the mice fed with a long term yoghrut suplemented diet showed an increased cell activity (Bcl-2(+) cells) and cytokine positve cells. Yogurt bacteria interact with Peyers's patches cells (inductor sites of the gut immune response) and the effect on the large intestine could be mediated by direct interaction with the immune cells or indirectly by cytokines produced in that inductor site of the intestine immune system which exert their functions at a distance (Barret, 1996).

This study allowed us to demonstrate that yogurt exerts a certain interaction directly with the large intestine cells, reinforcing or increasing the responce produced in the immune inductor site (Peyer's patch). This would be further evidence that yogurt can have an effect on pathologies affecting the mucose of the large intestine.

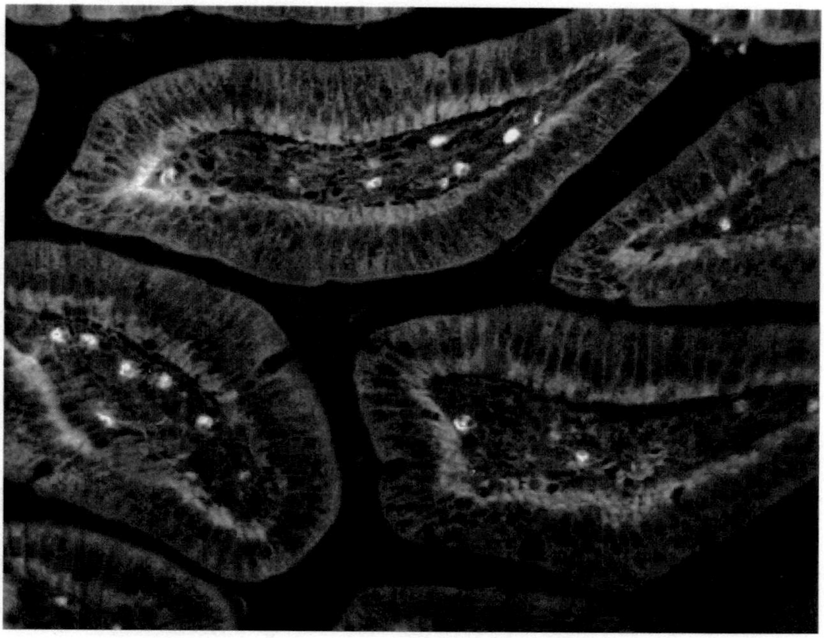

A

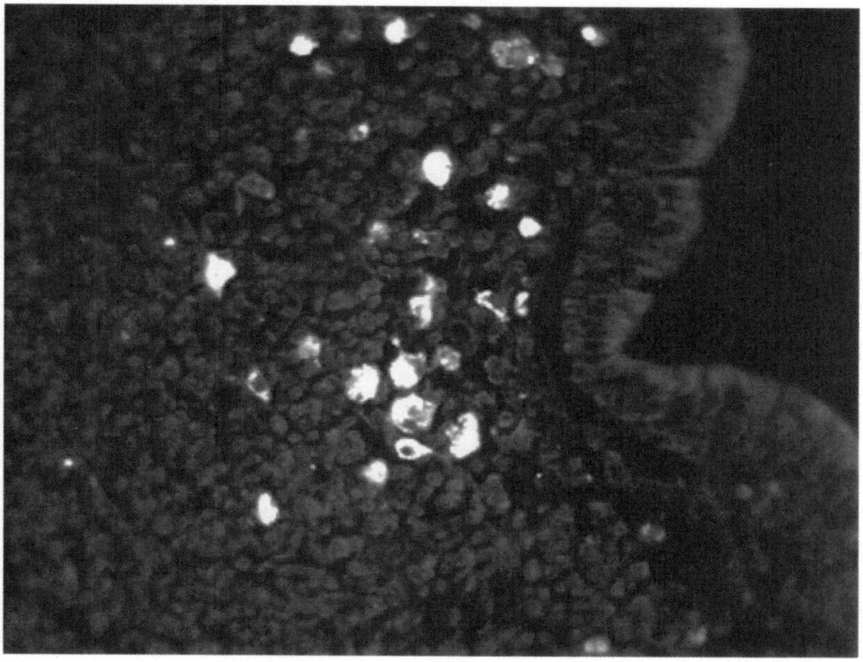

B

Figure 3. Continued on next page

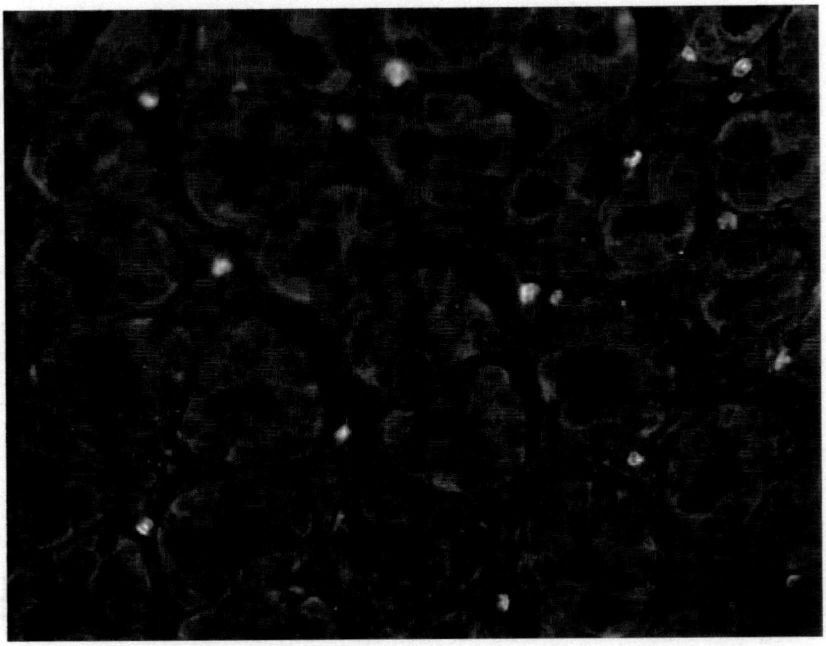

C

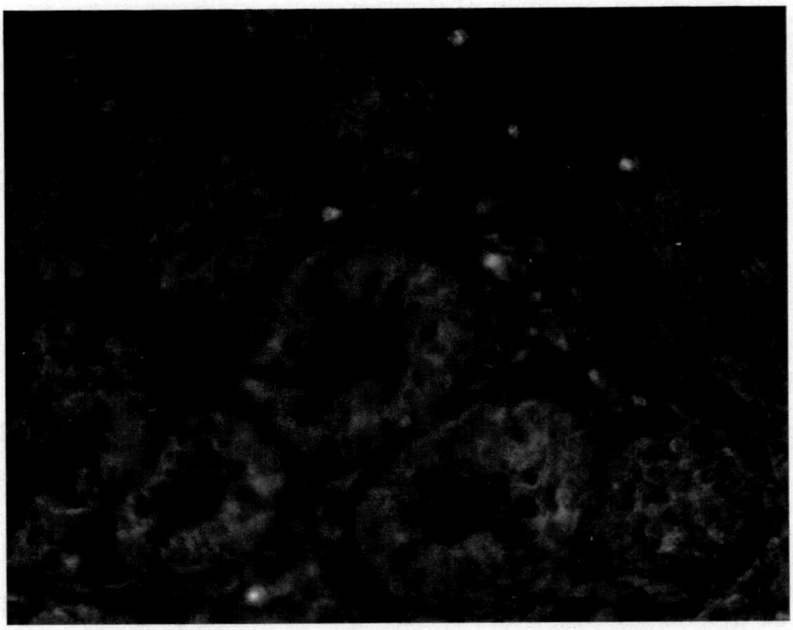

D

Figure 3. Continued on next page

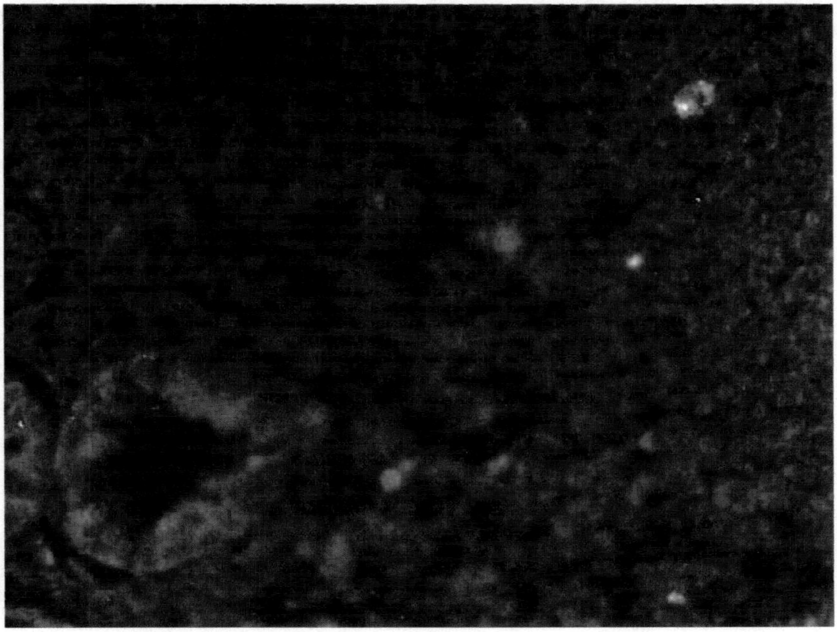

E

Figure 3. Interaction of yogurt bacteria antigens with the small and large intestine of the mice. Fluorescent cells were observed on histological sections from small and large intestine of the mice, 30 or 60 min after intragastric administration of yogurt bacteria labelled with FITC. A) Fluorescent cells in lamina propria of the small intestine at 30 min. B)Fluorescence observed in Peyers's patch at 30 min. C) Fluorescent cells in the lamina propria of the large intestine at 30 min. D) Bacteria interaction with large intestine cells at 60 min. E) Low fluorescence in the large intestine nodule at 60 min.

RELATIONSHIP BETWEEN INFLAMMATION AND TUMOUR

The association of chronic inflammation with several malignant diseases has been reported for a long time (Prescott and Fitzpatrick, 2000). There is also evidence that this relationship would be mediated by cytokines (Feghali and Wrigth, 1997) or by ROS generated by inflammatory phagocytes that can cause injury to target cells, contributing to cancer development (Weitzman and Gordon, 1990). Examples of the above include intestinal cancer after intestinal chronic inflammation (Korelitz, 1983; Collins *et al.*, 1987) and gastric cancer after atrophic gastritic (Correa, 1988). In addition to this, it seems clear that some carcinogens (such as tobacco in lung tumours) are also associated with a chronic inflammatory process. (Weitzman y Gordon, 1990). Patients with persistent ulcerative colitis have 5-7 times greater incidence of colon cancer development (Ekbom *et al.*, 1990).

As regards the relationdhip between inflammation and tumourthe oncology has recently, recognized that several drugs such as the inhibitors of the cyclooxygenase enzyme (COX) as the antiinflammatory drugs (NSAIDs), can delay or prevent certain cancers.

Evidence has shown that the NSAIDs these drugs block colon carcinogenesis in its early stages. The target for the study of NSAIDs is now COX-2, an inducible isoenzyme of cyclooxygenase which would be induce in the inflammatory sites by different factors such as cytokines.

A number of reports have indicated that the metabolites of arachidonic acid, especially prostaglandins of the E series, are involved in the initiation, promotion and progression of tumoral processes (Fischer, 1985; Trosko *et al.*, 1985; Fletcher, 1989). Several studies have demonstrated the beneficial effect of cyclooxygenase enzyme inhibitors on the therapy of a variety of tumours and metastases (Fulton, 1984; Lala *et al.*, 1986; Reddy *et al.,* 1987). In a murine fibrosarcoma, the antitumoral activity of antinflammatory drugs (piroxicam, indomethacin and aspirin) was correlated with the recovery of peritoneal macrophages activity and peripheral blood leukocytes level (Valdéz y Perdigón, 1991). Epidemiological evidence shows that people who take non steroidal antiinflammaories have less risk of developing colon cancer and its non malignant precursor, adenomatose polyps (Thun *et al.*, 1991).

On the basis of the thow previous results obtained in which the antitumour effect of yogurt on an induced colon cancer could be explained by a regulation of the inflammatory immune response exerted by the DMH carcinogen, with a significant increase in the activity and survival of the cells by long term feeding with yogurt, we analized the effect of an NSAID such as indomethacin on the inhibition of colon cancer to compare it with the antitumour activity of yogurt. A new group of mice to be treated with indomethacin was added (DMH-indomethacin group).

Histological observations showed that, during indomethacin administration, the immune cells infiltrated into the large intestine were smaller (de Moreno de LeBlanc *et al.*, 2004), different from those observed with the yogurt feeding, where a great increase in the number of immune cells infriltrating the lamina propria (yogurt-DMH-yogurt group) was found. However, no changes in the tissue was detected in relation to the carcinogen group. The cellular infiltration also occurred in the large intestine of long term yogurt fed mice, suggesting that these infiltrative cells would play an importat role in the antitumoral and antiinflammatory activity of yogurt.

During the fourth month of the indomethacin treatment, the histology of the large intestine from this group of mice was similar to the non-treatment control group. When indomethacin administration was stopped due to cachexia p in the animals, the tumour developed with the same characteristics as in the DMH group in the sixth month (de Moreno de LeBlanc *et al.* 2004).

This last observation showed different mechanisms for indomethacin and yogurt, since when the yogurt feeding was stopped at the end of the experiment (six months), the animals from the yogurt-DMH-yogurt group, which were observed until the ninth month did not develop tumour.

When we evaluated the CD4+ and CD8+ T lymphocytes from the large intestine in the DMH-indomethacin group, another difference with the yogurt feeding (yogurt-DMH-yogurt group) was observed. Mice treated with indomethacin increased the number of IgA+ cells only during the lst three months of the study, but they did not show a different balance between CD4+ or CD8+ populations as was reported for yogurt-DMH-yogurt and DMH groups when the inflammation decreased or increased (Table 1).

Another difference between indomethacin and yogurt treatment was found during the proinflamatory cytokines evaluation. Mice injected with the antiinflammatory drug presented fewer infiltrative cells in the large intestine with a low number of positive cells for TNFα and IFNγ. When the drug treatment was stopped, the cellularity and the proinflammatory cytokines increased and the tumour grew (Table 1).

For the purpose of demonstrating that the proinflammatory cytokines increase in the large intestine from mice fed to yogurt was not related with the development of a gut inflammatory response and that this cytokine response was being regulated, the nitric oxide synthase enzyme was studied.

The inducible oxide nitric synthase enzyme (iNOS) was evaluated in slices from the large intestine of different groups of mice (Table 1). INOS, which produces nitric oxide from L-arginin, is induced during the course of the immune response by microbial products and/or cytokines and plays a role in the antimicrobial effector mechanism of macrophages (Bogdan *et al.*, 2000). One of the Th1 effector mechanisms mediated by IFNγ is iNOS induction, where IL-4 plays an important role as a regulator (Patton *et al.*, 2002).

We demonstrated that tumour bearing mice (DMH group) presented high amounts of iNOS+ cells, suggesting an increase in nitric oxide production (NO) by these cells. The iNOS enzyme synthesis would be induced by IFNγ which was increased in the intestinal tissue from this group. In the group of mice injected with DMH and fed with yogurt, when the inflammation decreased, the iNOS+ cells also decreased. Long term yogurt adminstration showed an iNOS+ cells number similar to that of the non-treatment control group throughout the experiment. The DMH-indomethacin group an showed increased number of iNOS+ cells at the beginning of the antiinflamamtory treatment and at the end of the study, when the tumour grew. iNOS+ cells increase agreed with the IFNγ+ cell increase observed in the DMH-indomethacin group.

The lack of iNOS enzyme induction in the yogurt-DMH-yogurt and yogurt control groups demonstrated the way in which yogurt would regulate the immune system by modulating the inflammatory response. In spite of the increased number of IFNγ+ cells, these animals did not increase NO production and so did not present tumour, but only cellular infiltration. We thought that the large number of positive cells for in mice fed with yogurt would be related to the increase in the number of immune cells observed in the intestine; IFNγ would be regulated by other cytokines such as IL-10.

These results allow us to suggest that the immune mechanisms by which yogurt operates would be different for those induced with the antiinflammatory drug indomethacin, which did not show an increased activity of the infiltrative immune cells in the large intestine, where cytokine levels were lower than in the others groups and iNOS diminution was only evident during treatment. Yogurt exerted its antitumour activity by an antiinflammatory activity, down modulating the immune response principally through IL-10.

Stages of Colon Cancer in which Yogurt Acted

Most of the antiinflammatory drugs studied by different authors and using different models, exert their antitumor activity during the early stages of tumour development. It is known that the development of colon cancer presents a sequence of events that occurs in definable steps (initiation, promotion and progression). In the results described above mice fed with yogurt before and after DMH injections (yogurt-DMH-yogurt group) did not develop colon cancer throughout the period assayed (six months) in contrast with the tumour control group, which showed an intestinal tumour in the fifth or sixth month. In osder to find out during which stage of the tumour process yogurt acted (initiation, promotion or progression of tumour growth), we studied whether previous feeding with yogurt was sufficient by itself to reach the regulatory immune response observed, or whether cyclical administration of yogurt was necessary to prevent the effect of the DMH carcinogen.

Histological studies from the large intestine showed that previous yogurt feeding for 10 days before DMH injections only delayed tumour appearance (de Moreno de LeBlanc and Perdigón, 2004). Tumour tissue with the same characteristics as the DMH group was observed in the seventh month.. Thus yogurt administration before DMH injections was not enough to inhibit the tumour in the initiation stage. Cytokines studied in the large intestine of these mice showed that IFNγ and TNFα increased during all the periods assaye. IL-4 increased in the first months las in the yogurt-DMH-yogurt group. The number of IL-4+ cells decreased when yogurt feeding was stopped while the increase in IL-10 persisted in the large intestine cells after that time. In the same way as in the tumour control group, IL-4+ cells increased again at the end of the experience; however ,even when the number of IL-10+ cells increased, it was not enough to stop the inflammation and the tumour developed.

To study the effect of yogurt feeding in the promotion and progression of the tumour, a group of animals did not receive yogurt previous to DMH injection but were fed cyclically with this fermented milk after tumour induction following the same protocol as the yogurt-DMH-yogurt group. These animals presented amelioration in the large intestine when the yogurt was cyclically added to the diet after tumour induction with the carcinogen. This group of mice did not develop tumour and it was very similar to the yogurt-DMH-yogurt group previously described. In both groups, the number of immune cells increased in the lamina propria of the large intestine while cytokine production was similar to the one in the yogurt-DMH-yogurt group.

These results demonstrate that yogurt exerts its antitumour activity by inhibition of tumour progression and that this effect is achieved by long term cyclical yogurt consumption

Other Mechanisms Involved in the Antitumour Effect of Yogurt

The mechanisms of apoptosis or programmed cell death in the inhibition of tumour progression are well documented (Butler *et al.*, 1999). Apoptosis is a complex and active cellular process where individual cells are triggered to undergo self-destruction in a manner that will neither injure neighboring cells nor elicit an inflammatory reaction. The colonic epithelium is a tissue with a high cell turnover rate. The balance between cell proliferation and cell death is important to maintain the length of the crypts. A disturbance in this balance may lead to tumour development (Hao *et al.*, 1998), since the disruption of this type of regulation is a characteristic of the tumours.

Considering that cytokines such as TNFα could be involved in certain apoptotic pathways (Sellers and Fisher, 1999), and that an enhancement of this cytokinewas observed in our experimental model, apoptosis induction (Table 2) and the relationship between mitosis and apoptosis were studied in mice injected with DMH and in mice injected with DMH and fed with a diet supplemented with yogurt.

An increase in mitosis during the first four weeks of tumour was observed in the animals treated with the carcinogen. They presented an increase in the number of apoptotic cells during the second and third months in relation to the non-treatment control. These values decreased when the tumour grew. In the mice from the yogurt-DMH-yogurt group a moderate cell proliferation with a significant increase in the number of apoptotic cells was reported (Rachid *et al.*, 2002).

Yogurt feeding previous to carcinogen injection increased apoptosis until the fourth month (de Moreno de LeBlanc and Perdigón, sumitted). This observation and the enhancement of regulatory cytokines induced by the previous yogurt diet could explain the delay in the tumour appearance in this mice group. The behaviour of the mice that received yogurt only after DMH injections was similar to the yogurt-DMH-yogurt group, where the number of apoptotic cells increased throughout the experience (Table 2).

Long term feeding with yogurt increased the number of apoptotic cells, showing that yogurt favours cellular apoptosis in the large intestine (table 2). This fact demonstrates the importance of high TNFα levels in the mice given only yogurt as a dietary supplement, since yogurt could exert a control in the intestine by modulating the immune response and stimulating cell apoptosis, thus preventing the possible harmful effects of prolonged yogurt comsumption (Perdigon *et al.* 2003).

We cannot ignore the fact that the intestinal inflammatory process preceding tumour development may be due to changes in the epithelial cells induced by the carcinogen that enters the intestine as glucuronide. The normal microflora has the role of deconjugating this compound synthesized by gut microorganisms. Lactic acid bacteria present in yogurt could play a role in this process. Many authors have shown the influence of ingested LAB and fermented milk products on the activity of microbial flora enzymes associated with colon carcinogenesis. Bifidobacteria and lactobacillus have these enzyme activities lower than bacteroides, clostridia and enterobacteriaceae.

Since it has been demonstrated that yogurt bacteria interact in the large intestine and can affect the intestinal microflora, it is important to find out in our model whether other mechanisms such as a decrease in the activity of certain enzymes in the intestine can also be involved in the antitumour activity of the yogurt.

Table 2. Cellular apoptosis determination

Experimental group	Period of treatment	N° apoptotic cells/10 fields
DMH	1 month	ND
	2 months	43±5 *
	3 meses	26±2
	4 months	47±6 *
	5 months	ND
	6 months	ND
Y-DMH-Y	1 month	ND
	2 months	ND
	3 months	110±10 *
	4 months	60±9 *
	5 months	27±7
	6 months	33±6
Yogurt-DMH	1month	52±12 *
	2months	60±14 *
	3months	82±16 *
	4months	55±11 *
	5months	13±2
	6months	6±2
DMH-yogurt	1month	24±6
	2months	82±13 *
	3months	61±19 *
	4months	177±8 *
	5months	19±2
	6months	32±4
Yogurt	1month	ND
	2months	ND
	3months	114±13 *
	4months	50±9
	5months	99±12 *
	6months	62±11 *
Basal yogurt	10 days	34±6
Non-treatment control		25±3

The results are expressed as means ± SD of the number of apoptotic cells counted in ten fields of vision at 400X of magnification (Cells / 10 fileds) using slices from large intetsine.

* = significant differences between the sample of test groups and the non-treatment control group. $P < 0.001$.Y-DMH-Y= yogurt-DMH-yogurt; ND = Not determined.

CONCLUSIONS

The different studies carried out with the model of colon cancer inhibition through cyclic yogurt feeding demonstrate that yogurt modulates the immune system response and exerts its antitumour activity through its antiinflammatory capacity. Yogurt induces apoptosis and IL-10 production in the large intestine. This effect would be obtained by long term cyclic yogurt consumption, which inhibited promotion and progression in our experimental intestinal tumour.

In addition to this immunmodulator capacity, another mechanism by which yogurt could exert the antitumor activity observed in our model would be through yogurt bacteria interaction with the intestinal cells. These bacteria could induce decrease in the certain enzyme activities involved in the development of tumours in the intestine.

Numerous mechanisms in which the immune system plays a role can be involved in the antitumour activity of yogurt, which would be mediated by the bioactive peptides released during fermentation and by the microorganisms used as feremented starters. Our studies have demonstrated the immunoregulatory and antiinflammmatory effect of yogurt on the mucosal immune response as well as its capacity to induce cell apoptosis and thus prevent tumour growth.

REFERENCES

Abdelali, H., P. Cassand, V. Soussotte, M. Daubeze, C. Bouley, and J. F. Narbonne. 1995. Effect of dairy products on initiation of precursor lesions of colon cancer in rats. *Nutr Cancer* 24:121-32.

Ayebo, A. D., K. M. Shahani, R. Dam, and B. A. Friend. 1982. Ion exchange separation of the antitumor component(s) of yogurt dialyzate. *J Dairy Sci* 65:2388-90.

Barrett, K. E. 1996. Cytokines: sources, receptors and signalling. *Baillieres Clin Gastroenterol* 10:1-15.

Berg, D. J., N. Davidson, R. Kuhn, W. Muller, S. Menon, G. Holland, L. Thompson-Snipes, M. W. Leach, and D. Rennick. 1996. Enterocolitis and colon cancer in interleukin-10-deficient mice are associated with aberrant cytokine production and CD4(+) TH1-like responses. *J Clin Invest* 98:1010-20.

Biffi, A., D. Coradini, R. Larsen, L. Riva, and G. Di Fronzo. 1997. Antiproliferative effect of fermented milk on the growth of a human breast cancer cell line. *Nutr Cancer* 28:93-9.

Bogdan, C., J. Paik, Y. Yodovotz, and C. Nathan. 1992. Contrasting mechanisms for suppression of macrophage cytokine release by transforming growth factor and interleukin-10. *J. Biol. Chem.* 267:23301-09.

Bogdan, C., M. Rollinghoff, and A. Diefenbach. 2000. The role of nitric oxide in innate immunity. *Immunol Rev* 173:17-26.

Brady, L. J., D. D. Gallaher, and F. F. Busta. 2000. The role of probiotic cultures in the prevention of colon cancer. *J Nutr* 130:410S-414S.

Butler, L. M., P. J. Hewett, R. A. Fitridge, and P. A. Cowled. 1999. Deregulation of apoptosis in colorectal carcinoma: theoretical and therapeutic implications. *Aust. N. Zealand J. Surg.* 69:88.

Cebra, J. J. 1999. Influences of microbiota on intestinal imuune system development. *Am J Clin Nutr* 69 (suppl):1046-51.

Chang, T. L., X. Peng, and X. Fu. 2000. Interleukin-4 mediates cell growth inhibition through activation of Stat1. *J Biol Chem* 275:1012-17.

Collins, S. S., M. Feldman, and J. S. Fordtran. 1987. Colon cancer, sysplasia and surveillance in patients with ulcerative colitis: A critical review. *N. Engl. J. Med.* 316:1654.

Correa, P. 1988. A human model of gastric carcinogenesis. *Cancer Res* 48:3554-60.

Cummings, J. H. and S. A. Bingham. 1998. Diet and the prevention of cancer. *BMJ* 317:1636-40.

Curotto de Lafaille, M. A. and J. J. Lafaille. 2002. CD4(+) regulatory T cells in autoimmunity and allergy. *Curr Opin Immunol* 14:771-8.

de Moreno de LeBlanc, A. and G. Perdigón. Yogurt feeding inhibits promotion and progression of experimental colorectal cancer. *Medical Science Monitor,* 10(4):Br96-104.

de Moreno de LeBlanc, A., J. Valdéz, and G. Perdigón. 2003. Regulatory effect of yogurt on intestinal inflammatory immune response. *Eur J Inflamm* 2(1):21-61.

de Simone, C., B. B. Slavadori, R. Negri, M. Ferrazzi, L. Bladinelli, and R. Vesely. 1986. *The adjuvant effect of yogurt on production of gamma-interferon by con a-stimulated human peripheral blood lymphocytes*, abstr. pp. 419-433.

Ekbom, A., C. Helmick, M. Zack, and H. O. Adami. 1990. Ulcerative colitis and colorectal cancer. A population-based study. *N Engl J Med* 323:1228-33.

Feghali, C. A. and T. M. Wright. 1997. Cytokines in acute and chronic inflammation. *Front Biosci* 2:d12-26.

Fernandes, C. F. and K. M. Shahani. 1990. Anticarcinogenic and immunological propierties dietary lactobacilli. *J Food Prot* 53:704-10.

Ferrarini, M., E. Ferrero, L. P. A. Dagna, and M. R. Zocchi. 2002. Human γδ T cells: a nonredundant system in the immune-surveillance against cancer. *Trends Immunol* 23:14-18.

Fischer, S. M. Arachidonic acid metabolism and tumor promotion., p. 169. In: *Arachidonic acid metabolism and tumor promotion.* Fischer, S. M. and Slage, T. J. ed. Martinus Nijhoff, Boston.

Fletcher, J. R. Hematology/oncology, p. 59. In: *Prostaglandins in clinical practise.* Walkins, D. ed. Raven Press, New York.

Frucht, D. M., T. Fukao, C. Bogdan, H. Schindler, J. J. O'Shea, and S. Koyasu. 2001. IFN-gamma production by antigen-presenting cells: mechanisms emerge. *Trends Immunol* 22:556-60.

Fuller, R. 1989. Probiotics in man and animals. *J Appl Bacteriol* 66:365-78.

Fulton, A. M. 1984. In vivo effects of indomethacin on the growth of murine mammary tumors. *Cancer Res* 44:2416-20.

Goldin, B. R. and S. L. Gorbach. 1980. Effect of Lactobacillus acidophilus dietary supplements on 1,2-dimethylhydrazine dihydrochloride-induced intestinal cancer in rats. *J Natl Cancer Inst* 64:263-5.

Goldin, B. R. and S. L. Gorbach. 1984. The effect of milk and lactobacillus feeding on human intestinal bacterial enzyme activity. *Am J Clin Nutr* 39:756-61.

Goldin, B. R. and S. L. Gorbach. 1976. The relationship between diet and rat fecal bacterial enzymes implicated in colon cancer. *J Natl Cancer Inst* 57 [2], 371-5.

Goldin, B. R., L. J. Gualtieri, and R. P. Moore. 1996. The effect of Lactobacillus GG on the initiation and promotion of DMH-induced intestinal tumors in the rat. *Nutr Cancer* 25:197-204.

Goldin, B. R., L. Swenson, J. Dwyer, M. Sexton, and S. L. Gorbach. 1980. Effect of diet and Lactobacillus acidophilus supplements on human fecal bacterial enzymes. *J Natl Cancer Inst* 64:255-61.

Hao, X., M. Du, A. Bishop, and I. Talbot. 1998. Imbalance between proliferation and apoptosis in the development of colorectal carcinoma. *Virchows Arch* 433-523.

Hayashi, K. and M. Ohwaki. 1989. Antitumoor activity of *Lactobacillus casei* (LC 9018) in mic: T cell subset depletion. *Biotherapy* 3:1568-74.

Hughes, R. and I. Rowland. 2003. Nutritional and Microbial Modulation of carcinogenesis., pp In: *Gut Flora, nutrition, immunity and health*. R. Fuller and G. Perdigon ed Blackwell Publishing, Oxford, UK

Isaacson, P. 1982. Immunoperoxidase study of the secretory immunoglobulin system and lysozyme in normal and diseased gastric mucosa. *Gut* 23:578-88.

Kato, I. 2000. Antitumor activity of lactic acid bacteria., pp. 115-38. In: *Probiotics 3: Immunomodulation by the gut micgoflora and probiotics*. R. Fuller and G. Perdigón ed. Kluwer Academic Publishers, London.

Kato, I., T. Yokokura, and M. Mutai. 1984. Augmentation of mouse natural killer cell activity by Lactobacillus casei and its surface antigens. *Microbiol Immunol* 28:209-17.

Korelitz, B. I. 1983. Carcinoma of the intestinal tract in Crohn's disease: results of a survey conducted by the National Foundation for Ileitis and colitis. *Am J Gastroenterol* 78:44-6.

Lala, P. K., R. S. Parhar, and P. Singh. 1986. Indomethacin therapy abrogates the prostaglandin-mediated suppression of natural killer activity in tumor-bearing mice and prevents tumor metastasis. *Cell Immunol* 99:108-18.

LeBlanc, J. G., C. Matar, J. C. Valdez, J. LeBlanc, and G. Perdigon. 2002. Immunomodulatory effetcs of peptidic fractions issued from milk fermented with *Lactobacillus helveticus*. *J. Dairy Res.* 85:2733-42.

Ling, W. H., R. Korpela, H. Mykkanen, S. Salminen, and O. Hanninen. 1994. Lactobacillus strain GG supplementation decreases colonic hydrolytic and reductive enzyme activities in healthy female adults. *J Nutr* 124:18-23.

Matar, C., J. Amiot, L. Savoie, and J. Goulet. 1996. The effect of milk fermentation by Lactobacillus helveticus on the release of peptides during in vitro digestion. *J Dairy Sci* 79:971-9.

Matar, C., J. G. LeBlanc, L. Martin and G. Perdigon. 2003. Chapter 7. Biologically Active Peptides Released from Fermented Milk: Role and Functions. In: *Handbook of Fermented Functional Foods*. T. Farnworth ed. CRC Press, LLC, Boca Raton, Fl, USA.

Matar, C., S. S. Nadathur, A. T. Bakalinsky, and J. Goulet. 1997. Antimutagenic effects of milk fermented by Lactobacillus helveticus L89 and a protease-deficient derivative. *J Dairy Sci* 80:1965-70.

Matar, C., J. C. Valdez, M. Medina, M. Rachid, and G. Perdigon. 2001. Immunomodulating effects of milks fermented by Lactobacillus helveticus and its non-proteolytic variant. *J Dairy Res* 68:601-9.

Meydani, S. N. and W. K. Ha. 2000. Immunologic effects of yogurt. *Am J Clin Nutr* 71:861-72.

Mital, B. K. and S. K. Garg. 1995. Anticarcinogenic, hypocholesterolemic, and antagonistic activities of Lactobacillus acidophilus. *Crit Rev Microbiol* 21:175-214.

Nishihori, H., H. Tsuji, H. Wang, H. Tahara, M. Akiyama, Y. Ogawa, K. Matsushima, Y. Iwakura, and N. Mukaida. 2000. Participation of endogenously produced interferon gamma in interleukin 4-mediated tumor rejection. *Hum Gene Ther* 11:659-68.

Numata, A., T. Minagawa, M. Asano, A. Nakane, H. Katoh, and T. Tanabe. 1991. Functional evaluation of tumor-infiltrating mononuclear cells. etection of endogenous interferon- and tumor necrosis factor- in human colorectal adenocarcinomas . *Cancer* 68:1937-43.

Patton, E. A., A. C. La Flamme, J. A. Pedras-Vasoncelos, and E. J. Pearce. 2002. Central role for interleukin-4 in regulating nitric oxide-mediated inhibition of T-cell proliferation and gamma interferon production in schistosomiasis. *Infect Immun* 70:177-84.

Perdigón, G., A. de Moreno de LeBlanc, and M. Rachid. 2003. *Yogurt in the prevention of colon cancer*. Leatherhead Food Publishing, UK.

Perdigón, G., A. de Moreno de LeBlanc, J. Valdez, and M. Rachid. 2002. Role of yogurt in the prevention of colon cancer. *Eur J Clin Nutr* 56 Suppl 3:S65-8.

Perdigón, G., R. Fuller, and R. Raya. 2001. Lactic acid bacteria and their effect on the immune system. *Curr Issues Intest Microbiol* 2:27-42.

Perdigón, G., C. Maldonado Galdeano, J. C. Valdez, and M. Medici. 2002. Interaction of lactic acid bacteria with the gut immune system. *Eur J Clin Nutr* 56 Suppl 4:S21-6.

Perdigón, G., M. Medina, E. Vintiñi, and J. C. Valdéz. 2000. Intestinal pathway of internalization of lactic acid bacteria and gut mucosal immunostimulation. *Int J Immunopathol Pharmacol* 13:141.

Perdigón, G. and G. Oliver. 2000. Modulation of the immune response of the immusuppressed host by probiotics, pp 148-175. In: *Probiotics 3: Immunomodulation by the gut microflora and probiotics.* R. Fuller and G. Perdigón ed. Kluwer Academic Publisher, Netherlands.

Perdigón, G., M. Rachid, M. V de Budeguer, and J. C. Valdéz. 1994. Effect of yogurt feeding on the small and large intestine associated lymphoid cells in mice. *J.Dairy Res.* 61:553-62.

Perdigón, G., J. C. Valdez, and M. Rachid. 1998. Antitumour activity of yogurt: study of possible immune mechanisms. *J Dairy Res* 65:129-38.

Perdigón, G., E. Vintini, S. Alvarez, M. Medina, and M. Medici. 1999. Study of the possible mechanisms involved in the mucosal immune system activation by lactic acid bacteria. *J Dairy Sci* 82:1108-14.

Prescott, S. M. and F. A. Fitzpatrick. 2000. Cyclooxygenase-2 and carcinogenesis. *Biochim Biophys Acta* 1470:M69-78.

Rachid, M. M., N. M. Gobbato, J. C. Valdez, H. H. Vitalone, and G. Perdigon. 2002. Effect of yogurt on the inhibition of an intestinal carcinoma by increasing cellular apoptosis. *Int J Immunopathol Pharmacol* 15:209-216.

Read, S. and F. Powrie. 2001. CD4(+) regulatory T cells. *Curr Opin Immunol* 13:644-9.

Reddy, B. and A. Rivenson. 1993. Inhibitory effect of *Bifidobacterium longum* on colon, mammary, and liver carcinogenesis induced by 2-amino-3methylimidazo(4-5)quinoline, a food mutagen. *Cancer Res* 53:3914-18.

Reddy, B. S. 1998. Prevention of colon cancer by pre- and probiotics: evidence from laboratory studies. *Br J Nutr* 80:S219-23.

Reddy, B. S., H. Maruyama, and G. Kelloff. 1987. Dose-related inhibition of colon carcinogenesis by dietary piroxicam, a nonsteroidal antiinflammatory drug, during different stages of rat colon tumor development. *Cancer Res* 47:5340-6.

Rolfe, R. D. 2000. The role of probiotic cultures in the control of gastrointestinal health. *J Nutr* 130:396S-402S.

Saxelin, M. 1996. Colonizatiion of the human gastrointestinal tract by probiotic bacteria. *Nutr. Today* 31(suppl):5S.

Schiffrin, E. J., D. Brassart, A. L. Servin, F. Rochat, and A. Donnet-Hughes. 1997. Immune modulation of blood leukocytes in humans by lactic acid bacteria: criteria for strain selection. *Am J Clin Nutr* 66:515S-520S.

Schrezenmeir, J. and M. de Vrese. 2001. Probiotics, prebiotics, and synbiotics--approaching a definition. *Am J Clin Nutr* 73:361S-364S.

Sellers, W. R. and D. E. Fisher. 1999. Apoptosis and cancer drug targeting. *J Clin Invest* 104:1655-61.

Singh, J., A. Rivenson, M. Tomita, S. Shimamura, N. Ishibashi, and B. S. Reddy. 1997. Bifidobacterium longum, a lactic acid-producing intestinal bacterium inhibits colon cancer and modulates the intermediate biomarkers of colon carcinogenesis. *Carcinogenesis* 18:833-41.

Sreekumar, O. and A. Hosono. 2000. Immediate effect of Lactobacillus acidophilus on the intestinal flora and fecal enzymes of rats and the in vitro inhibition of Escherichia coli in coculture. *J Dairy Sci* 83:931-9.

Sydora, B. C., M. M. Tavernini, A. Wessler, L. D. Jewell, and R. N. Fedorak. 2003. Lack of Interleukin-10 leads to intestinal inflammation indepent of the time at which luminal microbial colonization occurs. *Inflamm Bow Dis* 9(2):87-97.

Thun, M. J., M. M. Namboodiri, and C. W. Heath Jr. 1991. Aspirin use and reduced risk of fatal colon cancer. *N Engl J Med* 325:1593-6.

Trosko, J. E., C. Aylsworth, and C. C. Chang. Possible in involvement of arachidonate products in tumor promoter inhibition of cell-cell communication., p. 22. In: *Arachidonic acid metabolism and tumor promotion.,* Fischer, S. M. and Slage, T. J. ed. Boston.

Valdéz, J. C. and G. Perdigon. 1991. Piroxicam, indomethacin and aspirin action on a murine fibrosarcoma. Effects on tumour-associated and peritoneal macrophages. *Clin Exp Immunol* 86:315-21.

Valdéz, J. C., M. Rachid, E. Bru, and G. Perdigon. 1997. *The effect of yogurt on the cytotoxic and phagocytic activity of macrophages in tumour-bearing mice*, abstr. pp. 299-308.

Vitini, E., S. Alvarez, M. Medina, M. Medici, M. V. de Budeguer, and G. Perdigon. 2000. Gut mucosal immunostimulation by lactic acid bacteria. *Biocell* 24:223-32.

Weitzman, S. A. and L. I. Gordon. 1990. Inflammation and cancer: role of phagocyte-generated oxidants in carcinogenesis. *Blood* 76:655-63.

Wollowski, I., G. Rechkemmer, and B. L. Pool-Zobel. 2001. Protective role of probiotics and prebiotics in colon cancer. *Am J Clin Nutr* 73(2):451S-55S.

In: Focus on Colorectal Cancer Research
Editor: Julia D. Martinez, pp. 123-141

ISBN #1-59454-101-9

Chapter VI

COX-2, PROSTAGLANDINS, AND COLON CANCER

Shinichi Ota[1,*] and Hiromi Bamba[2]

[1] Department of Gastroenterology and Hepatology, Internal Medicine, Saitama Medical School, Saitama, Japan

[2] First Department of Internal Medicine, Saitama Medical Center, Saitama Medical School, Saitama, Japan

ABSTRACT

Epidemiological, experimental, and clinical studies have demonstrated that colon carcinogenesis might be prevented by nonsteroidal anti-inflammatory drug (NSAID). Although there are some controversies, recent studies have revealed that NSAID suppresses colon carcinogenesis at adenoma stage where cyclooxygenase-2, a major molecular target in this action, is mainly expressed in interstitial cells but not in tumor cells. Therefore, it is unlikely that NSAID prevents colon cancer formation through modulating the functions of tumor cells. A more possible assumption is that NSAID suppresses colon carcinogenesis through the inhibition of prostaglandin formation. However, at present mechanisms by which how prostaglandins promote colon carcinogenesis have not been elucidated yet. Since prostaglandins act through both membrane receptors and nuclear receptors such as peroxisome proliferator receptor γ or δ, one of the focus in this area is to investigate their roles in colon carcinogenesis.

Key words: Colon Cancer, Prostaglandin, COX-2, PPARγ

* Address correspondence to: Shinichi Ota M.D., Ph.D., 38 Morohongo, Moroyama-machi, Iruma-gun, Saitama 350-0495, JAPAN, Phone: +81-492-76-1198, FAX: +81-492-76-1198, E-mail: ota@saitama-med.ac.jp

INTRODUCTION

Various studies have demonstrated that nonsteroidal anti-inflammatory drug (NSAID) prevents colon cancer formation. Epidemiological cancer prevention studies suggest that there may be a reduction in mortality from colorectal cancer in regular users of NSAID. [1] NSAID has also been shown to reduce the number and size of sporadic colon adenomas, [2] which are the precursor lesions of colon cancer. Some NSAIDs are also found to induce regression of adenomatous polyps in patients with familial adenomatous polyposis (FAP). [3] However there is no evidence showing that NSAID regresses or cures colon cancer. These findings in human studies suggest that NSAID suppresses colon carcinogenesis mainly at adenoma stage. It is controversial where cyclooxygenase-2 is expressed at this stage. Further, roles of prostaglandin (PG) in colon carcinogenesis have not been elucidated yet. In this review, we attempted to sort out controversies in this area and to discuss about the roles of PG in colon carcinogenesis.

PREVENTION OF COLON CANCER BY NSAID IN HUMANS

Since indomethacin, an NSAID, was found to suppress colon carcinogenesis in experimental animals in 1980, [4] various studies in human have demonstrated that NSAID prevents colon cancer. Kune *et al.* [5] first showed that regular aspirin or NSAID use was associated with reduced risk for the development of colorectal cancer. Subsequent epidemiological studies with a variety of designs have substantiated the original observation that NSAID prevents colorectal cancer and decrease the incidence and mortality of colorectal cancer. [6-10] Thun *et al.* [6] reported the largest study of chemoprevention of colon cancer by NSAID using about 600,000 individuals. The rate of colon cancer death was inversely correlated with aspirin use. This study showed a 40-50% reduction in the incidence of colon cancer among regular aspirin users. Most of the subsequent studies have obtained similar results, [7-10] although aspirin users showed a moderate increase in colon cancer among elderly Californians [11] and healthy male medical doctors, taking aspirin had a lower incidence of myocardial infarction but no decrease in the relative risk of colon cancer. [12]

FAP is an autosomal dominant disorder caused by a germline mutation of the adenomatous polyposis coli (*APC*) gene located at chromosome 5q21. [13-16] FAP is characterized by the formation of hundreds of colorectal adenomas and the development of colorectal cancer. Several studies have shown that sulindac, an NSAID, induces regression of colorectal polyp formation in FAP patients. [3, 17-19] Waddell and Loughry [17] first reported that use of sulindac induced regression of rectal adenomas in 4 patients with FAP. Thereafter, several cases of the resolution of adenomas in FAP patients by sulindac were reported. Giardiello *et al.* [3] conducted randomized, double-blinded, placebo-controlled trial in 40 patients with FAP. Patients receiving oral sulindac (300mg/day) exhibited decreases in the number (44%) and size (35%) of polyps, while there was no regression of polyps in the placebo group. No patient showed complete resolution of adenomas. However, they recently reported that sulindac did not inhibit the development of colorectal adenoma in FAP patients after 4 years. [20] In contrast another recent report suggested that long term treatment with sulindac significantly regresses, polyp number and prevents recurrence of high-grade adenomas in the retained rectal segment of most of FAP. [21] Therefore, sulindac may suppress colonic adenoma formation not at very early stage but at relatively late stage in FAP patients. Further studies are required to determine optimal dose, schedule, and duration of treatment with sulindac for FAP patients.

Somatic mutations in the *APC* gene have been reported in up to 50% of sporadic colorectal cancers. [22, 23] Conflicting results in the ability of NSAID to prevent sporadic adenomas of the colon have been reported. Seven cases of sporadic colonic adenomas did not regress after treatment with sulindac or piroxicam for 6 months. [24] Ladenheim *et al.* [25] performed a randomized, double-blinded, placebo-controlled trial in 44 patients with these lesions. Compared to the control group, the polyps did not significantly regress in the sulindac treated group after 4 months of treatment. However, Matsuhashi *et al.* [26] found that 13 of 20 polyps shrank or disappeared after treatment with sulindac for 4 months. One of the sulindac-treated patients developed rectal cancer 16 months after sulindac treatment, [27] suggesting that a careful follow-up is required in chemoprevention of colon cancer. These discrepancies between the study results might be caused by the small numbers of patients studied. A recent colonoscopy-based case control study by Sandler *et al.* [28] showed that NSAID use significantly reduced the incidence of colonic adenomas (odds ratio; 0.56). They therefore concluded that NSAID induce an early disruption of the adenoma-carcinoma sequence. More recent studies revealed that use of aspirin prevented colorectal adenomas in patients with or without previous history of adenomas or colorectal cancer. [29, 30] Recently, COX-selective inhibitors also reduced the incidence if colonic adenoma or cancer. [31]

Taken together, these findings suggest that treatment with sulindac causes the polyps of FAP patients and some sporadic polyps to regress. The difference in results for sporadic polyps might be associated with the presence of a mutation of the *APC* gene; the reason for these differences requires further investigations. However, these results suggest that NSAID may prevent the development of human colon cancer at the adenoma stage (Figure 1).

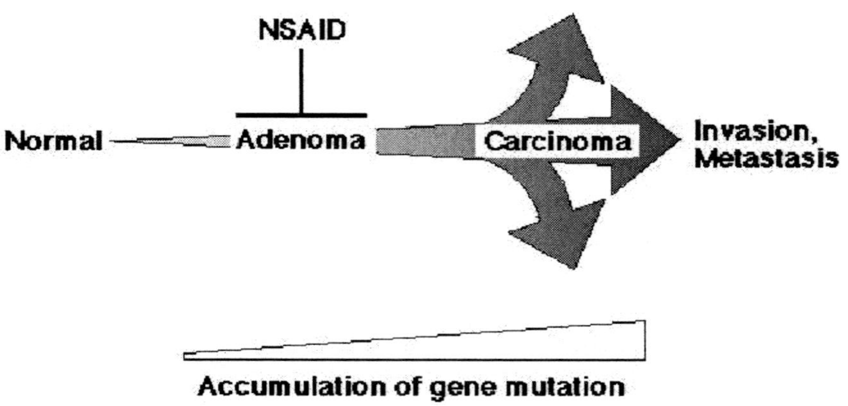

Figure 1. NSAID suppresses colon carcinogenesis at adenoma stage. NSAID, nonsteroidal anti-inflammatory drug.

Importance of Cox-2 in the Prevention of Colon Carcinogenesis by NSAID

There are at least two isoforms of cyclooxygenase (prostaglandin synthetase, COX) in humans. COX-1 is constitutively expressed in most tissues, whereas COX-2 is induced by cytokines, growth factors, and other agents. Several studies have shown that COX-2, but not COX-1 mRNA and/or protein expression is elevated in human colon cancers and adenomas, compared with that in normal mucosa. [32-34] Similarly, COX-2 mRNA and protein levels are markedly elevated in adenomas and cancers in carcinogen-induced rats, *Apc*^{Min} mice, [35, 36] a model of human FAP. Further, COX-2 inhibitors suppress the formation of intestinal tumors in these animal models. [37-41] These findings suggest the importance of COX-2 in NSAID-induced prevention of colon cancer. A study using *Apc*$^{\Delta 716}$ knockout mice, another model of human FAP, demonstrated functional evidence of the importance of COX-2 in intestinal polyp formation. [42] That study showed that inactivating the *Ptgs 2* (mouse COX-2) gene in *Apc*$^{\Delta 716}$ knockout mice or administration of a COX-2-selective inhibitor dramatically reduced the number and size of intestinal polyps. This is direct genetic evidence that COX-2 plays a key role in the early stage of intestinal polyp formation. Furthermore, a recent human study of FAP revealed that administration of celecoxib, a specific COX-2 inhibitor, significantly reduced colorectal adenomas after 6 months. [43]

These findings in animals and humans strongly support the importance of COX-2 at adenoma stage in colon carcinogenesis, although other factors might be involved in this step.

Expression of Cox-2 in the Adenoma-Carcinoma Sequence of Human Colon Cancer

Although COX-2 is up-regulated in colon cancer, an immunohistochemical study revealed that COX-2 is not diffusely expressed in cancer cells of these tumors. [33] As we described before, there is no evidence that NSAID has any therapeutic effects in established colon cancer, while they may induce regression of human colonic sporadic adenomas and those of FAP patients. [24-27, 43] Therefore it is more important to determine the expression of COX-2 in adenomas than in colon cancer.

COX-2 mRNA and/or protein level is elevated in adenomas of both humans and experimental animals. [22, 35, 36, 44] The location of expression of COX-2 in intestinal adenoma is controversial. Williams et al showed that COX-2 protein was over-expressed in epithelial cells of dysplastic and neoplastic foci in intestinal mucosa of *Apc*^{Min} mice by immunohistochemistry. [36] However, a study by Oshima *et al.* [42] using *Apc*$^{\Delta 716}$ knockout mice revealed inconsistent results. They showed that COX-2 plays an essential role in the very early stage of intestinal polyp formation, and that COX-2 expression is limited to interstitial cells. Additionally, Hull *et al.* [45] demonstrated that COX-2 protein is located in interstitial cells, mainly macrophages, at the base of and within adenomas of the small and large intestine of *Apc*^{Min} mice. It will thus be essential to study the localization of COX-2 in human colonic adenoma to sort out the differences in results of animal studies. Bamba *et al.* [46] examined the specificity of anti-human COX-2 antibody and performed immunostaining of human sporadic colon adenomas and cancer. They found that COX-2 was strongly expressed in subepithelial interstitial cells in surface area of human colonic adenomas. The localization of CD68 positive cells, i.e. macrophages, was similar to that of COX-2-positive cells in human colonic adenomas, consistent with the study of Apc^{Min} mice by Hull *et al.* [44]. Chappele *et al.* also performed immunohistochemical study including double staining with COX-2 and CD-68 antibody, which confirmed that COX-2 was mainly expressed in subepithelial macrophages of human sporadic colonic adenomas. [47] Furthermore, COX-2 mRNA detected by in-situ hybridization was localized in macrophages of these tumors. [48] Finally, expression of COX-2 in interstitial cells of intestinal tumors in APC^{Min} mice was approved by the group [49] who had reported that in epithelial tumor cells, [36] ß-catenin mutant mice confirmed this observation. [50] More recently, COX-2 expression was found in fibroblasts and endothelial cells in intestinal tumors of $Apc^{\Delta716}$ knockout mice and polyps of FAP patients, [51] although some studies revealed that COX-2 was was mainly expressed in tumor cells of sporadic human adenomas or those of FAP patients. [52, 53]

Table 1. Cyclooxugenase-2 expression in intestinal polyp

Authors	Year	Study	COX-2-expressing cell
		Animal model	
Oshima M *et al.* [42]	1996	$Apc^{\Delta716}$ KO mice	I*
Hull MA *et al.* [44]	1999	Apc^{Min} mice	I (M)
Harada N *et al.*	1999	ß-catenin mutant mice	I
Shattuck-Brandt RL *et al.*	2000	IL-10 KO mice	I (F)
		Apc^{Min} mice	I (F)
		AOM mice	I (F)
		Human	
Bamba H *et al.* [45]	1999	Sporadic adenoma	I (M)
Chapple KS *et al.* [46]	2000	Sporadic adenoma	I (M, F)
Sonoshita *et al.*	2002	Familial adenomatous polyp	I (F)
		Animal model	
Williams CS *et al.*	1996	Apc^{Min} mice	T
Shao J *et al.*	1999	AOM rat	T
		Human	
Khan KN *et al.*	2001	Familial adenomatous polyp	T > I
		Sporadic adenoma	T > I
Sato S *et al.*	2003	Sporadic adenoma	T > I

Abbreviations: I, interstitial cells; T, tumor cells; M, macrophages; F, fibroblasts; AOM, azoxymethane; KO, knockout.

*These are characterized as fibroblasts by Sonoshita *et al.*

Differences in results might be caused by tissue preparation and/or specificity of COX-2 antibodies. However most of the studies supported that COX-2 is mainly expressed in interstitial cells, although further characterization of COX-2-expressing interstitial cells in colonic tumors is required in humans and experimental animals (Table 1). Interestingly, recent reports revealed that COX-2 is expressed in human gastric hyperplastic polyps. [54, 55] The pattern of COX-2 expression in human hyperplastic gastric polyps was similar to that in human colonic adenoma. Therefore, COX-2 might be involved not only in colon carcingenesis but also gastric carcinogenesis through the development from benign polyps to cancer.

ROLES OF PGs IN COLON CARCINOGENESIS

Next important question is what is the role of COX-2 in colon carcinogenesis. Since it is expressed mainly in interstitial cells, it is unlikely that COX-2 directly modulates the function of tumor cells. It is reasonable to assume that PG produced by COX-2-expressing interstitial cells accelerates colon carcinogenesis. How PG positively regulates this step? There are several possibilities as described below (Figure 2).

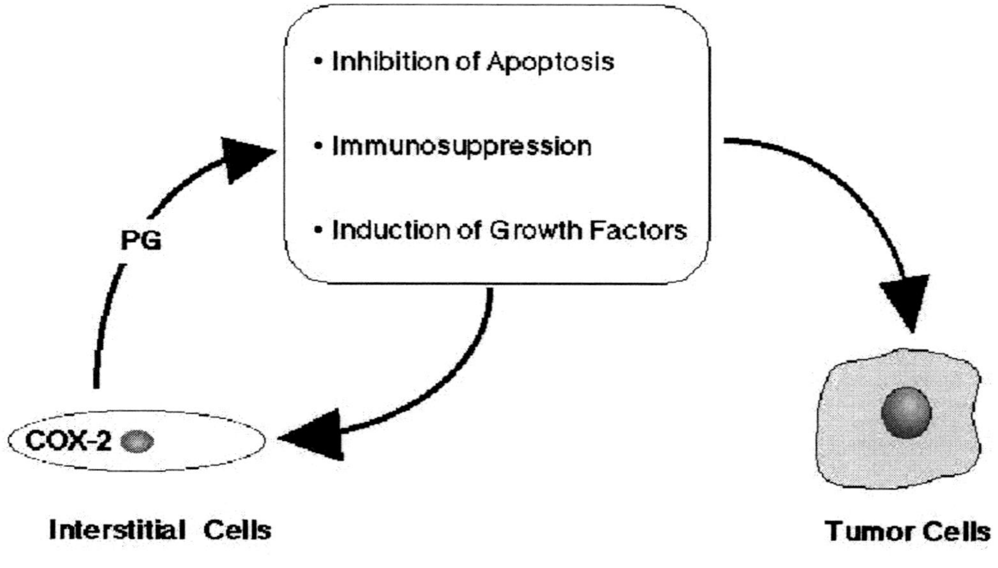

Figure2. Possible roles of prostaglandins in colon carcinogenesis. Prostaglandins produced by COX-2 expressing interstitial cells modulate colon cancer formation and coordinate signaling between the cell of origin (autocrine), and neighboring cells (paracrine) . PG, prostaglandin; COX-2, cyclooxygenase-2.

Apoptosis

Effects of PG on apoptosis have been controversial. Hanif *et al.* [56] reported that PG stimulated cancer cell proliferation, but did not have any effect on NSAIDs-induced apoptosis of these cells. However, Sheng *et al.* [57] demonstrated that PGE_2 induced Bcl-2, an anti-apoptotic protein and decreased cell death by SC-52125, a specific COX-2 inhibitor. The reason for the discrepancy in results is not known. Further studies are required to establish the action of PG on apoptosis.

Immune Suppression

Tumor immune response is an interaction of tumor and stroma. PG can modify the immune response. Especially, PGs of E-series stimulate B- and T-cell by enhancing immunoglobulin-class switching and antibody production. [58] Tumor-associated macrophages are a major target of this response. Macrophage-derived PGE_2 also appears to be responsible for immunosuppression. [59] By contrast, human lung cancer cell-derived, PGE_2 can orchestrate an imbalance in IL-10 and IL-12 production by lymphocytes and macrophages.[60] This group further suggested that specific COX-2 inhibition, genetically and/or pharmacologically, serves to restore the tumor-induced imbalance in IL-10 and IL-12 production and then suppress tumor growth in an immunocompetent murine lung cancer model.[61] PGs produced by both COX-2-expressing interstitial cells and tumor epithelial cells modify the immune response. Accordingly, NSAID may activate host immune response by decreasing PG-induced immune suppression.

Induction of Growth Factor

Various growth factors play important roles in tumor - stromal (mesenchymal) interaction and are thereby involved in proliferation, mitosis, angiogenesis, carcinogenesis, invasion, and metastasis. [62] Recent studies suggested that COX-2 plays a key role in tumor angiogenesis, as was first reported by Tsujii *et al.* [63] They suggested that a specific COX-2 inhibitor suppressed the production of vascular endothelial growth factor (VEGF), a known tumor angiogenesis factor, by COX-2-overexpressing Caco-2 cells, although the role of endogenous PG in this step was not fully studied. Selective COX-2 inhibitors blocked the growth factor such as VEGF and/or basic-fibroblast growth factor (bFGF)-mediated angiogenesis in rat corneal or rat sponge implant models *in –vivo*. [64, 65]

PG is a potent inducer of growth factors in interstitial cells, such as skin fibroblasts, gastric fibroblasts, and colon fibroblasts. [65-69] It has been demonstrated that hepatocyte growth factor (HGF) production is markedly increased in COX-2-expressing human colonic fibroblasts via a PG-mediated pathway, and that indomethacin, suppresses PG-mediated HGF production in human colonic fibroblasts. [69] PGs also stimulated the expression of VEGF in interstitial cells. [70, 71] PGE_1 has been shown to increase VEGF production dramatically by human macrophages but modestly by human colon cancer cell line T84. [72] PGE_1 dramatically induced VEGF production by human macrofages, but modestly that by T84. This step was mediated by cAMP, an important second messenger of cellular signal transduction, since exogenous cAMP showed similar effects and PGE_1 significantly increased cellular cAMP. EP_2 and EP_4 (PGE specific membrane receptors) whose second messenger is cAMP (Table 2) mRNA was expressed in both cells. These observations suggest that PG dramatically increases VEGF production by activated macrophages, but not by cancer cells, through specific PGE receptor-mediated process. NSAID, therefore, may suppress colon carcinogenesis, in part, through the suppression of VEGF expression by inhibiting endogenous PG production induced by the expression of COX-2 in macrophages.

Importance of the relation between COX-2 expressed in interstitial cells and VEGF production was genetically studied by Willams *et al.* [73] Using mouse Lewis lung carcinoma cells (LLC) implant models, they demonstrated that the growth of LLC is markedly attenuated in COX-2 null mice or in LLC tumors bearing mice treated with a selective COX-2 inhibitor, but not COX-1 null mice or wild-type mice. Their study further revealed that COX-2 null mouse fibroblasts and a selective inhibitor treated wild-type mouse fibroblasts cause a decreased ability to produce VEGF compared with their wild-type. These results suggested that host COX-2 modulates tumor growth through VEGF production. Sonoshita *et al.* [74] showed that the levels of VEGF mRNA and angiopoietin-2, another angiogenic factor, were completely suppressed in the polyps of both EP_2, a cell surface receptor of PGE_2,-deficient and COX-2-deficient $Apc^{\Delta 716}$ mice, when they were compared with $Apc^{\Delta 716}$ mice. Seno *et al.* [75] further demonstrated that the expression of COX-2, VEGF and bFGF increased in the polyps of $Apc^{\Delta 716}$ mice, although these were suppressed in the polyps of COX-2 deficient $Apc^{\Delta 716}$ mice. These results suggest that PG produced by COX-2 expressing interstitial cells might stimulate tumor angiogenesis through VEGF production via specific membrane PG receptor, leading to promote the development of intestinal polyps.

MEMBRANE PG RECEPTORS AND COLON CARCINOGENESIS

Eight prostanoid G protein-coupled cell surface receptors, membrane receptors, have been cloned; the four subtypes EP_1 to EP_4 for PGE_2; DP for PGD_2; FP for $PGF_{2\alpha}$; IP for PGI_2; and TP for thromboxane A_2 (Table 2). These are leading to changes in the cellular levels of cAMP and Ca^{2+}. [76] The distribution of these receptors is well established in rodent gastrointestinal tracts. [77, 78] The cell surface receptors modulated gastrointestinal tract function. Watanabe *et al.* [79] first approached genetic and pharmacological studies in mice for the understanding of the relationship between PG receptor and colon carcinogenesis. Their results suggest that PGE_2 promotes colon carcinogenesis through EP_1 receptor, but not EP_3 receptor. Introduction of the deletion of the EP_1 gene and EP_1 selective antagonist reduced azoxymethane (AOM)-induced aberrant crypt foci (ACF, a putative precursor of colonic adenoma) formation, although the inactivation of EP_3 gene did not have an affect. Sonoshita *et al.* [74] found that EP_2 -deficient, but not EP_1-or EP_3-dificient, $Apc^{\Delta 716}$ mice showed decreases in the number and size of intestinal polyps when compared with $Apc^{\Delta 716}$ mice. A study by Mutoh *et al.* [80] revealed that introduction of deletion of the EP_4 gene and EP_4-selective antagonist decreased the formation of AOM-induced colon ACFs.

Table 2 Classification of prostanoid receptors

Natural ligands	Receptor Type				
	Membrane				Nuclear
	Type	Subtype	G-protein*	Second messenger*	
PGD_2	DP		Gs	cAMP ↑	
15d-PGJ_2	-	-	-	-	PPARγ
PGE_2	EP				
		EP_1	G (?)	Ca^{2+} ↑	
		EP_2	Gs	cAMP ↑	
		EP_3	Gi, Gs, Gq	cAMP ↓, cAMP ↑ Ca^{2+}	
		EP_4	Gs	cAMP ↑	
$PGF_{2\alpha}$	FP		Gq	Ca^{2+} ↑	
PGI_2	IP		Gs, Gq	cAMP ↑, Ca^{2+} ↑	PPARδ
TXA_2	TP		Gq, Gs, Gi	Ca^{2+}↑, cAMP ↓, cAMP ↑	

Abbreviations: PG, prostaglandin; 15d-PGJ_2, 15-deoxy-$\Delta^{12,14}$-PGJ_2; TXA_2, thromboxane A_2; PPAR, peroxisome proliferator receptor;↑, increae; ↓, decrease.
*Data were obtained mainly murine receptors.

Recently, expression of EP receptors in human FAP was studied by using in situ-hybridization. Takafuji *et al.* [81] showed that the cell-specific prostanoid receptors, EP_3 and EP_4, prominently expressed epithelial and lamina propria mononuclear cells in FAP, respectively.

These studies provide information for the understanding of the involvement of PGs and their receptors in carcinogenesis. The data mentioned above were mainly focused EP receptors, since PGE_2 is increased in colorectal tumor tissue, [82, 83] although production of other PGs has not been fully studied yet. These results may be obtained by relatively crude measurements of PG concentrations in human colon tissues and tumors, because PGs are either chemically or metabolically unstable. In addition, these data should be interpreted carefully, since PGs partly share their receptors.

Taken together, membrane PGE receptors might contribute to the development of intestinal polyps, although further studies using different experimental models and in humans are necessary to elucidate the role of membrane PG receptors in colon carcinogenesis.

PPARs and Colon Carcinogenesis

Physiological effects of PGs appear to be mediated by two distinct pathways involving G protein-coupled cell surface receptors such as EP receptors, [76] and nuclear receptors such as peroxisome proliferator receptor (PPAR) γ and δ [84-86] Recently, attention has focused on the roles of these receptors in colon carcinogenesis. Both PGI_2 and metabolites of PGD_2 can transactivate members of the PPAR family. [87] PPAR is a member of the nuclear receptor superfamily of ligand-dependent transcription factors. [88] The PPAR family is subdivided into three subtypes:PPARα, PPARδ (PPARβ, or NUC-1), and PPARγ. (Table 3) [89] PPAR heterodimerizes with the retinoid X receptor and binds to specific peroxisome proliferator response element (PPRE) located within the promoters of target genes (Figure 3). [90, 91] PPAR raised a new insights into the physiological actions of PG.

Table 3. Ligands and function of PPARs.

PPARs	Ligands	Function
α	Fatty acids Fibrates Leukotriene B_4 ?	β-oxidation, Lipid metabolism
δ *	Fatty acids Carbaprostacyclin	Lipid metabolism Colon carcinogenesis?
γ	15-deoxy-$\Delta^{12, 14}$-PGJ_2 Thiazolidinediones	Foam cell formation Adipocyte differentiation Anti-inflammation Colon carcinogenesis?

Abbreviations:PPAR, peroxisome proliferator receptor; PG, prostaglandin.
* This also called ß, FAAR, or NUC-1.

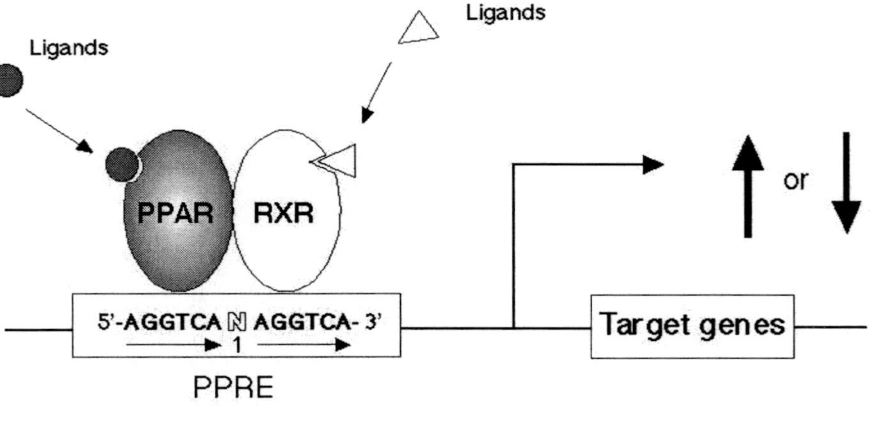

Figure3. Transcriptional regulation of target gene by PPARγ. Transcriptional regulation of target gene by PPARs. PPARs heterodimerize RXR and regulate transcription of the target genes after binding to specific DNA sequence elements. These elements consist of a direct repeat of two conserved AGGTGA hexamers separeted by one nucleotide. PPAR, peroxisome proliferator receptor; RXR, retinoid X receptor; PPRE, peroxisome proliferator response element.

PPARγ

15-deoxy-$\Delta^{12,14}$-PGJ_2 (15d-PGJ_2), a metabolite of PGD_2, has been identified as a natural ligand for PPARγ [84, 85] PPARγ. is expressed in adipocyte, macrophages and cells in neoplasms such as those of the breast, prostate, colon, and stomach. This receptor also regulates the differentiation and/or growth of these cells. [92-97] Activation of PPARγ might therefore be a useful target for the treatment of human cancers.

However, several more recent studies on the role of PPARγ in colon carcinogenesis have yielded conflicting results. In APC^{Min} mice, a mouse model of the human genetic disease FAP, treatment with a synthetic PPARγ ligand increased the number of polyps, [98, 99] whereas human colon carcinoma cell lines responded to the same ligand with a reduced growth rate and induction of cell differentiation. [100] Additionally, several reports demonstrated that AOM-induced formation of ACF was suppressed by the administration of PPARγ ligands. [101-103] A genetic approach was performed to resolve these conflicting results. [104] PPARγ wild type $^{+/+}$mouse and heterozygous deficient mice$^{+/-}$ were treated with AOM. PPARγ $^{+/-}$mice showed significantly low survival rates compared with PPARγ $^{+/+}$mice. There were significantly greater number of polyps in PPARγ$^{+/-}$ mice compared with PPARγ $^{+/+}$mice. Up-regulation of β-catenin by the defect of *APC* protein has been shown to influence the development of colon cancer at an early stage. In the absense of carcinogen, β-catenin levels of in colonic epithelium were significantly higher in PPARγ$^{+/-}$ mice compared with PPARγ$^{+/+}$ mice, although in tumors of both types of mice, β-catenin levels showed no difference. Finally, PPARγ$^{+/-}$mice were crossed with mice heteroxygous for a truncating mutation in the *APC* gene. There were no differences in either suvival or the number of colonic tumors between PPARγ$^{+/-}$: $APC^{+/1638}$ mice and PPARγ$^{+/+}$ $APC^{+/1638}$ mice. These results suggest that PPARγ can suppress beta-catenin levels and colon carcinogenesis but only before damage to the APC/β-catenin pathway, although the reason why increrase of in tumor formation observed in APC^{Min} mice by PPARγ ligands is not clear. Furhter, a study with human colon cancer cell lines demonstrated growth inhibition by PPARγ ligands even in the cell lines with mutant *APC*. [100] Therefore, controversies can not be solved completely and further studies are required in this area, but recent data supported that PPARγ might be a possible target of colon cancer prevention.

Is there a possible explanation of the increase of tumor formation by PPARγ ligands in vivo? Both COX-2 and PPARγ are expressed in macrophages. [46-48, 92] As we described before, PGs dramatically increased VEGF production by activated macrophages through specific PGE receptors -mediated process. [105] 15d-PGJ_2 also dramatically stimulated the production of VEGF by these cells, while mRNAs of both PGE specific receptors and PPARγ were detected in these cells. The effect of PPARγ ligands on the production of VEGF by interstitial cells was confirmed by another study using vascular smooth muscle cells, [106] although a study demonstrated that PPARγ negatively regulates angiogenesis *in vivo*. [107] Further studies are required to clarify the roles of PPARγ in angiogenesis. However, if PPARγ is a negative regulator of colon carcinogenesis, endogenous ligand for PPARγ such as 15d-PGJ_2 might not have a significant role in human colon carcinogenesis, since NSAID suppresses the formation of endogenous PGs and acts as a tumor suppressive agent.

As we described, recent reports support the hypothesis that PPARγ is a useful target in the prevention of colon carcinogenesis, although further studies will be necessary to establish the role of this nuclear receptor in human colon carcinogenesis. Synthetic ligands for PPARγ are currently being widely used to treat patients with type 2 diabetes mellitus. These patients should be followed up carefully.

PPARδ

PPARδ, another nuclear receptor of PPAR family, is induced by APC/ β-catenin/ T-cell factor 4 (Tcf-4) pathway and thereby may associate with colon carcinogenesis. [108] PPARδ mRNA has been frequently overexpressed in many colorectal cancers. [108, 109] Park *et al.* [110] showed that PPARδ null cells decreased the ability to form tumors compared with wild-type cells by using the nude mice xenograft assay. Because PGI_2 has been found to act as a ligand for PPARδ [111] and the expression of PPARδ is similar to that of COX-2 in human colorectal cancer, [109] PG may modulate colon cancer formation through this receptor. However, a more recent study showed that the introduction of the deletion of PPARδ gene to Apc^{Min} mice did not modulate the number of intestinal polyps, although large size polyps, in excess of a diameter of 1 mm, were insignificantly decreased, suggesting that PPARδ is dispensable for colorectal polyp formation. [112]

Taken together, signals through PPARδ either stimulate or have no effects on colon carcinogenesis. Further studies will be necessary the roles of PPARδ in colon carcinogenesis.

Future Prospects

Based on the evidence described above, COX-2 expressed in colonic adenomas may play important roles in the maintenance and development of these tumors, NSAIDs and a specific COX-2 inhibitor inhibited the growth of colonic adenomas. However, it remains unclear what induces COX-2 in interstitial cells. Further studies in this initial step is required. Accumulating evidence suggests that the importance of PG derived from COX-2 expressing interstitial cells. However, the roles of membrane and nuclear PG receptors is really controversial. One of the important focus in this is to study the significance of PG and their receptors in colon carcinogenesis.

Acknowledgement

This study was supported in part by a grant from the Japanese Ministry of Education, Science and Culture (KAKEN NO. 14570502 to S.A.).

References

[1] Smalley W, Dubois RN. Colorectal cancer and nonsteroidal anti-inflammatory drugs. *Adv Pharmacol.* 1997;39:1-20.

[2] Shiff SJ, Basil R. Nonsteroidal anti-inflammatory drugs and colorectal cancer:Evolving concepts of their chemopreventive actions. *Gastroenterology*. 1997;113:1992-1998.
[3] Giardielo FM, Hamilton SR, Krush AJ, et al. Treatment of colonic and rectal adenomas with sulindac in familial adenomatous polyposis. *New Engl J Med*. 1993;328:1313-1316.
[4] Kudo T, Narisawa T, Abo S. Anti-tumor activity of indomethacin on methylazoxymethanol-induced large bowel tumors in rats. *Gann*. 1980;71:260-264.
[5] Kune GA, Kune S, Watson LF. Colorectal cancer risk, chronic illnesses, operations, and medications: case control results from the Melbourne Colorectal Cancer Study. *Cancer Res*. 1988;48: 4399-43404.
[6] Thun MJ, Namboodiri MM, Heath CW. Aspirin use and reduced risk of colon cancer. *New Engl J Med*. 1991;325:1593-1596.
[7] Peleg II, Maiboch HT, Brown SH, Wilcox CM. Aspirin and non-steroidal anti-inflammatory drug use and the risk of subsequent colorectal cancer. *Arch Int Med*. 1994;154:394-399.
[8] Suh O, Mettlin C, Petrelli NJ. Aspirin use, cancer, and polyps of the large bowel. *Cancer*. 1993;72:1171-1177.
[9] Gridley G, Meloughlin JK, Ekbom A, et al. Incidence of cancer among patients with rheumatoid arthritis. *J Natl Cancer Inst*. 1993;85:307-311.
[10] Schreinemacher DM, Everson RB. Aspirin use and lung, colon, and breast cancer incidence in a prospective study. *Epidemiology* 1994;5:138-146.
[11] Paganini-Hill A, Chao A, Ross RK, Henderson BEl. Aspirin use and chronic disease: a cohort study of elderly. *Br Med J*. 1989;229:1247-1250.
[12] Giovanucci E, Rimm EB, Stampfer MJ, Colditz GA, Ascherio A, Willett WC. Aspirin use and the risk for colorectal cancer and adenoma in male health professionals. *Ann Int Med*. 1994;121;241-246.
[13] Kinzler KW, Nilbert MC, Su LK, et al. Identification of FAP locus genes from chromosome 5q21. *Science*. 1991;253: 661-665.
[14] Nishisho I, Nakamura Y, Miyoshi Y, et al. Mutations of chromosome 5q21 genes in FAP and colorectal cancer patients. *Science*. 1991;253:665-669.
[15] Groden J, Thliveris A, Samowitz W, et al. Identification and characterization of the familial adenomatous polyposis coli gene. *Cell*. 1991;66:589-600.
[16] Joslyn G, Carlson M, Thliveris A, et al. Identification of deletion mutations and three new genes at the familial polyposis locus. *Cell*. 1991;66:601-613.
[17] Waddel WR, Laughry RW. Sulindac for polyposis of the colon. *J Surg Oncol*. 1983;24:83-87.
[18] Rigau J, Pique JM, Rubio E, Planas R, Tarrech JM, Bordas JM. Effect of long-term sulindac therapy on colonic polyposis. *Ann Int Med*. 1991;115:952-954.
[19] Labayle D, Fischer D, Vielh P, et al. Sulindac causes regression of rectal polyps in familial adenomatous polyposis. *Gastroenterology*. 1991, 101, 635-639.
[20] Nugent KP, Farmer KC, Spigelman AD, Williams CB, Phillips RK. Randomized control trial of the effect of sulindac on duodenal and rectal polyposis and cellproliferation in patients with familial adenomatous polyposis. *Br J Surg*. 1993;80:1618-1619.

[21] Giardiello FM, Yang VW, Hylind LM, et al. Primary chemoprevention of familial adenomatous polyposis with sulindac. *N Engl J Med.* 2002;346:1054-1059.

[22] Cruz-Correa M, Hylind LM, Romans KE, Booker SV, Giardiello FM. Long-term treatment with sulindac in familial adenomatous polyposis: a prospective cohort study. *Gastroenterology.* 2002;122:641-645.

[23] Powell SM, Zilz N, Beazer-Barclay Y, et al. APC mutation occur early during colorectal tumorigenesis. *Nature (Lond.)* 1992;359:235-237.

[24] Hixson LJ, Earnest DL, Fennerty MB, Sampliner RE. NSAID effect on sporadic colon polyps. *Am J Gastroenterology.* 1993;88:1652-1656.

[25] Ladenheim J, Garcia G, Titzer D, et al. Effects of sulindac on sporadic colonic polyps. *Gastroenterology.* 1995;108:1083-1087.

[26] Matsuhashi N, Nakajima A, Fukushima Y, Yazaki Y, Oka T. Effects of sulindac on sporadic colorectal adenomatous polyps. *Gut.* 1977;40:344-349.

[27] Matsuhashi N, Nakajima A, Shinohara K, Oka T, Yazaki Y. Rectal cancer after sulindac therapy for a sporadic adenomatous colonic polyp. *Am J Gastroenterology.* 1998;93:2261-2266.

[28] Sandler RS, Galanko JC, Murray SC, Helm JF, Woosley JT. Aspirin and nonsteroidal anti-inflammatory agents and risk for colorectal adenomas. *Gastroenterology.* 1998;114:441-447.

[29] Baron JA, Cole BF, Sandler RS, et al. A randomized trial of aspirin to prevent colorectal adenomas. *N Engl J Med.* 2003;348:891-899.

[30] Sandler RS, Halabi S, Baron JA, et al. A randomized trial of aspirin to prevent colorectal adenomas in patients with previous colorectal cancer. *N Engl J Med.* 2003;348:883-890.

[31] Rahme E, Barkun AN, Toubouti Y, Bardou M. The cyclooxygenase-2-selective inhibitors rofecoxib and celecoxib prevent colorectal neoplasia occurrence and recurrence. *Gastroenterology.* 2003;125:404-412.

[32] Eberhart CE, Coffey RJ, Radhika A, Giardiello FM, Ferrenbach S, DuBois RN. Up-regulation of cyclooxygenase 2 gene expression in human colorectal adenomas and adenocarcinomas. *Gastroenterology.* 1994;107, 1183-1188.

[33] Sano H, Kawahito Y, Wilder RL, et al. Expression of cyclooxygenase-1 and -2 in human colorectal cancer. *Cancer Res.* 1995;55, 3785-3789.

[34] Kargman SL, O'Neill GP, Vickers PJ, Evans JF, Mancini JA, Jothy S. Expression of prostaglandin G/H synthase-1 and 2 protein in human colon cancer. *Cancer Res.* 1995;55:2556-2559.

[35] Dubois RN, Radhika A, Reddy BS, Entingh AJ. Increased cyclooxygenase-2 levels in carcinogen-induced rat colonic tumors. Gastroenterology 1996:110:1252-62

[36] Williams CS, Luongo C, Radhika AA, et al. Elevated cyclooxygenase-2 levels in Min mouse adenomas. *Gastroenterology.* 1996;111:1134-1140.

[37] Kawamori T, Rao CV, Seibert K, Reddy BS. Chemopreventive activity of celecoxib, a specific cyclooxygenase-2 inhibitor, against colon carcinogenesis. *Cancer Res.* 1998;58:409-412.

[38] Yoshimi N, Kawabata K, Hara A, Matsunaga K, Yamada Y, Mori H. Inhibitory effect of NS-398, a selective cyclooxygenase inhibitor, on azoxymethane-induced aberrant crypt foci in colon carcinogenesis of F344 rats. *Jpn J Cancer Res.* 1997;88:1044-1051.

[39] Yoshimi N, Shimizu M, Matsunaga K, et al. Chemopreventive effect of N-(2-cyclohexy-4-nitrophenyl) methanesulfonamide (NS-398), a selective cyclooxygenase inhibitor, in rat colon carcinogenesis induced by azoxymethane. *Jpn J Cancer Res.* 1999;90:406-412.

[40] Fukutake M, Nakatsugi S, Isoi T, Takahashi M, Ohta T, Mamiya. Suppressive effects of nimesulide, a selective inhibitor of cyclooxygenase-2, on azoxymethane-induced coloncarcinogenesis in mice. *Carcinogenesis.* 1998;19:1939-1942.

[41] Jacoby RF, Seibert K, Cole CE, Kelloff G, Lubet RA. The cyclooxygenase-2 inhibitor celecoxib is a potent preventive and therapeutic agent in the min mouse model of adenomatous polyposis. *Cancer Res.* 2000;60:5040-5044.

[42] Oshima M, Dinchuk JE, Kargman SL, et al. Suppression of intestinal polyposis in $APC^{\Delta 716}$ knockout mice by inhibition of cyclooxygenase 2 (COX-2). *Cell.* 1996;87:803-809.

[43] Steinbach G, Lynch PM, Phillips RK, et al. The effect of celecoxib, a cyclooxygenase-2 inhibitor, in familial adenomatous polyposis. *N Engl J Med.* 2000,342:1946-1952.

[44] Shao J, Sheng H, Aramandla R, et al. Coordinate regulation of cyclooxygenase-2 and TGF-beta1 in replication error-positive colon cancer and azoxymethane-induced rat colonic tumors. *Carcinogenesis.* 1999;20:185-191.

[45] Hull MA, Booth JK, Tisbury A, Scott N, et al. Cyclooxygenase-2 is up-regulated and localized to macrophages in the intestine of Min mice. *Br J Cancer.* 1999;79:1399-1405.

[46] Bamba H, Ota S, Kato A, Adachi A, Itoyama S, Matsuzaki F. High expression of cyclooxygenase-2 in macrophages of human colonic adenoma. *Int J Cancer.* 1999; 83:470-475.

[47] Chapple KS, Cartwright EJ, Hawcroft G, et al. Localization of cyclooxygenase-2 in human sporadic colorectal adenomas. *Am J Pathol.* 2000;156:545-553.

[48] Hull M, Chapple K, Coletta L, Poulsom R. COX-2 in murine intestinal tumors. *Gastroenterology.* 2000;119:600-602.

[49] Shattuck-Brandt RL, Varilek GW, Radhika A, et al: Cyclooxygenase 2 expression is increased in the stroma of colon carcinomas from IL-10 (-/-) mice. *Gastroenterology.* 2000;118:337-345.

[50] Harada N, Tamai Y, Ishikawa T, et al. Intestinal polyposis in mice with a dominant stable mutation of the beta-catenin gene. *EMBO J.* 1999,18:5931-5942.

[51] Sonoshita M, Takaku K, Oshima M, Sugihara K, Taketo MM. Cyclooxygenase-2 expression in fibroblasts and endothelial cells of intestinal polyps. *Cancer Res.* 2002;62:6846-6849.

[52] Sato T, Yoshinaga K, Okabe S, et al. Cyclooxygenase-2 expression in colorectal adenomas. *Dis Colon Rectum.* 2003;46:786-792.

[53] Khan KN, Masferrer JL, Woerner BM, Soslow R, Koki AT. Enhanced cyclooxygenase-2 expression in sporadic and familial adenomatous polyposis of the human colon. *Scand J Gastroenterol.* 2001;36:865-869.

[54] Kawada M, Seno H, Wada M, et al. Cyclooxygenase-2 expression and angiogenesis in gastric hyperplastic polyp - association with polyp size. *Digestion*. 2003;67:20-24.

[55] Bamba H., Ota S., Arai S., et al. Expression of COX-2 in human gastric hyperplastic polyps. *J. Exp. Clin. Cancer Res*. In press 2003.

[56] Hanif R, Pittas A, Feng Y, et al. Effects of nonsteroidal anti-inflammatory drugs on proliferation and on induction of apoptosis in colon cancer cells by a prostaglandin-independent pathway. *Biochem Pharmacol*.1996;52,:237-245.

[57] Sheng H, Shao J, Morrow JD, Beauchamp RD, DuBois RN. Modulation of apoptosis and Bcl-2 expression by prostaglandin E2 in human colon cancer cells. *Cancer Res*. 1998;58:362-366.

[58] Phipps RP, Stein SH, and Roper RL, A new view of prostaglandin E regulation of the immune response. *Immunol. Today*. 1991;12:349-352.

[59] Marnett LJ. Aspirin and the potential role of prostaglandins in colon cancer. *Cancer Res*. 1992;52: 5575-5589.

[60] Huang M, Stolina M, Sharma S, et al. Non-small cell lung cancer cyclooxygenase-2-dependent regulation of cytokine balance in lymphocytes and macrophages: up-regulation of interleukin 10 and down-regulation of interleukin 12 production. *Cancer Res*. 1998;58:1208-1216.

[61] Stolina M, Sharma S, Lin Y, et al. Specific inhibition of cyclooxygenase 2 restores antitumor reactivity by altering the balance of IL-10 and IL-12 synthesis. *J Immunol*. 2000;164:361-370.

[62] Hong W, Sporn MB. Recent advances in chemoprevention of cancer. *Science*. 1997;278:1073–1077.

[63] Tsujii M, Kawano S, Tsuji S, Sawaoka H, Hori M, DuBois RN. Cyclooxygenase regulates angiogenesis induced by colon cancer cells. *Cell*. 1998;93:705-716.

[64] Masferrer JL, Leahy KM, Koki AT, et al. Antiangiogenic and antitumor activities of cyclooxygenase-2 inhibitors. *Cancer Res*. 2000;60:1306-1311.

[65] Majima M, Hayashi I, Muramatsu M, Katada J, Yamashina S, Katori M. Cyclo-oxygenase-2 enhances basic fibroblast growth factor-induced angiogenesis through induction of vascular endothelial growth factor in rat sponge implants. *Br J Pharmacol*. 2000;130:641-649.

[66] Matsumoto K, Okazaki H, Nakamura T. Novel function of prostaglandins as inducers of gene expression of HGF and putative mediators of tissue regeneration. *J Biochem (Tokyo)* 1995;117:458-464.

[67] Takahashi M, Ota S, Hata Y, et al. Hepatocyte growth factor as a key to modulate anti-ulcer action of prostaglandins in stomach. *J Clin Invest*. 1996;98:2604-2611.

[68] Bamba H, Ota S, Kato A, Matsuzaki F. Nonsteroidal anti-inflammatory drugs may delay the repair of gastric mucosa by suppressing prostaglandin-mediated increase of hepatocyte growth factor production. *Biochem Biophys Res Commun*. 1998;245: 567-571.

[69] Ota S, Tanaka Y, Bamba H, Kato A, Matsuzaki F. Nonsteroidal anti-inflammatory drugs may prevent colon cancer through suppression of hepatocyte growth factor expression. *Eur J Pharmacol*. 1999;367:131-138.

[70] Harada S, Nagy JA, Sullivan KA, Thomas KA, Endo N, Rodan GA, Rodan SB. Induction of vascular endothelial growth factor expression by prostaglandin E2 and E1 in osteoblasts. *J Clin Invest.* 1994;93:2490-2496.

[71] Ben-Av P, Crofford LJ, Wilder RL, Hla T. Induction of vascular endothelial growth factor expression in synovial fibroblasts by prostaglandin E and interleukin-1: a potential mechanism for inflammatory angiogenesis. *FEBS Lett.* 1995;372:83-87.

[72] Bamba H, Ota S, Kato A, Kawamoto C, Matsuzaki F. Effect of prostaglandin E1 on vascular endothelial growth factor production by human macrophages and coloncancer cells. *J Exp Clin Cancer Res.* 2000;19:219-223.

[73] Williams CS, Tsujii M, Reese J, Dey SK, DuBois RN. Host cyclooxygenase-2 modulates carcinoma growth. *J Clin Invest.* 2000;105:1589-1594.

[74] Sonoshita M, Takaku K, Sasaki N, et al. Acceleration of intestinal polyposis through prostaglandin receptor EP2 in $Apc^{\Delta 716}$ knockout mice. *Nat Med.* 2001;7:1048-1051.

[75] Seno H, Oshima M, Ishikawa T, et al. Cyclooxygenase 2- and prostaglandin E_2 receptor EP_2-dependent angiogenesis in $Apc^{\Delta 716}$ mouse intestinal polyps. *Cancer Res.* 2002;62:506-511.

[76] Coleman RA, Smith WL, Narumiya S. International Union of Pharmacology classification of prostanoid receptors: properties, distribution, and structureof the receptors and their subtypes. *Pharmacol Rev.* 1994;46:205-229.

[77] Morimoto K, Sugimoto Y, Katsuyama M, et al Cellular localization of mRNAs for prostaglandin E receptor subtypes in mouse gastrointestinal tract. 1997, *Am J Physiol.* 272, G681-G687.

[78] Ding M. Kinoshita Y, Kishi K, et al. Distribution of prostaglandin E receptors in the rats gastrointestinal tract. *Prostaglandins.* 1997; 53: 199-216.

[79] Watanabe K, Kawamori T, Nakatsugi S, et al. Role of the prostaglandin E receptor subtype EP1 in colon carcinogenesis. *Cancer Res.* 1999;59:5093-5096.

[80] Mutoh M, Watanabe K, Kitamura T, et al. Involvement of prostaglandin E receptor subtype EP_4 in colon carcinogenesis. *Cancer Res.* 2002;62:28-32.

[81] Takafuji V, Lublin D, Lynch K, Roche JK. Mucosal prostanoid receptors and synthesis in familial adenomatous polyposis. *Histochem Cell Biol.* 2001;116:171-181.

[82] Rigas B, Goldman IS, Levine L. Altered eicosanoid levels in human colon cancer. *J Lab Clin Med.* 1993;122:518-523.

[83] Yang VW, Shields JM, Hamilton SR, et al. Size-dependent increase in prostanoid levels in adenomas of patients with familial adenomatous polyposis. *Cancer Res.* 1998;58:1750-1753.

[84] Forman BM, Tontonoz P, Chen J, Brun RP, Spiegelman BM, Evans RM. 15-Deoxy-delta 12, 14-prostaglandin J2 is a ligand for the adipocyte determination factor PPAR gamma. *Cell.* 1995;83:803-812.

[85] Kliewer SA, Lenhard JM, Willson TM, Patel I, Morris DC, Lehmann JM.. A prostaglandin J2 metabolite binds peroxisome proliferator-activated receptor gamma and promotes adipocyte differentiation. *Cell.* 1995;83:813-819.

[86] Hertz R, Berman I, Keppler D, Bar-Tana J. Activation of gene transcription by prostacyclin analogues is mediated by the peroxisome-proliferators-activated receptor (PPAR). *Eur J Biochem.* 1996;235:242-247.

[87] Forman BM, Chen J, Evans RM. Hypolipidemic drugs, polyunsaturated fatty acids, and eicosanoids are ligands for peroxisomeproliferator-activated receptors α and δ. *Proc Natl Acad Sci U S A*. 1997;94:4312-4317.

[88] Mangelsdorf DJ, Thummel C, Beato M, et al. The nuclear receptor superfamily: the second decade. *Cell*. 1995;83:835-839.

[89] Kliewer SA, Forman BM, Blumberg B, et al.Differential expression and activation of a family of murine peroxisome proliferator-activated receptors. *Proc Natl Acad Sci U S A*. 91:7355-7359.

[90] Kliewer SA, Umesono K, Noonan DJ, Heyman RA, Evans RM. Convergence of 9-cis retinoic acid and peroxisome proliferator signalling pathways through heterodimer formation of their receptors. *Nature*. 1992;358:771-774.

[91] Palmer CN, Hsu MH, Griffin HJ, Johnson EF. Novel sequence determinants in peroxisome proliferator signaling. *J Biol Chem*. 1995;270:16114-16121

[92] Tontonoz P, Hu E, Graves RA, Budavari AI, Spiegelman BM. mPPAR gamma 2: tissue-specific regulator of an adipocyte enhancer. *Genes Dev*. 1994 ;8:1224-1234.

[93] Tontonoz P, Nagy L, Alvarez JG, Thomazy VA, Evans RM. PPARgamma promotes monocyte/macrophage differentiation and uptake of oxidized LDL. *Cell*. 1998 ;93:241-252.

[94] Mueller E, Sarraf P, Tontonoz P,et al. Terminal differentiation of human breast cancer through PPAR gamma. *Mol Cell*. 1998;1:465-470.

[95] Kubota T, Koshizuka K, Williamson EA, et al. Ligand for peroxisome proliferator-activated receptor gamma (troglitazone) has potent antitumor effect against human prostate cancer both in vitro and in vivo. *Cancer Res*. 1998;58:3344-3352.

[96] Takahashi N, Okumura T, Motomura W, Fujimoto Y, Kawabata I, Kohgo Y. Activation of PPARgamma inhibits cell growth and induces apoptosis in human gastric cancer cells. *FEBS Lett*. 1999;455:135-139.

[97] Rumi MA, Sato H, Ishihara S, et al. Peroxisome proliferator-activated receptor gamma ligand-induced growth inhibition of human hepatocellularcarcinoma. *Br J Cancer*. 2001 15;84:1640-1647.

[98] Lefebvre AM, Chen I, Desreumaux P, et al. Activation of the peroxisome proliferator-activated receptor γ promotes the development of colon tumors in C57BL/6J-APC^{Min}/+ mice. *Nat Med*. 1998;4:1053-1057.

[99] Saez E, Tontonoz P, Nelson MC, et al. Activators of the nuclear receptor PPARγ enhance colon polyp formation. *Nat Med*. 1998;4:1058-1061.

[100] Sarraf P, Mueller E, Jones D, et al. Differentiation and reversal of malignant changes in colon cancer through PPARγ. *Nat Med*. 1998;4:1046-1052.

[101] Tanaka T, Kohno H, Yoshitani S, et al. Ligands for peroxisome proliferator-activated receptors alpha and gamma inhibit chemically induced colitis and formation of aberrant crypt foci in rats. *Cancer Res*. 2001;61:2424-2428.

[102] Kohno H, Yoshitani S, Takashima S, et al. Troglitazone, a ligand for peroxisome proliferator-activated receptor gamma, inhibits chemically-induced aberrant crypt foci in rats. *Jpn J Cancer Res*. 2001;92:396-403.

[103] Osawa E, Nakajima A, Wada K, et al. Peroxisome proliferator-activated receptor gamma ligands suppress colon carcinogenesis induced by azoxymethane in mice. *Gastroenterology*. 2003;124:361-367.

[104] Girnun GD, Smith WM, Drori S, et al. APC-dependent suppression of colon carcinogenesis by PPARgamma. *Proc Natl Acad Sci U S A*. 2002;99:13771-13776.

[105] Bamba H, Ota S, Kato A, Kawamoto C, Fujiwara K. Prostaglandins up-regulate vascular endothelial growth factor production through distinct pathways in differentiated U937 cells. *Biochem Biophys Res Commun*. 20005;273:485-491.

[106] Yamakawa K, Hosoi M, Koyama H, et al. Peroxisome proliferator-activated receptor-gamma agonists increase vascular endothelial growth factor expression in human vascular smooth muscle cells. *Biochem Biophys Res Commun*. 2000;271:571-574.

[107] Panigrahy D, Singer S, Shen LQ, et al..PPARγ ligands inhibit primary tumor growth and metastasis by inhibiting angiogenesis. *J Clin Invest*. 2002;110:923-32.

[108] He TC, Chan TA, Vogelstein B, Kinzler KW. PPARδ is an APC-regulated target of nonsteroidal anti-inflammatory drugs. *Cell*. 1999;99:335-345.

[109] Gupta RA, Tan J, Krause WF, et al. Prostacyclin-mediated activation of peroxisome proliferator-activated receptor δ in colorectal cancer. *Proc Natl Acad Sci U S A*. 2000;97:13275-13280.

[110] Park BH, Vogelstein B, Kinzler KW. Genetic disruption of PPARδ decreases the tumorigenicity of human colon cancer cells. *Proc Natl Acad Sci U S A*. 2001 ;98:2598-25603.

[111] Lim H, Gupta RA, Ma WG, et al. Cyclo-oxygenase-2-derived prostacyclin mediates embryo implantation in the mouse via PPARδ. *Genes Dev*. 1999;13:1561-1574.

[112] Barak Y, Liao D, He W, et al. Effects of peroxisome proliferator-activated receptor δ on placentation, adiposity, and colorectal cancer. *Proc Natl Acad Sci U S A*. 2002;99:303-308.

In: Focus on Colorectal Cancer Research
Editor: Julia D. Martinez, pp. 143-170
ISBN #1-59454-101-9

Chapter VII

EARLY COLORECTAL CANCER: NEW DIAGNOSTIC METHODS AND COLONOSCOPIC THERAPEUTIC TECHNIQUES

David P. Hurlstone* and Jackie Kelly
Royal Hallamshire Hospital
Sheffield, United Kingdom

ABSTRACT

The recognition of flat colorectal lesions and the use of chromoscopy as a diagnostic tool in colonoscopy has followed a similar evolution to gastric and early oesophageal cancers. Hence, concepts and diagnostic techniques that were used only for malignancies of the stomach and oesophagus have now been applied in colorectal cancer. Kariya *et al* reported the first case of a depressed lesion in 1977, but until 1994, when Kudo *et al* reported their flat adenoma cohort and classification, flat and depressed lesions were thought to be a unique Japanese phenomena (phantom carcinoma or Akita disease). Studies from Western groups now prove this to be incorrect.

For the detection of large polyps and advanced colorectal cancers, chromoendoscopy and magnification colonoscopy is not required. The strength of the techniques are essentially in identification of flat and diminutive colorectal lesions whose detection with conventional colonoscopy is sub-optimal. Current data proposes flat adenomas may account for in excess of 30% of all colorectal lesions. In addition, malignant potential conferred in this group may be significantly higher compared to conventional colorectal polypoid lesions. Magnification colonoscopy complemented by mucosal dye spraying may therefore be a helpful diagnostic tool.

Most flat colorectal lesions are small and have an innocent appearance at initial colonoscopy. Macroscopic non-magnified views commonly reveal only subtle architectural deviation, such as a modest colour change (discolour and faint redness) or a

* Address for correspondence: David P Hurlstone*, MRCP MD (Dist), Consultant Endoscopist/Gastroenterologist, Room P39/Ward P2, The Gastrointestinal and Liver Unit, Royal Hallamshire Hospital, Glossop Road, Sheffield S10, United Kingdom, Email: p.hurlstone@shef.ac.uk

loss of the vascular net. The use of stains such as indigo carmine in addition to magnification colonoscopy can offer a quick and simple diagnostic tool in this group.

This chapter explores new colonoscopic diagnostic and therapeutic techniques now available in Western practice, previously developed by Japanese groups. We discuss the controversies surrounding the diagnosis and therapeutic strategies involved in flat and depressed colorectal lesions and explore the concept of 'virtual biopsy' techniques as applicable to high-magnification chromoscopic colonoscopy. Finally, new and evolving diagnostic colonoscopic techniques using autofluorescence are discussed.

INTRODUCTION

Colorectal cancer (CRC) is the most common malignant lesion of the gastrointestinal tract in the United Kingdom being responsible for 20,000 deaths per year [1-5]. It is the most common fatal malignancy among non-smokers in North America and Europe and is the second most common cause of cancer mortality in the United States (US) and UK after lung cancer [6]. In the UK and US there are approximately 32,000 and 160,000 new cases of CRC per annum respectively with an estimated 500,000 new cases of CRC annually worldwide[6]. The estimated cost to the National Health Service in the UK is £1 million/year/250,000 population [7].

Although improvements in peri-operative care, surgical procedures and healthcare provision for colorectal cancer in Western countries has improved, the prognosis for CRC remains poor with an average survival of 3-years following diagnosis, with approximately 50% of all patients diagnosed with CRC dyeing from their disease [8]. There is also evidence to suggest that the 5-year survival of CRC may be worse in the UK than other European countries [6, 9]. This reflects the fact that a large proportion of patients who present with CRC have advanced disease at initial investigations [7]. However, if malignancy can be detected at an earlier stage prognosis improves significantly, with reported 5-year survival rates for early CRC being in excess of 97% [10].

CRC is therefore a major health problem where early detection and treatment is essential to improve outcome. The strong relationship between stage and prognosis [11], coupled with the natural history of CRC [12-14] has provided a rationale for the introduction of population screening programmes [15-17]. This is now the subject of much international research and debate with trials now underway in the UK to establish the most cost effective modality, appropriate population target groups, patient acceptability, compliance, manpower and health economics [16, 18, 19].

Given the importance of early CRC detection [20] Japanese investigators have developed new technologies in the form of magnification colonoscopies [21]. When used in conjunction with colonic dye spray techniques (chromoscopy) [22, 23] magnification chromoscopy may permit earlier and more accurate diagnosis of CRC and its associated precursor lesions [21, 24-27]. This technology may also allow the *in vivo* prediction of histology [27-30] and depth of submucosal invasion [21, 31] while enhancing the safety and efficacy of colonoscopic luminal therapeutic techniques such as endoscopic mucosal resection (EMR) [32]. Such techniques are of importance when applied to the diagnosis and treatment of flat and depressed colorectal lesions, whose detection with conventional colonoscopy is inadequate

[20, 23, 26, 27, 33, 34]. Until recently such lesions were considered irrelevant to Western populations and thought to represent a phenomena unique to Japan termed 'phantom carcinoma' or 'Akitas' disease [20]. However, data from numerous Western groups now suggests that flat and depressed colorectal lesions account for more than 30% of all colorectal lesions where their malignant potential may be significantly higher than that of polypoid lesions [35-39]. Given these data, our approach to the secondary prevention of CRC is evolving, as is our understanding of the pathogenesis of colorectal cancer.

PATHOGENESIS OF COLORECTAL CANCER

Approximately 70% of colorectal cancers develop from sporadic adenomatous polyps where post-mortem studies have shown the incidence of sporadic adenomas to be 30-40% in Western populations [40, 41]. Recognised familial syndromes account for 5% of CRC [42, 43] with the most common being familial adenomatous polyposis (FAP) [44] and hereditary non-polyposis colon cancer (HNPCC) [45]. Clusters of CRC also occur in families more often than would be expected by chance alone. This group is known as the family cancer syndrome (FCS) [43].

The Adenoma Carcinoma Sequence

The adenoma carcinoma sequence as proposed by Morson in 1974 [13] constitutes the rationale for current endoscopic diagnostic and therapeutic interventions, namely polypectomy, to prevent eventual progression to CRC [46-48]. According to Morson's hypothesis, progressive dysplasia in adenomatous polyps occurs as they enlarge with progression to carcinoma in situ and ultimately invasive neoplasia when the submucosal and muscularis propria are infiltrated [13, 49]. Miller observed that the risk of developing CRC increases with age, with reported incidence rates of 19 per 100,000 and 337 per 100,000 in patients under the age of 65 years and those over 65 years of age respectively [50]. This data reflects the time course required for the adenoma carcinoma sequence to be completed [51]. Further confirmation of this hypothesis comes from Crohn and Rosenberg who first described the association between CRC and chronic ulcerative colitis (CUC) [52].

Although there are a large number of data supporting the validity of the adenoma-carcinoma sequence it has now been demonstrated that colonoscopic polypectomy of exophytic lesions results in a higher than expected incidence of colorectal cancer at follow-up [46, 47]. Winawer et al in the National Polyp Study reported on the 6-year surveillance of 1418 patients following repeated colonoscopy and polypectomy for a median of 5.9 years [47]. A reduction in CRC incidence when compared to 3 reference populations of 76-90% was demonstrated [47]. However, in this population there were 5 interval cancers [47]. The Veterans Affairs study of 32,702 patients found only 50% of cancers were prevented, but not all patients had received total colonoscopy [46].

Reasons for the inability of conventional colonoscopy and polypectomy to prevent subsequent CRC are numerous [53-55]. Endoscopic experience is an important issue [53, 56]. Indeed, both of the large polyps missed in Rex's 'back-to-back' colonoscopy study were by the least experienced endoscopists [56]. Other factors such as inadequate bowel preparation and prolonged, difficult intubation may result in inadequate mucosal views [20]. In addition, the morphology of polyps may influence miss rates [20, 57]. Many authors suggest that flat lesions can be difficult to detect using conventional colonoscopy alone and that chromoscopy is useful to improve detection [24, 34-36, 57-61]. Furthermore, traditional colonoscopic training and education has focused on the diagnosis of polypoid lesions with little emphasis given to flat and depressed types [60]. It is therefore plausible that a number of cancers may develop from flat lesions and include a *de novo* pathogenic group [62-65]. Such lesions can demonstrate only subtle changes endoscopically [62]. It is therefore plausible that the interval CRCs in both Winawer's [47] and Muller's [46] series may have derived from flat and depressed lesions which were not detected or if so inadequately treated.

The Flat Adenoma-Carcinoma Concept

Although up to two-thirds of CRCs are assumed to develop from the exophytic (sessile and pedunculated) adenoma-carcinoma sequence [66], data from Japanese [67] and recently Western groups [35-38, 68] suggest that the 'missing' one third of lesions may develop from morphologically distinct lesions that assume a flat or depressed appearance. Following the initial report of a flat depressed lesion by Kariya in 1977 [69], Kudo in a large series of 17,000 adenomas reported the prevalence of flat colorectal lesions to be 45% [67]. Muto's description of 33 such lesions describes the essential endoscopic features; a flat or slightly elevated lesion, usually less than 10 mm in diameter, sometimes associated with an area of central depression and often 'reddish' in colour [70]. Histologically, most flat adenomas have a tubular as opposed to villous architecture [71, 72].

The prevalence and clinicopathological characteristics of flat and depressed colorectal lesions in Western studies have shown much variability [22, 26, 34-37, 39, 73]. In part this is related to the variable definitions of endoscopic morphology used, differences in case mix and colonoscopic diagnostic techniques [32]. Hence, colorectal lesions which may be classed as flat non-polypoid lesions in Japan may be described as sessile in the West. This has been shown when the results of the National Polyp Survey were re-analysed [25]. Of the 703 lesions diagnosed that were originally described as sessile, 32% subsequently met the definition for diagnosis as flat [25]. Furthermore, variability in histological diagnostic criteria used by Western and Japanese pathologists make comparative studies difficult [74].

Several Western studies have now addressed the prevalence of flat and depressed colorectal lesions. Lanspa *et al* (USA) [73] demonstrated that 48% of all adenomas assumed a flat morphology with Smith *et al* (UK) [75] reporting 50% of early colorectal cancers assumed a flat or depressed appearance at colonoscopy. In contrast, Wolber *et al* (Canada) [39] and Saitoh (North America) [37] established lower prevalence rates of 8.6% and 22% respectively.

Two prospective UK based trials have now addressed the prevalence and clinicopathological characteristics of flat and depressed colorectal lesions [35, 36]. The Sheffield group reported a total of 458 flat lesions in a cohort of 850 patients of which 38% were hyperplastic and 62% adenomatous or beyond [35]. Twenty five percent of the flat adenomas had foci of high-grade dysplasia (HGD) with 82% of these lesions clustering in the right-hemi-colon [35]. Ten flat invasive adenocarcinomas were diagnosed of which 9 also were proximal to the hepatic flexure [35]. In contrast, HGD was evident in only 12% of protuberant (sessile / pedunculated) adenomas of which 95% were located in the left colon [35]. HGD was present in 17% of all sessile adenomas vs. 44% of flat lesions exceeding 8 mm in diameter [35]. These data confirmed the findings of the Leeds group where the prevalence of flat and depressed neoplastic lesions was 22% [36]. Depressed lesions and larger flat adenomas were similarly more likely to contain HGD with 54% of early carcinomas assuming a flat or depressed appearance [36]. Flat adenomas >10 mm in diameter were almost twice as likely as protuberant lesions of a similar size to have HGD or foci of invasive carcinoma [36].

The malignant potential of flat and depressed colorectal lesions is controversial. Adachi [72], Wolber [39] and Tada [76, 77] all suggest that the small flat adenoma has a malignant potential in excess of that expected by size. HGD has been reported in 40% of such lesions in Teixeira's series [78]. Western studies suggest that the incidence of HGD in flat lesions is not as common, with data from Sheffield and Leeds reporting HGD in 25% and 10% of flat adenomas respectively [35, 36]. Importantly, Saito *et al* found flat and depressed lesions contained invasive cancer more often than polypoid lesions (4.5% vs. 0%; p=0.04) where the average size of all flat and depressed lesions with HGD or invasive cancer were significantly smaller than that of polypoid advanced lesions (10.75+/-2.7 mm vs. 20+/- 2.9 mm; p<0.05 respectively) [37]. Furthermore, the stage of flat and depressed cancers was more advanced than their size (as compared to protuberant lesions) would suggest, with extension to the subserosa and local lymph node metastasis in two cases [37]. Significantly, the presence of HGD and carcinoma appears dependent on whether there is a depressed component within the lesion [33, 37, 67, 72, 79].

Invasive Potential and Risk of Metastasis in Flat and Depressed Colorectal Lesions

Many studies have reported an increased propensity of small, flat and depressed colorectal cancers for submucosal invasion [20]. Fourteen cases of advanced cancer in flat lesions less than 10 mm in diameter have now been reported, with the Sheffield group reporting a 1 mm depressed adenocarcinoma at stage T2 (invading the muscularis propria) [80]. Shimoda *et al* in a series of 32 'non-polypoid growth pattern carcinomas' (NPG-Ca) found intramucosal carcinoma in 10 lesions (31%) with a mean size of 5.1 mm [81]. The remaining 22 lesions (69%) demonstrated invasion to the level of the submucosal layer 3 with marked lymphatic and venous infiltration with a mean lesional diameter of 10.3 mm [81]. In comparison, only 35% of sessile and broad-based early polypoid carcinomas in this series invaded the submucosa with accompanying lower lympho-vascular invasion rates (32%) [81]. Tada's series of 15 flat rectal carcinomas showed 9 (60%) lesions had invaded the deep submucosal layer with 7 (47%) lesions demonstrating lympho-vascular involvement [77]. Furthermore, 2 lesions of 10 mm had metastasised to peri-rectal lymph nodes [77]. All lesions in this series were less than 20 mm in diameter [77]. Matsumoto *et al* also found flat tumours were smaller than polypoid cancers (median 9.5 mm vs. 14.5 mm) with submucosal invasion diagnosed more commonly in flat/depressed as compared to exophytic cancers (87.5% vs. 9.1%; $p=0.032$) [82]. The data of Iishi [33], Minamoto [83] and Kasumi [84] corroborate these findings.

In a similar manner to polypoid colorectal lesions, the risk of nodal metastasis in flat and depressed colorectal lesions is dependent on the depth of vertical submucosal invasion [85-87]. This fact explains why many authors have reported such detailed data. At the present time, the depth of submucosal invasion is the best clinical indicator or lympho-vascular and nodal metastatic disease [88] which ultimately determines stage and hence prognosis [23, 89]. For flat and depressed colorectal lesions the risk of nodal metastasis for lesions invading the submucosal layer 1-2 (2-400um; stage T1) is 2-3% as compared to 8-12% for those invading the submucosal layer 3 or beyond to the muscularis propria (4-600um; stage T2) [86, 87]. Nodal metastasis were found in 3 depressed type carcinomas found in the Sheffield study where invasion to the submucosal layer 2 had occurred [35], with Tada [77] and Minamoto [83] both reporting nodal disease in 2 and 3 flat lesions less than 10 mm in diameter respectively.

NON-ADENOMATOUS OR *DE NOVO* PATHOGENESIS

Neoplastic lesions, which have no concomitant adenomatous component, are described as *de novo* lesions [62]. Shimoda *et al* found intramucosal carcinoma without adenoma in 10 lesions that were morphologically flat with depression (average size 5.1 mm) [81]. They concluded that non-polypoid early colorectal carcinomas rapidly progressed to invasive, advanced carcinoma where *de novo* carcinoma accounted for 80% of all depressed type colorectal carcinomas [81]. Data from Wada *et al* also suggested that 70-80% of superficial type early colorectal cancers develop from a *de novo* carcinoma pathogenic sequence with only 20% from pre-existing adenomas [63]. Such lesions have now been reported in Western studies [64], corroborating the data of Japanese authors [62, 90].

The exact molecular mechanisms operative in depressed-type *de novo* colorectal cancers are poorly defined. Morita *et al* analysed the genetic alterations of K-*ras* and p53 expression in 81 flat/depressed lesions that are known to be operative in the adenoma-carcinoma sequence [91]. Additionally, the expression of COX-2 and Ki-67 index was measured as a marker of tissue proliferation [91]. No flat lesions with central depression were positive for the p53 protein with the proportion of specimens with K-*ras* codon 12 mutation being 13.4% in diminutive adenomas as compared to 8.6% in flat/depressed lesions ($p=0.073$) [91]. The median (interquartile range) of the Ki-67 index of the flat/depressed lesions also tended to be lower than that of polypoid lesions without depression (0.0 [0.0-5.9] vs. 4.5 [0.0-17.1]; $p=0.0281$) respectively [91]. Furthermore, COX-2 over-expression was observed in 15.6% of depressed lesions [91]. This data demonstrated low rates of the genetic alterations associated with malignant progression associated with the adenoma-carcinoma pathogenic sequence and hence suggests that a different neoplastic mechanism is operative for cancers showing *de novo* pathological characteristics [91]. Further studies are required to clarify this observation.

Definitions and Morphological Classification of Flat and Depressed Colorectal Lesions

As previously described, there is controversy regarding the endoscopic diagnosis between flat and sessile colorectal lesions. Clinically, flat colorectal lesions are defined as mucosal change with a flat or rounded surface combined with a height of less than half the diameter [70, 92]. In practice, most flat adenomas have a height of less than 2 mm [36]. Depression within a flat colorectal lesion is defined as a constant concavity whether air is insufflated or deflated [23]. Histologically, flat adenomas are defined as lesions with a height, as measured from the muscularis mucosa to the apex of the lesions, of less than twice the height of the adjacent mucosa [70].

At present no standardised endoscopic reporting criteria for flat colorectal lesions exists in Western practice. However, the Japanese Research Society for Cancer of the Colon and Rectum (JRSC) has provided a detailed macroscopic classification system derived from that used for gastric neoplasia [93, 94]. Lesion morphology is divided into exophytic (class I) or flat (class II) [93, 94]. By using a sub-classification of each morphological group, a detailed, standardised and reproducible method of reporting endoscopic morphology is achievable (see table 1) [24]. This has major implications to ongoing endoscopic research, where standardisation in both morphological and histopathological reporting is required between Western and Japanese groups.

Table 1. The Japanese Research Society Classification for colorectal lesions.

Endoscopic appearance	JRSC class		Description
Protruded lesions	Ip	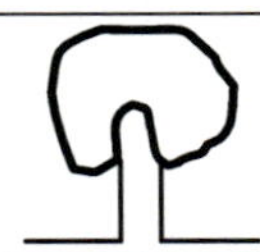	Pedunculated polps
	Ips	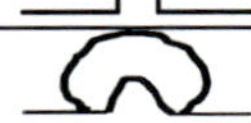	Subpedunculated polyps
	Is	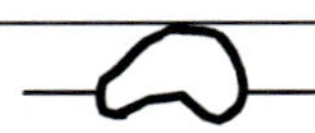	Sessile polyps
Flat elevated lesions	IIa	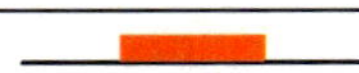	Flat elevation of mucosa
	IIa / IIc	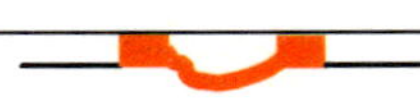	Flat elevation with central depression
Flat lesions	IIb	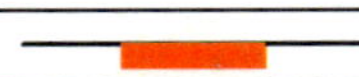	Flat mucosal change
	IIc	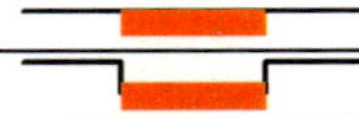	Mucosal depression
	IIc / IIa	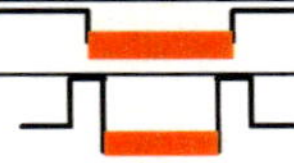	Mucosal depression with raised edge

Histopathological Classification

Translation of the Japanese pathological and molecular experience to Western practice has been difficult due to disparity in reporting and classification, a problem that mirrors that of endoscopic practice [74]. Schlemper *et al* assessed differences in the diagnostic criteria used by Japanese and Western pathologists to diagnose colorectal carcinoma [95]. Within this study, 8 expert pathologists from Japan (4), North America (2) and Europe (2) individually reviewed microscopic slides of 20 colorectal lesions from Japanese patients who had undergone EMR or surgery when early stage CRC or adenoma was clinically suspected [95]. In 11 cases where the Western pathologist diagnosed adenoma with low-grade dysplasia (LGD), the Japanese diagnosed definite carcinoma with or without adenoma in 4 cases, adenoma in 5 and were equally divided between a diagnosis of adenoma and carcinoma in 2 cases [95]. For 5 cases reported as adenoma with HGD by Western pathologists, the Japanese diagnosed definite carcinoma with adenoma in 3 cases, adenoma in 1 and again were equally divided between a diagnosis of adenoma and carcinoma in a further case [95]. For one case in which the Western pathologists were equally divided between a diagnosis of carcinoma and adenoma with HGD, all Japanese pathologists diagnosed definitive carcinoma with or without adenoma [95]. Furthermore, the presence of invasion was the most important diagnostic criterion of colorectal cancer for Western pathologists, with the Japanese favouring nuclear features and glandular structures [95]. Hence, in Japan colorectal carcinoma may be diagnosed on the basis of nuclear and structural criteria, even in cases considered by Western pathologists to be non-invasive lesions with LGD [95]. Therefore, this important study showed that this diagnostic practice might contribute to the high incidence of early stage colorectal carcinoma reported in early Japanese series.

Given these data, the Vienna criteria were proposed to bridge the East-West discrepancies in histopathological reporting, based on clinically meaningful categories from which patient management options could be focused [96]. Using the Vienna system, which includes LGD and HGD categories in addition to invasive carcinoma as a specific subset separate from HGD, marked improved levels of agreement between Japanese and Western pathologists have been achieved, while affording a system that clinicians can use to rationalise therapeutic options and compare outcome data between the two cultures [96]. The Sheffield study examining the prevalence and clinicopathological characteristics of flat and depressed colorectal lesions in the UK [35] was the first study to use both standardised Vienna histopathological criteria [96] combined with the JRSC endoscopic classification system [93, 94].

New Techniques for the Colonoscopic Detection of Flat Colorectal Lesions

Using chromoscopic colonoscopic techniques to aid the detection of flat colorectal lesions, an increasing proportion of colorectal cancers are being diagnosed at an early stage in Japan with similar results in the UK [97]. In 2001, 18% or colorectal cancers detected at the National Cancer Centre Tokyo were staged at T1 (confined to the mucosa or submucosa) at index diagnosis [97]. A similar trend has now been shown in both Leeds and Sheffield [35, 36].

High-Magnification Colonoscopy: The Optical Biopsy Hypothesis

In 1993, the Olympus 200Z series colonoscope was introduced which permitted *in vivo* magnification of up to 100x normal. Using high-magnification colonoscopy and colonic chromoscopy it is therefore possible to examine the colonic pit or crypt patterns previously described using *ex vivo* stereomicroscopy [21]. Kudo has proposed a clinical classification system for the *in vivo* pit pattern classification using HMCC (see table 2) [21]. The premise of this technology is to provide an *in vivo* optical biopsy that can be used at the time of colonoscopy to enhance diagnostic precision and help guide subsequent therapeutic strategies [21, 27, 32, 98]. Such strategies are highly dependent on the detailed morphological appearance and pit pattern in flat and depressed colorectal lesions, where early submucosal invasion, lympho-vascular invasion and nodal metastatic disease can occur even when the lesion is small [70] (figure 1 a-e).

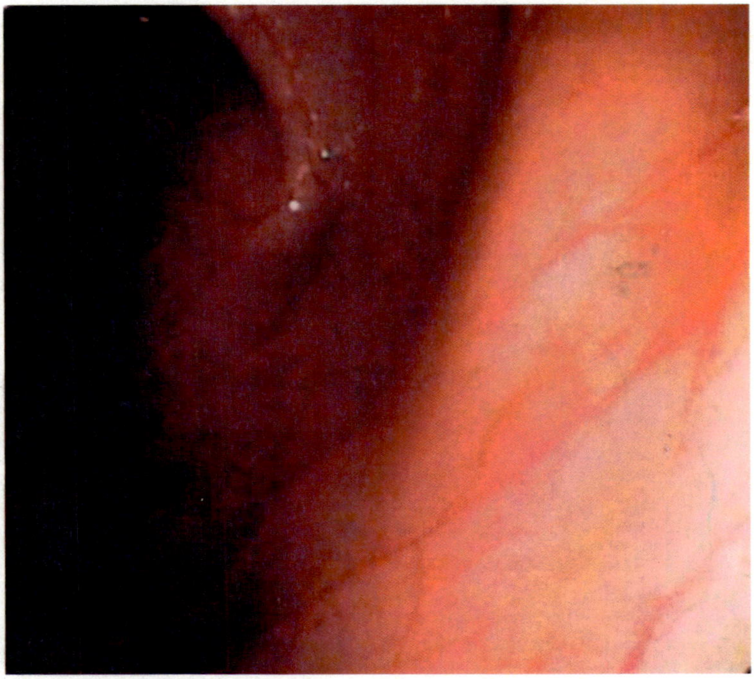

Figure 1a. Subtle erythema and vascular net loss implies the presence of a lesion

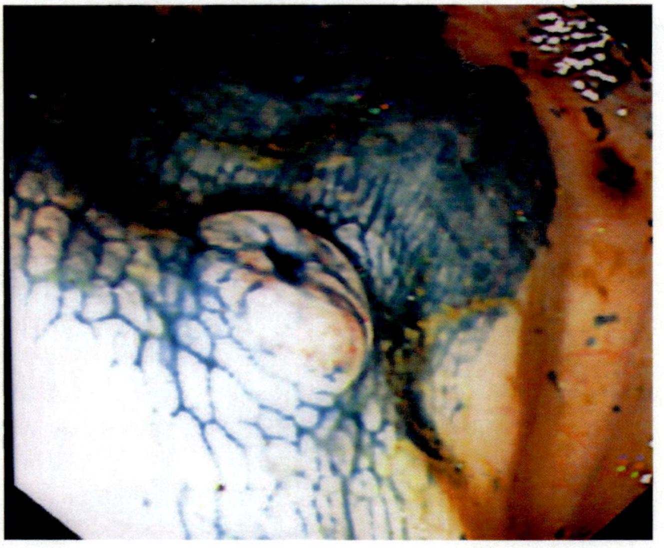

Figure 1b. Indigo carmine chromoscopy 0.5% clearly delineates the margin of the lesion. This is a JRSC class IIa/c (flat with central depression).

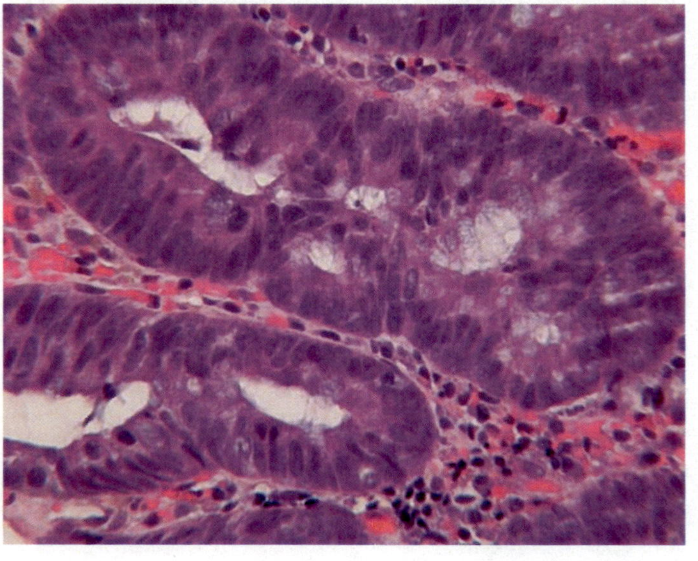

Figure 1c. Haematoxylin and eosin-stained section of an area of high grade dysplasia in an adenomatous polyp. There is an abnormal architecture with internal 'bridging' of epithelial cells in crypt lumina to produce 'back to back' glands. There is extensive stratification of epithelial cell nuclei, with many mitotic figures in cells which are not in contact with the basement membrane. There is also hyperchromatism and pleomorphism of the epithelial cell nuclei.

Table 2. The modified Kudo criteria for colorectal pit pattern classification

PIT TYPE	CHARACTERISTICS	APPEARANCE USING HMCC	PIT SIZE (mm)
I	Normal round pits	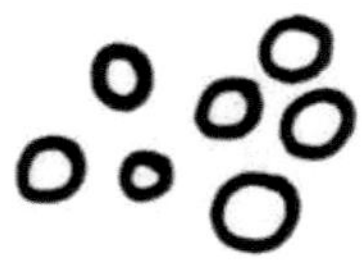	0.07+/- 0.02mm
II	Stella or papillary		0.09 +/- 0.02mm
IIIs	Tubular / round pits Smaller than pit type I	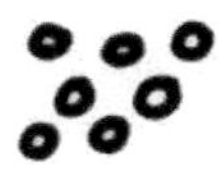	0.03 +/- 0.01mm
IIIL	Tubular / large	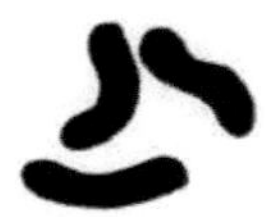	0.22+/- 0.09mm
IV	Sulcus / gyrus	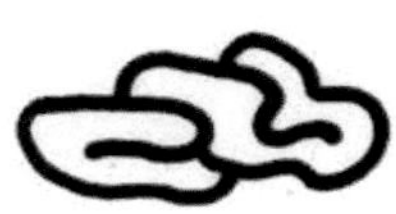	0.93 +/- 0.32mm
V(a)	Irregular arrangement and sizes of IIIL, IIIs, IV type pit	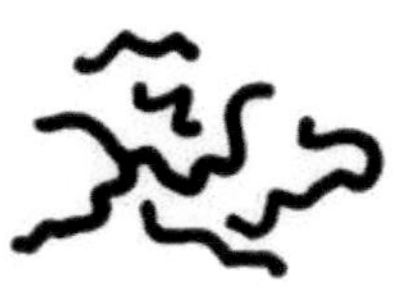	N/A
V(n)	Non discernable		N/A

Kato's retrospective review of 4445 patients undergoing HMCC examined 3438 lesions (classified according to modified Kudo criteria) and compared them to either endoscopic or surgically resected specimens [27]. Diagnostic accuracy rates in this series for non-neoplastic lesions, adenomas and invasive carcinomas were 75%, 94% and 85% respectively [27]. However, despite the large numbers of lesions examined translation to Western practice was complicated by an adapted Vienna criterion for histopathological classification, which failed to differentiate the grade of dysplastic change in lesions examined [27].

Only two prospective studies have addressed the efficacy of HMCC at differentiating neoplastic from non-neoplastic colorectal lesions [28, 29]. Tung's group showed a sensitivity and specificity for the differentiation of neoplastic and non-neoplastic lesions of 93.8% and 64.6% respectively [28]. Furthermore, 6 neoplastic lesions in this small cohort of 175 lesions were miss-classified [28, 99]. Togashi *et al* in the second prospective analysis showed improved sensitivity (92%) and specificity (73%) for the differentiation of neoplastic from non-neoplastic lesions using HMCC (see figure 2 a-d), with both groups concluding that inadequate operator experience may be responsible for low overall specificity rates [29].

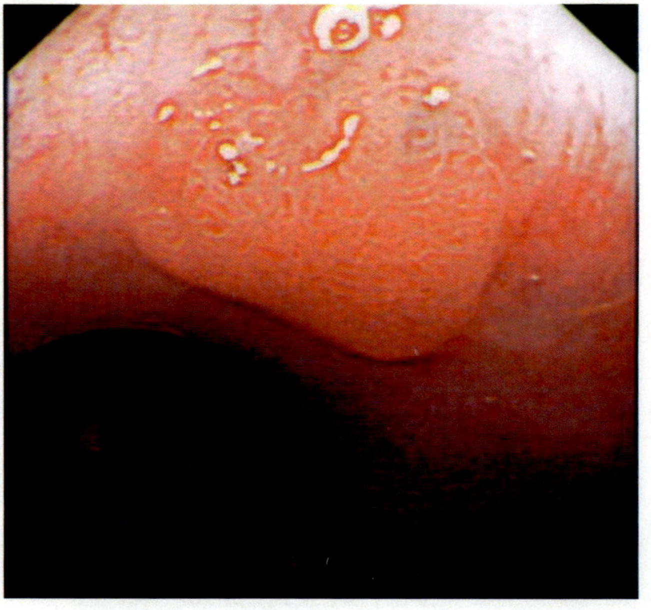

Figure 2a. A flat JRSC class IIa lesion of the distal ascending colon.

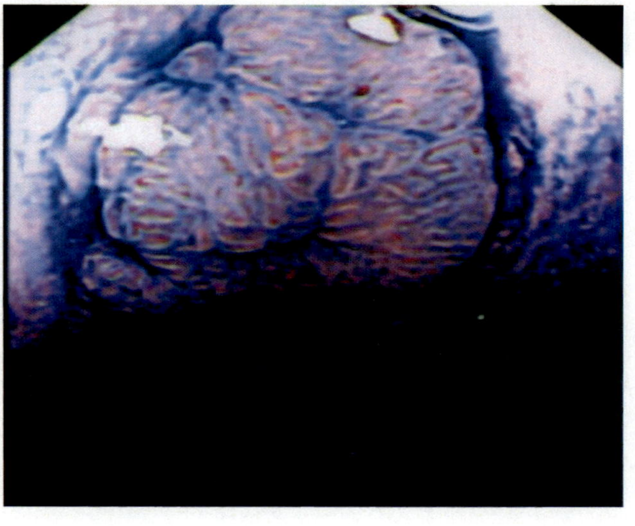

Figure 2b. Indigo carmine 0.5% chromoscopy shows the margin contour clearly with no evidence of a depressed component.

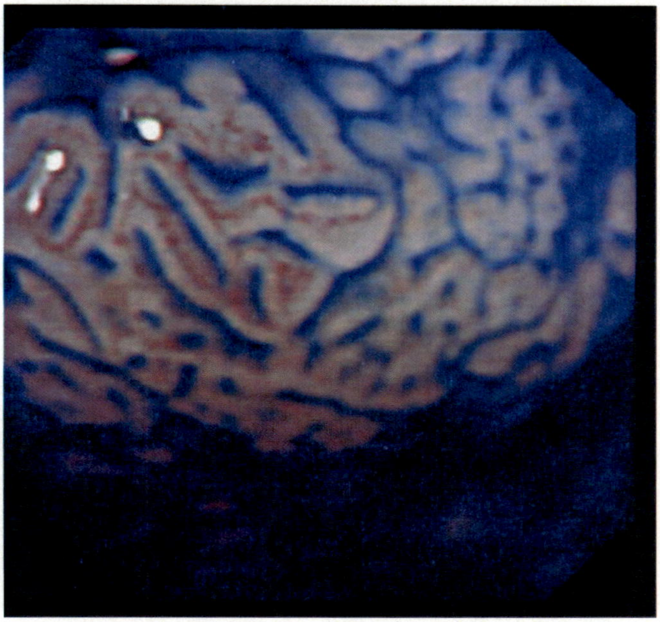

Figure 2c. High-magnification views (x100). The surface pit pattern is a Kudo type IIIL.

Further large prospective studies are required to assess the accuracy of HMCC as an optical biopsy tool. At the present time, it is not 100% sensitive or specific and although a helpful diagnostic tool *in vivo* is not a replacement for histopathology [20]. However, the technology represents a significant advance in colonoscopic practice as it may improve diagnostic yield of significant lesions while lowering the burden of insignificant biopsies interpreted by pathologists. Further studies are underway in the UK assessing a further novel application of HMCC for the *in vivo* assessment of resection completeness post EMR [100]. All these features are useful tools to the endoscopists given the imminent introduction of a nationwide CRC screening programme in the UK [17].

In Vivo Staging of Colorectal Lesions Using Magnification-Chromoscopy

As previously described, flat focal submucosal invasive CRCs which are limited to the submucosal layer 1 (i.e. stage T1), can be managed by EMR as the risk of lympho-venous invasion and nodal metastasis is rarev [101-103]. For lesions with deeper vertical invasion into the submucosal layer 3 or beyond (stage T2) the risk of nodal disease increases to 10-15% [104]. EMR in this group is therefore undesirable due to a higher risk of perforation, non-curative excision and untreated nodal disease [105]. Surgical excision is recommended is this group [97, 105].

Chromoscopic colonoscopy used as an *in vivo* staging tool has been reported by Saitoh *et al* [31]. In this retrospective analysis of depressed type early CRCs, combined videoendoscopy and chromoscopy was used to characterise the essential endoscopic features favoured by lesions with submucosal layer 1 and 2 invasion, which at the time of endoscopy may be used as a tool to guide the colonoscopists management (i.e. attempted EMR or biopsy alone with surgical referral) [31]. Using Saitoh's criteria (expansion appearance, present; surface depression, deep; irregularity of depressed surface, uneven; and converging folds toward the tumour) the sensitivity and specificity for determining submucosal layer 2 disease was 90% [31]. However, when 21 lesions showing intramucosal carcinoma were excluded from the analysis, specificity rates fell to 70% [31]. In the clinical context such results imply a trend to over-stage lesions, which may deprive some patients the opportunity of curative local excision with EMR. Similar problems have been encountered using the 7.5Mhz ultrasound probe in the staging of rectal carcinoma, with variable accuracy rates reported from 60-79% according to the T stage system [106, 107]. The introduction of high-frequency 'mini probe' ultrasound has now been reported by one group to have a high overall accuracy (88%) when used to determine submucosal invasion for flat and depressed lesions [108]. Again, more prospective studies are required to validate this initial data and to clarify the optimal tool used for the staging of such lesions. Ultrasound imaging requires further training, has significant expense and may prolong the procedure. Chromoscopic colonoscopy with high-magnification would therefore be a useful tool to the endoscopist should further data validate its efficacy for *in vivo* staging.

The Detection of Flat and Diminutive Colorectal Lesions Using Chromoscopic Colonoscopy

Chromoscopic colonoscopy may improve the detection of diminutive (<5 mm) and flat colorectal lesions by highlighting subtle changes in mucosal architecture [57, 59, 61, 109]. Such changes include loss of vascular nett pattern, focal pallor, fold convergence and marginal irregularity [23]. Many authors advocate 'selective' chromoscopy upon the detection of such subtle mucosal signs using conventional colonoscopy [35, 36, 38]. This involves a localised application of 2-5 ml of indigo carmine (IC) 0.5% sprayed onto the lesion via the side port of the colonoscope (chromoscopic techniques are discussed in the following section) [28]. Other groups have advocated total colonic mucosal chromoscopy using a 'through-the-scope' diffusion catheter [57]. Studies addressing the efficacy of IC capsules taken prior to colonic lavage have also been described [109]. Brooker *et al* conducted the only randomised control trial of pan-mucosal chromoscopy using a colonic diffusion spray catheter for the detection of sporadic neoplastic lesions of the colorectum [57]. Both studies from Mitooka [61] and Brooker [57] showed a significant increase in the detection of diminutive neoplastic lesions in the right colon. In the latter study extubation time was uncontrolled with no control volume of normal saline used in the conventional colonoscopy group (controls) to remove the potential bias of the effect of lavage [57]. Furthermore, extubation times in the chromoscopy group were twice that of the conventional colonoscopy group [57]. However, 3% of diminutive lesions in Brooker's cohort showed moderate dysplastic histology with 2% having a villous component [57]. Despite their small size (< 5 mm) such lesions are of clinical significance with a high risk of progression to carcinoma [48]. Significantly more diminutive adenomas were found proximal to the sigmoid colon in the chromoscopy group as compared to controls, which is consistent with reports of higher miss-rates for diminutive lesions proximal to the sigmoid colon as well as supporting the observations of other groups describing a 'shift' in adenoma distribution toward the right colon at follow-up colonoscopy [110, 111]. Chromoscopy also identified more patients with multiple (> 3) adenomas, which is a group at increased risk for advanced neoplasia during follow-up [48, 112]. However, at present it remains unclear whether the advantages of pan-colonic chromoscopy are resultant from the technique or a reflection of the endoscopic withdrawal time. Further randomised control trials are required to clarify this issue.

In addition to the detection of sporadic neoplastic lesions of the colorectum, chromoscopic colonoscopy has now been described for the detection of intraepithelial neoplasia (IN) in chronic ulcerative colitis (CUC) [113]. This group is at high risk of CRC with current incidence rates reported between 7-30% [114-116]. CRC complicating ulcerative colitis accounts for 33% of colitis related deaths [114], which forms the rational for CRC surveillance in patients with longstanding colitis.

As intraepithelial neoplasia and colitis-associated cancer can occur in macroscopically normal mucosa [117, 118], random biopsies at 10 cm interval throughout the colorectum are currently recommended during screening colonoscopy [114]. The probability for detection of neoplastic change also correlates with the numbers of biopsies taken [119]. Recent data suggests that pan-chromoscopy using methylene-blue can improve the detection of flat and diminutive lesions in CUC when compared to conventional colonoscopic screening protocols alone [113]. Kiesslich et al showed that chromoscopy permitted a more accurate diagnosis of extent and inflammatory activity in CUC but also enhanced the detection of IN and CRC in colitis ($p=0.0002$ and $p=0.003$) respectively [113].

Hurlstone *et al* have now validated this data using a selective IC chromoscopic technique [120]. In this series of CUC screening, chromoscopic colonoscopy significantly improved the detection of IN and flat colorectal lesions as compared to conventional colonoscopic screening protocols ($p<0.001$) [120]. In this series chromoscopy increased the diagnostic yield of IN by 4-fold [120]. Furthermore, differentiation of neoplastic from non-neoplastic mucosal change was possible with a high sensitivity, specificity and overall accuracy (96%) [120]. This data suggests that chromoscopic colonoscopy is a valid tool for the detection and *in vivo* classification of IN in CUC [120].

CHROMOSCOPIC TECHNIQUES

Contrast dyes are used commonly in colonic chromoscopy [20]. IC is a non-toxic and inexpensive agent, normally used at a concentration of 0.5% [20]. However, concentrations of IC used vary, ranging from 0.2-2% [20]. The method of delivery is usually to draw up 3-5 mls of solution in a 20 ml syringe along with 20 ml of air. The syringe is then pushed through the biopsy channel along with the air to create a spray effect on the colonic wall [20, 24, 121]. Meticulous mucosal cleaning prior to chromoscopy is essential, as faecal fluid and debris can distort the chromoscopic effect [99]. Following aspiration of any excess dye, the contours of abnormal mucosa become clearly delineated.

An alternative to the syringe push technique, which is used to delineate a single discrete lesion after initial identification of subtle mucosal changes such as fold convergence, erythema or loss of vascular net pattern, is the chromoscopy diffusion catheter [57]. The catheter is placed through the biopsy channel, which has a sprinkler device at the proximal end. A syringe of IC can then be pushed through the catheter. This allows diffuse mucosal coverage using only a relative small volume of dye and is used when numerous lesions are anticipated (i.e. suspected attenuated familial adenomatous polyposis). Studies using IC capsules taken orally with bowel preparation have proved unhelpful due to proximal colonic dye loading and minimal left-hemi-colonic coverage [61, 109].

Selective Chromoscopic Techniques

IC is used to initially delineate lesion contour and morphology. Enhanced views of a lesion's pit pattern using high-magnification, in particular those present in neoplastic invasive disease, requires a second line reactive dye such as crystal violet (CV) [21, 99]. Although there are no known case reports from the Japanese literature describing adverse reactions when CV is used in the setting of colonoscopy, *in vitro* and animal studies suggest possible long-term toxicity [122]. Therefore, it should be used selectively for the identification of invasive pit patterns (Kudo type V) at subsequent magnification imaging. Prior to CV chromoscopy the lesion should first be prepared with a proteinase solution (N-acetyl-cysteine 2 mg/ml) to remove adherent mucous with small drops applied using a steel tipped non-traumatic catheter (Olympus Keymed UK 2.45mm PW5V-1) [123]. A 'fixing' phase of between 2-3 minutes should then be observed followed by a final saline mucosal wash prior to high-magnification views being obtained [105].

Often subtle endoscopic signs such as mucosal erythema, paleness, haemorrhagic spots, absence of vascular network pattern, unevenness or mucosal deformity initially detect flat, depressed and superficial elevated type colorectal lesions [71, 72, 88, 124]. It is following detection of such mucosal abnormalities in any patient group that magnification-chromoscopy becomes a useful tool. Qualitative diagnosis of early cancer is often reflected by endoscopic features of marginal irregularity, 'star-shaped' depression, air induced deformation (under altered air volume) and the absence of inominate grooves [24]. Such endoscopic abnormalities should prompt localised dye spraying or chromoscopy to aid visualisation of the lesion [109]. Subsequent magnifying views can then determine abnormal pit pattern structure; particularly pit types IIIs and V (Vn), which may signify overt neoplastic change with deep invasive mucosal characteristics [21, 28].

Colonoscopic Resection Techniques-Endoscopic Mucosal Resection

Following the initial description of EMR or the 'strip biopsy technique' by Dehyle *et al* [125], EMR has been developed by Japanese endoscopists for the resection of sessile and flat lesions of the stomach, oesophagus and colorectum [126]. For pedunculated lesions this technique is not required, as simple snare resection is adequate. EMR permits the resection of flat and sessile lesions by longitudinal section through the submucosal layer [105]. In the colorectum, EMR may provide curative resection for flat and sessile adenomas in addition to early colorectal cancer [105]. EMR facilitates complete histological analysis of the resected lesion and makes it possible to determine precisely the completeness of excision in both the horizontal and vertical resection planes [127]. Such a technique is preferable to primary tissue ablative techniques such as argon plasma coagulation [128] and electrocoagulation [25]. Numerous EMR techniques have now been described using transparent caps fitted to the proximal aspect of the endoscope [129] and that using an insulation tipped cutting knife [97]. With the exception of submucosal posterior rectal tumours, these techniques are reserved for oesophageal and gastric resection with the strip biopsy technique used routinely in the colorectum [126].

The technique of EMR comprises 4 stages:

1. Diagnosis and localisation of the lesion.
2. Evaluation of invasive depth to exclude lesions invading the deep submucosal layer 3 or beyond (i.e. T2 disease) using HMCC or ultrasound techniques.
3. Excision procedure.
4. Post resection evaluation.

Initial diagnosis and location of flat and sessile lesion of the colorectum is facilitated by the use of IC and allows the observation of detailed morphology [23]. *In vivo* staging of identified lesions can then be achieved using high-magnification [21] or ultrasound techniques as previously described [130]. Flat and sessile lesions up to 20 mm in diameter can be resected by *en block* or by 'single pass' resection with larger lesions requiring a piecemeal approach [127]. A needle catheter is then inserted through the side port of the colonoscope with sterile saline injected around the lesion and surrounding mucosa. A cleavage of the submucosa (having the effect of raising the lesion) then permits simple snare resection. A single cannulation can be used for small lesions (< 10 mm) diameter with multiple cannulation usually required for lesions of 20 mm or larger [127]. Some authors advocate the use of Adrenaline (1/100,000) mixed with saline or the use of twice-normal saline at submucosal injection [131]. However, there are no randomised controlled trials proving superiority with regard to resection clearance, post EMR haemorrhage or perforation. Whatever injection medium used it is essential to maintain a sufficient mucosal lift or detachment throughout the EMR, which minimised the risk of muscularis mucosa entrapment and subsequent perforation [126].

The Sheffield group advocate peripheral margin tattoos prior to saline submucosal injection that delineates the normal mucosal boundaries around the lesion prior to snaring [132]. This is a helpful technique, as at submucosal lift, the lesion can become distorted and indistinct from the surrounding normal mucosa [132]. If the lesion fails to lift (the non-lifting sign of Uno) or has an asymmetrical appearance then the resection should be abandoned as this indicates tethering to the underlying muscularis mucosa [133]. Perforation and risk of non-curative resection can occur in this scenario [24, 133].

Following successful submucosal lift, a spiked or 'barbed' snare is applied over the lesion and slowly closed under gentle suction [126]. This permits the lesion to be retained within the snare boundaries before final resection [126]. Prior to final cutting (usually using a 25W coagulation current) the snare should be relaxed slightly to allow any entrapped muscularis mucosa to retract [126]. Following resection, the lesion is retrieved using a pronged grasping forcep, followed by immediate fixation in 10% Formalin solution. Japanese endoscopists ‘pin out’ the lesion onto a solid cork or polystyrene plate prior to fixation that limits shrinkage of the resection specimen and permits easier and more accurate histopathological sectioning [97].

Following resection, it is important to re-evaluate the cut margin of the mucosa and if necessary use IC chromoscopy to delineate any remnant or unsuccessfully resected tissue [32]. An extended EMR can therefore be performed at the same treatment session that limits the risk of recurrent disease at the resection site [32]. Should a further EMR be unsuccessful APC of any remnant tissue, including application to the entire circumference of the cut margin should be applied [128]. All lesions should have an adjacent submucosal tattoo applied using Indian ink to facilitate localisation at follow-up colonoscopy [134].

The main complications of EMR are haemorrhage, perforation and stenosis [134, 135]. The immediate and early complications (10% of cases) described in the first 12 hours post resection are principally haemorrhage and rarely perforation [135]. The Sheffield group reported bleeding complications in only 2% of patients undergoing EMR in their cohort of 599 lesions [32], which was significantly lower than that reported in Ahmed’s retrospective analysis (22%) [136]. However, other Japanese authors have reported haemorrhage rates post colonic EMR of 1.16% (10/863) [137]. comparable to that observed in the Sheffield series [32]. Okamoto’s review of interventional colonoscopic resections also reports a perforation rate secondary to EMR of only 0.35% [135] with Kaneko’s multi-centre analysis of endoscopic mortality showing rates of less than 0.0001% for this procedure [138]. EMR may therefore be a safe and effective endoscopic therapy that may enhance our current strategies aimed at the secondary prevention of colorectal cancer.

Evolving Technology for the Future-Autoflurescence Colonoscopy

Chromoscopic and high-magnification techniques have been introduced in an attempt to improve the sensitivity and specificity of ‘white-light’ colonoscopy. However, a new endoscopic technology that is fluorescence-based is under evaluation by many groups [139, 140]. This technology exploits either the ‘autofluorescence’ of naturally occurring molecules such as collagen, NAD-H, flavins and porphyrins or fluorescence caused by exogenously administered fluorescent drugs.

The detection of neoplastic lesions using autoflurescence depends on subtle changes in the concentration or distribution in depth of endogenous fluorophores, changes in tissue micro-architecture and altered mucosal thickness or blood concentrations [141]. All these factors affect the fluorescence intensity or spectrum due to wavelength-specific light absorption [141]. Using exogenous fluorophores, the detection of lesions is based on selective drug uptake or target tissue retention relative to uptake by normal tissue [141].

Kapadia *et al* using ultraviolet (UV) light in the colon were able to discriminate normal mucosa, adenomas and hyperplastic lesions with accuracies of 100%, 100% and 94% respectively [140]. In the first *in vivo* human colonic spectroscopic study by Cothren *et al*, differentiation between adenoma and non-adenomatous lesions was achieved in 97% of cases

[142]. Cotheran *et al* in the first blinded study also identified colonic dysplasia with 90% sensitivity and 95% specificity [143].

However, the clinical potential of spectroscopy in routine endoscopic practice has not yet been clarified. Chwirot *et al* performed multi-spectral autoflurescence imaging in the colon of polyps *ex vivo* [144], with Wang recently describing a prototype fluorescence imaging system applied *ex vivo* to detect and localise adenomas in colectomy specimens from patients with FAP [145]. A second generation fluorescence imaging system was described by Wang in 1999 for the *in vivo* detection of colorectal adenomas in which UV light was transmitted through a fibre-optic bundle inserted through the side port of the endoscope [146]. A videocolonoscope was then used to capture the fluorescence light within the wavelength band 400-700 nm [146]. False-colour images were then overlaid onto the conventional white-light images, displaying regions where the fluorescence intensity exceeded threshold values relative to a moving image [146]. In this study of 30 patients, 18 lesions visible with white-light imaging were examined where all 6 hyperplastic lesions were correctly identified with sensitivity for dysplasia reported as 83% [146]. However, despite these encouraging initial data, further studies are required before such technology can be implemented to routine endoscopic clinical practice.

CONCLUSIONS

The data presented in this chapter has shown that emerging concepts in endoscopic detection and therapeutic techniques, initially pioneered by the Japanese are applicable to Western practice. We have demonstrated the apparent clinicopathological significance of diminutive and flat colorectal lesions and explored the safety and efficacy of EMR. We hope that chromoscopic colonoscopy and magnification imaging in addition to EMR will now be more widely practiced by both surgical and medical gastroenterologists. However, while differences remain between Japanese and Western classification systems it is difficult to extrapolate endoscopic and pathological data reported in Japanese studies to our practice. Furthermore, additional studies are required to clarify the role of chromoscopic colonoscopy and magnification imaging in routine clinical practice. Finally, all practitioners require further education and training, if new diagnostic techniques and therapeutic procedures are going to be adopted.

AUTHOR NOTES

No conflicts of interest declared.

Grant Support

The Smith and Nephew Research Foundation (UK). BRET Research Foundation (UK). Butterfield 'Sasakawa' Research Foundation (UK). Mason Medical Research Foundation (UK). Keymed (UK).

REFERENCES

[1] HMSO. Office of Population Censuses and Surveys. *Cancer statistics.* Registration 1989. Series MBI; No 22. London 1994.

[2] Sharp LS, Black RJ, Harkness EF, Finlayson A, Muir CS. *Cancer registration statistics. Scotland 1981-90.* Edinburgh: Information and Statistics Division. 1995.

[3] NHS Centre for Reviews and Dissemination, York. Effective Health Care: The management of colorectal cancer. *Financial Times Healthcare* 1997;3:1-12.

[4] American Cancer Society. *Cancer Facts and Figures.* American Cancer Society 1995.

[5] Anonymous. *Registration of cases of diagnosed cancer registered in England and Wales 1986.* Office of Population Censuses and Surveys. Cancer Statistics. 1986.

[6] World Health Organisation International Agency for Research on Cancer, European Commission. *Survival of cancer patients in Europe: the Eurocare study.* Lyons: International Agency for Research on Cancer Scientific Publications.

[7] Mountney L, Sanderson H, Harris J. Colorectal cancer. In: Stevens A, Raftery J, eds. *Health care needs assessment.* Oxford: Radcliffe. Chapter 7. 1994.

[8] Parkin DM, Muir CS, Whelan SL, Gao YT, Ferlay J, Powell J. *Cancer Incidence in Five Continents.* Lyons: International Agency for Research on Cancer. 1992;4.

[9] Peipins LA, Sandler RS. Epidemiology of colorectal adenomas. *Epidemiology Reviews* 1994;16:273-297.

[10] Moreaux J, Catala M. Carcinoma of the colon: long-term survival and prognosis after surgical treatment in a series of 798 patients. *World J Surg* 1987;11:804-809.

[11] NHS-executive. *Guidance on Commisioning Cancer Services. Improving Outcomes in Colorectal Cancer.* Wetherby - UK. NHS Executive 1997.

[12] Morson BC. Precancerous and early malignant lesions of the large intestine. *Br J Surg* 1968;55:725-731.

[13] Morson BC. Evolution of cancer of the colon and rectum. *Cancer* 1974;34:suppl:845-849.

[14] Muto T, Nagawa H, Watanabe T, Masaki T, Sawada T. Colorectal carcinogenesis: historical review. *Dis Colon Rectum* 1997;40:S80-85.

[15] Byers T, Levin B, Rothenberger D, Dodd GD, Smith RA. American Cancer Society guidelines for screening and surveillance for early detection of colorectal polyps and cancer: update 1997. *CA Cancer J Clin* 1997;47:154-160.

[16] Atkin WS. Implementing screening for colorectal cancer. *BMJ* 1999;319:1212-1213.

[17] Joint Position Statement by the British Society of Gastroenterology, The Royal College of Physicians and the Association of Coloproctology of Great Britain and Ireland. Colorectal cancer screening in the UK. *Gut* 2000;46:746-748.

[18] Atkin WS, Hart AR, Edwards R. Uptake, yield of neoplasia, and adverse effects of flexible sigmoidoscopy screening. *Gut* 1998;42:560-565.

[19] Atkin WS, Cuzick J, Northover JMA, Whynes DK. Prevention of colorectal cancer by once-only sigmoidoscopy. *Lancet* 1993;341:736-740.

[20] Hurlstone DP, Fujii T, Lobo AJ. Early detection of colorectal cancer using high-magnification chromoscopic colonoscopy. *Br J Surg* 2002;89:272-282.

[21] Kudo S, Rubio CA, Teixeira CR, Kashida H, Kogure E. Pit pattern in colorectal neoplasia: endoscopic magnifying view. *Endoscopy* 2001;33:367-373.

[22] Jaramillo E, Watanabe M, Slezak P, Rubio C. Flat neoplastic lesions of the colon and rectum detected by high-resolution video endoscopy and chromoscopy. *Gastrointest Endosc* 1995;42:114-122.

[23] Kudo S, Kashida H, Tamura T, Kogure E, Imai Y, Yamano H, Hart AR. Colonoscopic diagnosis and management of nonpolypoid early colorectal cancer. *World J Surg* 2000;24:1081-1090.

[24] Kudo S, Kashida H, Nakajima T, Tamura S, Nakajo K. Endoscopic diagnosis and treatment of early colorectal cancer. *World J Surg* 1997;21:694-701.

[25] Lambert R, Provenzale D, Ectors N, Vainio H, Dixon MF, Atkin WS, Werner M, Franceshi S, Watanabe H, Tytgat GN, Axon AT, Neuhaus H. Early diagnosis and prevention of sporadic colorectal cancer. *Endoscopy* 2001;33:1042-1064.

[26] Kiesslich R, Jung M. Magnification endoscopy: does it improve mucosal surface analysis for the diagnosis of gastrointestinal neoplasias? *Endoscopy* 2002;34:819-822.

[27] Kato S, Fujii T, Koba I, Sano Y, Fu KI, Parra-Blanco A, Tajiri H, Yoshida S, Rembacken B. Assessment of colorectal lesions using magnifying colonoscopy and mucosal dye spraying: can significant lesions be distinguished? *Endoscopy* 2001;33:306-310.

[28] Tung SY, Wu CS, Su MY. Magnifying colonoscopy in differentiating neoplastic from nonneoplastic colorectal lesions. *Am J Gastroenterol* 2001;96:2628-2632.

[29] Togashi K, Konishi F, Ishizuka T, Sato T, Senba S, Kanazawa K. Efficacy of magnifying endoscopy in the differential diagnosis of neoplastic and non-neoplastic polyps of the large bowel. *Dis Colon Rectum* 1999;42:1602-1608.

[30] Fujii T, Nagata K, Saito Y. The correspondence of magnifying endoscopic diagnosis and pathological diagnosis. *Stomach and Intestine* 1999;34:1653-1664.

[31] Saitoh Y, Obara T, Watari J, Nomura M, Taruishi M, Orii Y, Taniguchi M, Ayabe T, Ashida T, Kohgo Y. Invasion depth diagnosis of depressed type early colorectal cancers by combined use of videoendoscopy and chromoendoscopy. *Gastrointest Endosc* 1998;48:362-370.

[32] Hurlstone DP, Cross SS, Adam I, Shorthouse AJ, Brown S, Sanders DS, Lobo AJ. An evaluation of colorectal endoscopic mucosal resection using high-magnification chromoscopic colonoscopy: a prospective study of 1000 colonoscopies. *Endoscopy* 2003:in press.

[33] Iishi H, Tatsuta M, Tsutsui S, Imanishi K, Otani T, Okuda S, Ishiguro S, Taniguchi H. Early depressed adenocarcinomas of the large intestine. *Cancer* 1992;69:2406-2410.

[34] Fujii T, Rembacken BJ, Dixon MF. Flat adenomas in the United Kingdom: are treatable cancers being missed? *Endoscopy* 1998;30:437-443.

[35] Hurlstone DP, Cross SS, Adam I, Shorthouse AJ, Brown S, Sanders DS, Lobo AJ. A prospective clinicopathological and endoscopic evaluation of flat and depressed colorectal lesions in the UK. *Am J Gastroenterol* 2003:in press.

[36] Rembacken BJ, Fujii T, Cairns A, Dixon MF, Yoshida S, Chalmers DM, Axon AT. Flat and depressed colonic neoplasms: a prospective study of 1000 colonoscopies in the UK. *Lancet* 2000;355:1211-1214.

[37] Saito Y, Waxman I, West AB, Popnikolov NK, Gatalica Z, Watari J, Obara T, Kohgo Y, Pasricha PJ. Prevalence and Distinctive Biological Features of Flat Colorectal Adenomas in a North American Population. *Gastroenterology* 2001;120:1657-1665.

[38] Tsuda S, Veress B, Toth E, Fork FT. Flat and depressed colorectal tumours in a southern Swedish population: a prospective chromoendoscopic and histopathological study. *Gut* 2002;51:550-555.

[39] Wolber RA, Owen DA. Flat adenoma of the colon. *Hum Pathol* 1991;22:70-74.

[40] Kuramoto S, Oohara T. How do colorectal cancers develop? *Cancer* 1995;75:1534-1538.

[41] Robbins DH, Itzkowitz SH. The molecular and genetic basis of colon cancer. *Med Clin North Am* 2002;86:1467-1495.

[42] Kurahashi T, Kaneko K, Makino R, Mitamura K. Colorectal carcinoma with special reference to growth pattern classifications: clinicopathological characteristics and genetic changes. *Journal of Gastroenterology* 2002;37:354-362.

[43] Church J, Lowry A, Simmang C. Practice parameters for the identification and testing of patinets at risk for dominantly inherited colorectal cancer-supporting documentation. Prepared by the Standards Task Force, The American Society of Colon and Rectal Surgeons. *Dis Colon Rectum* 2001;44:1403-1412.

[44] Guillem JG, Smith AJ, Culle J, Ruo L. Gastrointestinal polyposis syndromes. *Curr Prob Surg* 1999;36:219-323.

[45] Marra G, Boland CR. Hereditary nonpolyposis colorectal cancer: The syndrome, the genes and historical perspective. *J Natl Cancer Inst* 1995;87:1114-1125.

[46] Muller AD, Sonnenberg A. Prevention of colorectal cancer by flexible endoscopy and polypectomy. A case-control study of 32,702 veterans. *Ann Intern Med* 1995;123:904-910.

[47] Winawer SJ, Zauber AG, Ho MN, O'Brien MJ, Gottlieb LS, Sternberg SS, Waye JD, Schapiro M, Bond JH, Panish JF. Prevention of colorectal cancer by colonoscopic polypectomy. The National Polyp Study Workgroup. *N Engl J Med* 1993;329:1977-1981.

[48] Atkin WS, Morson BC, Cuzick J. Long-term risk of colorectal cancer after excision of rectosigmoid adenomas. *N Engl J Med* 1992;326:658-662.

[49] Morson B. President's address. The polyp-cancer sequence in the large bowel. *Proc R Soc Med* 1974;67:451-457.

[50] Miller BA, Ries LAG, Hankey BF. *Cancer Statistics Review*. National Cancer Institute; NIH Publication 1992.

[51] Hamilton SR. The adenoma-adenocarcinoma sequence in the large bowel: variations on a theme. *J Cell Biochem Suppl* 1992;16:41-46.

[52] Crohn B, Rosenberg H. The sigmoidoscopic picure of chronic ulcerative colitis (non-specific). *Am J Med Sci* 1925;170:220-228.

[53] Neale AV, Demers RY, Budev H, Scott RO. Physician accuracy in diagnosing colorectal polyps. *Dis Colon Rectum* 1987;30:247-250.

[54] Hixson LJ, Fennerty MB, Sampliner RE, Garewal HS. Prospective blinded trial of the colonoscopic miss-rate of large colorectal polyps. *Gastrointest Endosc* 1991;37:125-127.

[55] Hixson LJ, Fennerty MB, Sampliner RE, McGee D, Garewal H. Prospective study of the frequency and size distribution of polyps missed by colonoscopy. *J Natl Cancer Inst* 1990;82:1769-1772.

[56] Rex DK, Cutler CS, Lemmel GT, Rahmani EY, Clark DW, Helper DJ, Mark DG. Colonoscopic miss rates of adenomas determined by back-to-back colonoscopies. *Gastroenterology* 1997;112:24-28.

[57] Brooker JC, Saunders BP, Shah SG, Thapar CJ, Thomas HJ, Atkin WS, Cardwell CR, Williams CB. Total colonic dye-spray increases the detection of diminutive adenomas during routine colonoscopy: a randomized controlled trial. *Gastrointest Endosc* 2002;56:333-338.

[58] Jiang B. Chromoendoscopy and high-magnification colonoscopy in early detection of colorectal cancer. *Di Yi Jun Yi Da Xue Xue Bao* 2002;22:385-387.

[59] Keisslich R, von Bergh M, Hahn M, Hermann G, Jung M. Chromoendoscopy with indigocarmine improves the detection of adenomatous and nonadenomatous lesions in the colon. *Endoscopy* 2001;33:1001-1003.

[60] Kobayashi K, Sivak MV. Flat adenoma: are western colonoscopists careful enough? *Endoscopy* 1998;30:487-489.

[61] Mitooka H, Fujimori T, Ohno S, Morimoto S, Nakashima T, Ohmoto A, Okano H, Miyamoto M, Oh T, Saeki S. Chromoscopy of the colon using indigo carmine dye with electrolyte lavage solution. *Gastrointest Endosc* 1992;38:373-374.

[62] Kudo S, Tamura S, Hirota S, Sano Y, Yamano H, Serizawa M, Fukuoka T, Mitsuoka H, Nakajima T, Kusaka H. The problem of de novo colorectal carcinoma. *Eur J Cancer* 1995;31:1118-1120.

[63] Wada R, Matsukuma S, Abe H, Kuwabara N, Suda K, Arakawa A, Kitamura S. Histopathological studies of superficial- type early colorectal carcinoma. *Cancer* 1996;77:44-50.

[64] Stolte M, Bethke B. Colorectal mini-de novo carcinoma: a reality in Germany too. *Endoscopy* 1995;27:286-290.

[65] Bedenne L, Faivre J, Boutron MC, Piard F, Cauvin JM, Hillon P. Adenoma--carcinoma sequence or "de novo" carcinogenesis? A study of adenomatous remnants in a population-based series of large bowel cancers. *Cancer* 1992;69:883-888.

[66] Muto T, Bussey HJ, Morson BC. The evolution of cancer of the colon and rectum. *Cancer* 1975;36:2251-2270.

[67] Kudo S, Hayashi S, Miura K, Takano M, Saito M, Kubuta Y. The clinicopathological features of flat and depressed type of early colorectal cancer [in Japanese with English abstract]. *Stomach and Intestine* 1989;24:317-329.

[68] Owen DA. Flat adenoma, flat carcinoma, and de novo carcinoma of the colon. *Cancer* 1996;77:3-6.

[69] Kariya A. A case of early colonic cancer type IIc associated with familial polyposis coli [English abstract]. *Stomach and Intestine* 1977;12:1359-1364.

[70] Muto T, Kamiya J, Sawada T, Konishi F, Sugihara K, Kubota Y, Agawa S, Saito Y, Morioka Y. Small 'flat' adenoma' of the large bowel with special reference to its clinicopathological feature. *Dis Colon Rectum* 1985;28:857-851.

[71] Adachi M, Muto T, Okinaga K, Morioka Y. Clinicopathologic features of the flat adenoma. *Dis Colon Rectum* 1991;34:981-986.

[72] Adachi M, Okinaga K, Muto T. Flat adenoma of the large bowel: re-evaluation with special reference to central depression. *Dis Colon Rectum* 2000;43:782-787.

[73] Lanspa SJ, Rouse J, Smyrk T, Watson P, Jenkins JX, Lynch HT. Epidemiologic characteristics of the flat adenoma of Muto. A prospective study. *Dis Colon Rectum* 1992;35:543-546.

[74] Willis J, Riddell RH. Biology versus terminology: East meets West in surgical pathology. *Gastrointest Endosc* 2003;57:369-376.

[75] Smith GA, Oien KA, O'Dwyer P. Frequency of early colorectal cancer in patients undergoing colonoscopy. *Br J Surg* 1999;86:1328-1331.

[76] Tada S, Yao T, Iida M, Koga H, Hizawa K, Fujishima M. A clinicopathologic study of small flat colorectal carcinoma. *Cancer* 1994;74:2430-2435.

[77] Tada S, Iida M, Matsumoto T, Yao T, Aoyagi K, Koga H, Tanoue Y, Fujishima M. Small flat cancer of the rectum: clinicopathological and endoscopic features. *Gastrointest Endosc* 1995;42:109-113.

[78] Teixeira CR, Tanaka S, Haruma K, Yoshihara M, Sumii K, Kajiyama G, Shimamoto F. Flat-elevated colorectal neoplasms exhibit a high malignant potential. *Oncology* 1996;53:89-93.

[79] Colton CG, Sivak MVJ. Flat adenomas and cancers. *Gastrointest Endosc* 1995;42:182-184.

[80] Hurlstone DP, Cross SS, Lobo AJ. A 1mm depressed type IIc minute colorectal cancer: first reported case and discussion of clinical relevance, with special reference to endoscopic diagnosis. *J Gastro Hepatol* 2003;in press.

[81] Shimoda T, Ikegami M, Fujisaki J, Matsui T, Aizawa S, Ishikawa E. Early colorectal carcinoma with special reference to its development de novo. *Cancer* 1989;64:1138-1146.

[82] Matsumoto T, Iida M, Kuwano T, Tada S, Yao T, Fujishima M. Small nonpolypoid neoplastic lesions of the colon: endoscopic features with emphasis on their progression. *Gastrointest Endosc* 1995;41:135-140.

[83] Minamoto T, Sawaguchi K, Ohta T, Itoh T, Mai M. Superficial-type adenomas and adenocarcinomas of the colon and rectum: a comparative morphological study. *Gastroenterology* 1994;106:1436-1443.

[84] Kasumi A, Kratzer GL. Fast-growing cancer of the colon and rectum. *Am Surg* 1992;58:383-386.

[85] Haggitt RC, Glotzbach RE, Soffer EE, Wruble LD. Prognostic factors in colorectal carcinomas arising in adenomas: implications for lesions removed by endoscopic polypectomy. *Gastroenterology* 1985;89:328-336.

[86] Wilcox GM, Anderson PB, Colacchio TA. Early invasive carcinoma in colonic polyps. A review of the literature with emphasis on the assessment of the risk of metastasis. *Cancer* 1986;57:160-171.

[87] Kikuchi R, Takano M, Takagi K, Fujimoto N, Nozaki R, Fujiyoshi T, Uchida Y. Management of early invasive colorectal cancer. Risk of recurrence and clinical guidelines. *Dis Colon Rectum* 1995;38:1286-1295.

[88] Kudo S. Endoscopic mucosal resection of flat and depressed types of early colorectal cancer. *Endoscopy* 1993;25:455-461.

[89] Kosaka T. Clinico-pathological study of the minute elevated lesion of the colorectal mucosa. *Journal of the Japanese Society of Coloproctology* 1975;28:218-226.

[90] Kuramoto S, Oohara T. Flat early cancers of the large intestine. *Cancer* 1989;64:950-955.

[91] Morita T, Tomita N, Ohue M, Sekimoto M, Yamamoto H, Ohnishi T, Tada M, Ikenaga M, Miyake Y, Sakita I, Tamaki Y, Matsuura N, Ito M, Monden M. Molecular analysis of diminutive, flat, depressed colorectal lesions: Are they precursors of polypoid adenoma or early stage carcinoma? *Gastrointest Endosc* 2002;56:663-671.

[92] Sawada T, Hojo K, Moriya Y. Colonoscopic management of focal and early colorectal carcinoma. *Bailliere's Clinical Gastroenterology* 1989;3:627-645.

[93] Anonymous. General rules for clinical and pathological studies on cancer of the colon, rectum and anus. Part I. Clinical classification. Japanese Research Society for Cancer of the Colon and Rectum. *Jpn J Surg* 1983;13:557-573.

[94] Anonymous. General rules for clinical and pathological studies on cancer of the colon, rectum and anus. Part II. Histopathological classification. Japanese Research Society for Cancer of the Colon and Rectum. *Jpn J Surg* 1983;13:574-598.

[95] Schlemper RJ, Itabashi M, Kato Y, Lewin KJ, Riddell RH, Shimoda T, Sipponen P, Stolte M, Watanabe H. Differences in the diagnostic criteria used by Japanese and Western pathologists to diagnose colorectal carcinoma. *Cancer* 1998;82:60-69.

[96] Schlemper RJ, Riddell RH, Kato Y, Borchard F, Cooper HS, Dawsey SM, Dixon MF, Fenoglio-Preiser CM, Flejou JF, Geboes K, Hirota T, Itabashi M, Iwafuchi M, Kim YI, Kirchner T, Klimpfinger M, Koike M, Lauwers GY, Lewin KJ, Oberhuber G, Price AB, Rubio CA, Shimoda T, Sipponen P, Stolte M, Watanabe H, Yamabe H. The Vienna classification of gastrointestinal neoplasia. *Gut* 2000;47:251-255.

[97] Rembacken BJ, Fujii T, Kondo H. The recognition and endoscopic treatment of early gastric and colonic cancer. *Best Practice & Research Clinical Gastroenterology* 2001;15:317-336.

[98] Nagata S, Tanaka S, Haruma K, Yoshihara M, Sumii K, Kajiyama G, Shimamoto F. Pit pattern diagnosis of early colorectal carcinoma by magnifying colonoscopy: clinical and histological implications. *Int J Oncol* 2000;16:927-934.

[99] Hurlstone DP. High-resolution magnification chromoendoscopy: common problems encountered in "pit pattern" interpretation and correct classification of flat colorectal lesions. *Am J Gastroenterol* 2002;97:1069-1070.

[100] Hurlstone DP, Lobo AJ. Assessing resection margins using high-magnification chromoscopy: a useful tool after colonic endoscopic mucosal resection. *Am J Gastroenterol* 2002;97:2143-2144.

[101] Shida H, Ban K, Matsumoto M, Masuda K, Imanari T, Machida T, Yamamoto T. Prognostic significance of location of lymph node metastases in colorectal cancer. *Dis Colon Rectum* 1992;35:1046-1050.

[102] Newland RC, Chapuis PH, Pheils MT, MacPherson JG. The relationship of survival to staging and grading of colorectal carcinoma: a prospective study of 503 cases. *Cancer* 1981;47:1424-1429.

[103] Newland RC, Chapuis PH, Smyth EJ. The prognostic value of substaging colorectal carcinoma. A prospective study of 1117 cases with standardized pathology. *Cancer* 1987;60:852-857.

[104] Tanaka S, Haruma K, Teixeira CR, Tatsuta S, Ohtsu N, Hiraga Y, Yoshihara M, Sumii K, Kajiyama G, Shimamoto F. Endoscopic treatment of submucosal invasive colorectal carcinoma with special reference to risk factors for lymph node metastasis. *J Gastroenterol* 1995;30:710-717.

[105] Kudo S, Tamegai Y, Yamano H, Imai Y, Kogure E, Kashida H. Endoscopic mucosal resection of the colon: the Japanese technique. *Gastrointest Endosc Clin N Am* 2001;11:519-535.

[106] Roseau G, Palazzo L, Amouyal P. Endoscopic ultrasonography in the preoperative evaluation of rectal cancer. *Presse Med* 1990;19:1450-1453.

[107] Roubein LD, David C, DuBrow R. Endoscopic ultrasonography in staging rectal cancer. *Am J Gastroenterol* 1990;85:1391-2394.

[108] Oohara N, Murata Y, Kawanami C. Ultrasonography in the colorectal lesion: a comparison between endoscopic ultrasonography (7.5 MHz) and sonoprobe system (20MHz) [in Japanese with English abstract]. *Progress of gastrointestinal endosonography* 1991;39:221-225.

[109] Mitooka H, Fujimori T, Maeda S, Nagasako K. Minute flat depressed neoplastic lesions of the colon detected by contrast chromoscopy using an indigo carmine capsule. *Gastrointest Endosc* 1995;41:453-459.

[110] Woolfson IK, Eckholdt GJ, Wetzel CR, Gathright JB, Ray JE, Hicks TC. Usefulness of performing colonoscopy one year after endoscopic polypectomy. *Dis Colon Rectum* 1990;33:389-393.

[111] Hofstad B, Vatn M, Larsen S, Osnes M. Growth of colorectal polyps: recovery and evaluation of unresected polyps of less than 10 mm, 1 year after detection. *Scand J Gastroenterol* 1994;29:640-645.

[112] Winawer SJ, Zauber AG, O'Brien MJ. Randomised comparison of surveillance intervals after colonoscopic removal of newly diagnosed adenomatous polyps. The National Polyp Study Workgroup. *N Engl J Med* 1993;328:901-906.

[113] Kiesslich R, Fritsch J, Holtmann M, Koehler HH, Stolte M, Kanzler S, Nafe B, Jung M, Galle PR, Neurath MF. Methylene Blue-Aided Chromoendoscopy for the Detection of Intraepitheial Neoplasia and Colon Cancer in Ulcerative Colitis. *Gastroenterology* 2003;124:880-888.

[114] Eaden JA, Mayberry JF. Colorectal cancer complicating ulcerative colitis: a review. *Am J Gastroenterol* 2000;95:2710-2719.

[115] Shelton AA, Lehman RE, Schrosck TR, Welton ML. Retrospective review of colorectal cancer in ulcerative colitis at a tertiary centre. *Arch Surg* 1996;131:806-810.

[116] Eaden JA, Abrams KR, Mayberry JF. The risk of colorectal cancer in ulcerative colitis: a meta-analysis. *Gut* 2001;48:526-535.

[117] Fogt F, Urbanski SJ, Sanders ME, Furth EE, Zimmerman RL, Noffsinger AE, Vortmeyer AO, Hartmann CJ, Odze RL, Brown CA. Distinction between dysplasia-associated lesion or mass (DALM) and adenoma in patinets with ulcerative colitis. *Hum Pathol* 2000;31:288-291.

[118] Tytgat GN, Dhir V, Gopinath N. Endoscopic appearances of dysplasia and cancer in inflammatory bowel disease. *Eur J Cancer* 1995;31:1174-1177.

[119] Rubin CE, Haggit RC, Burmer GC, Brentnall TA, Stevens AC, Levine DS, Dean PJ, Kimmey M, Perera DR, Rabinovitch PS. DNA aneuploidy in colonic biopsies predicts future development of dysplasia in ulcerative colitis. *Gastroenterology* 1992;103:1611-1620.

[120] Hurlstone DP, McAlindon ME, Sanders DS, Lobo AJ. Further validation of high-magnification-chromoscopic colonoscopy for the detection of intraepithelial neoplasia and colon cancer in ulcerative colitis. *Gastroenterology* 2003:in press.

[121] Kudo S. [*Endoscopic mucosal resection*]. *Nippon Geka Gakkai Zassh*i 1999;100:776-781.

[122] Au W, Pathak S, Collie CJ, Hsu TC. Cytogenetic toxicity of gentian violet and crystal violet on mammalian cells in vitro. *Mut Res* 1978;58:269-276.

[123] Hurlstone DP, Brown S. Evidence to support high-magnification chromoscopic colonoscopy: evaluation of the Kudo type V crypt pattern with reference to flat and depressed colorectal lesions and screening implications for the UK. *Gastrointest Endosc* 2003;58:164.

[124] Kudo S, Tamure S, Nakajima T, Hirota S, Asano M, Ito O, Kusaka H. Depressed type of colorectal cancer. *Endoscopy* 1995;27:54-57.

[125] Deyhle P, Largader F, Jenny S, Fumagalli I. A method for endoscopic electroresection of sessile colonic polyps. *Endoscopy* 1973;5:38-40.

[126] Rembacken BJ, Gotoda T, Fujii T, Axon AT. Endoscopic mucosal resection. *Endoscopy* 2001;33:709-718.

[127] 1Kudo S, Tamura S, Kashida H, Nakajima T, Kusaka H, Fukuoka T, Hirayama K, Tasaka K, Nakajo K. [Endoscopic treatment in colorectal lesions--especially on endoscopic mucosal resection]. *Nippon Rinsho* 1996;54:1298-1306.

[128] Brooker JC, Saunders BP, Shah SG, Thapar CJ, Suzuki N, Williams CB. Treatment with argon plasma coagulation reduces recurrence after piecmeal resection of large sessile colonic polyps: a randomised trial and recommendations. *Gastrointest Endosc* 2002;55:371-375.

[129] Inoue H, Takeshita K, Hori H, Muraoka Y, Yoneshima H, Endo M. Endoscopic mucosal resection with a cap-fitted panendoscope for esophagus, stomach, and colon mucosal lesions. *Gastrointest Endosc* 1993;39:58-62.

[130] Saitoh Y, Obara T, Einami K, Nomura M, Taruishi M, Ayabe T, Ashida T, Shibata Y, Kohgo Y. Efficacy of high-frequency ultrasound probes for the preoperative staging of invasion depth in flat and depressed colorectal tumors. *Gastrointest Endosc* 1996;44:34-39.

[131] Palazzo MGL, Canard PJM. Guidelines of the French Society of Digestive Endoscopy: Endoscopic Mucosectomy. *Endoscopy* 2001;33:187-190.

[132] Hurlstone DP, Lobo AJ. Resection margin 'thermal tattooing' for lateral spreading tumour resection using endoscopic mucosal resection: a new technique for assisting complete horizontal clearance. *World J Surg* 2003:(in press).

[133] Uno Y, Munakata A. The non-lifting sign of invasive colon cancer. *Gastrointest Endosc* 1994;40:485-489.

[134] Ponchon T. Endoscopic mucosal resection. *J Clin Gastroenterol* 2001;32:6-10.

[135] Okamoto H, Tanaka S, Haruma K. Japanese review of complications and measure by endoscopic treatment for colorectal tumor between 1989-1993 [in Japanese with English abstract]. *Hiroshimaigaku* 1996;49:585-591.

[136] Ahmad NA, Kochman ML, Long WB, Furth EE, Ginsberg GG. Efficacy, safety, and clinical outcomes of endoscopic mucosal resection: a study of 101 cases. *Gastrointest Endosc* 2002;55:390-396.

[137] Kaneko E, Harada H, Kasugai T, Sakita T. The results of a multi-centre analysis from 1988-1992. *Gastroenterol Endosc* 1995;37:642-652.

[138] Kaneko E, Hanada H, Kasugai T. The survey of gastrointestinal endoscopic complications in Japan (1993-1997). *Gastroenterol Endosc* 2000;42:308-313.

[139] Wagnieres GA, Star WM, Wilson BC. In vivo fluorescence spectroscopy and imaging for oncological applications. *Photochem Photobiol* 1998;68:603-632.

[140] Kapadia CR, Cutruzzola FW, O'Brien KM, Stetz M, Enriquez R, Deckelbaum L. Laser-induced fluorescence spectroscopy of human colonic mucosa. Detection of adenomatous transformation. *Gastroenterology* 1990;99:150-157.

[141] Haringsma J, Tytgat GNJ, Yano H, Iishi H, Tatsuta M, Ogihara T, Watanabe H, Sato N, Marcon N, Wilson BC, Cline RW. Autofluorescence endoscopy: feasibility of detection of GI neoplasms unapparent to white light endoscopy with an evolving technology. *Gastrointest Endosc* 2001;53:642-650.

[142] Cothren RM, Richards-Kortum R, Sivak MV, Van Dam J, Petras R, Fitzmaurice M. Gastrointestinal tissue diagnosis by laser-induced fluorescence spectroscopy at endoscopy. *Gastrointest Endosc* 1990;36:105-111.

[143] Cothren RM, Sivak MV, Van Dam J, Petras R, Fitmaurice M, Crawford J. Detection of dysplasia at colonoscopy using laser-induced fluorescence: a blinded study. *Gastrointest Endosc* 1996;44:168-176.

[144] Chwirot BW, Kowalska M, Sypniewska N, Michniewicz Z, Gradziel M. Spectrally resolved fluorescence imaging of colonic adenomas. *J Photochem Photobiol* 1999;50:174-183.

[145] Wang TD, Van Dam J, Crawford JM, Preisinger EA, Wang Y, Feld MS. Fluorescence endoscopic imaging of human colonic adenomas. *Gastroenterology* 1996;111:1182-1191.

[146] Wang TD, Crawford JM, Feld MS, Wang Y, Itzkan I, Van Dam J. In vivo identification of colonic dysplasia using fluorescence endoscopic imaging. *Gastrointest Endosc* 1999;49:447-455.

In: Focus on Colorectal Cancer Research
Editor: Julia D. Martinez, pp. 171-208
ISBN #1-59454-101-9

Chapter VIII

TREATMENT OF ADVANCED COLORECTAL CANCER: CURRENT STATUS AND FUTURE PERSPECTIVES

I. Grivicich[1,2,3,*], A. B. da Rocha[1,3,4], G. J. Peters[5] and G. Schwartsmann[1,2]

[1]South-American Office for Anticancer Drug Development, Porto Alegre, RS, Brazil
[2]Programa de Pós-Graduação em Genética e Biologia Molecular, Universidade Federal do Rio Grande do Sul, Porto Alegre, RS, Brazil
[3]Laboratório de Marcadores de Estresse Celular, Centro de Pesquisas em Ciências Médicas, Universidade Luterana do Brasil, Canoas, RS, Brazil
[4]Programa de Pós Graduação em Diagnóstico Genético e Molecular, Universidade Luterana do Brasil, Canoas, RS, Brazil
[5]Department of Medical Oncology, VU University Medical Center, Amsterdam, The Netherlands

ABSTRACT

Colorectal cancer is a common disease with high rate of mortality and very well understood genetics. The majority of patients are diagnosed in an advanced stage of the disease, thus requiring chemotherapy. The prognosis and treatment modality for advanced colorectal cancer depends on the tumor stage, since the accumulation of molecular alterations has been commonly associated with poor prognosis and treatment failure. Although there is evidence of benefit of chemotherapy in adjuvant and metastatic settings, its use still remains unsatisfactory because of intrinsic or acquired drug resistance. The most commonly used protocols in advanced colorectal carcinoma include the antimetabolite 5-fluorouracil (5-FU). Several effective alternative treatment options became available for patients with colorectal cancer who relapse after a 5-FU-based

* Corresponding author: Centro de Pesquisa em Ciências Médicas, Universidade Luterana do Brasil, Rua Miguel Tostes, 101, Prédio 22, 5° andar, 92420-280 – Canoas – RS, Brazil, Tel: 55 51 477 9219, Fax: 55 51 478 1747, e-mail: grivicich@terra.com.br

chemotherapy. The introduction of irinotecan and oxaliplatin to the therapy with 5-FU/leucovorin has contributed to increase therapeutic options and to improve response rates and survival. The development of oral agents broadened the treatment options available for patients with this disease. Based on the diversity of molecular behavior of advanced colorectal cancer, a number of new agents entered clinical trials. Among others, cyclooxygenase-2 inhibitors, vascular endothelial growth inhibitors and epidermal growth factor inhibitors, are under investigation. Furthermore, the knowledge of the genetics characteristics can be useful to identify prognostic differences, tumor molecular staging and patient stratification, leading to elect a better treatment modality.

INTRODUCTION

Epidemiology and Etiology

Colorectal cancer is the third most common cancer mortality in both sexes in the western world [1,2]. Incidence rates vary about 20-fold around the world, with the highest rates being noted in industrialized countries such as Australia and Germany, and the lowest in India and Greece [3]. Despite the equivalent frequency observed in men and women, in areas with high incidence such as North America and Australia, rates in men exceed those in women by 20% [4]. In 2003, 105,500 new cases of colorectal cancer were expected to occur and approximately 57,000 deaths, accounting for 10% of cancer deaths. In spite of this, incidence rates of colorectal cancer declined by 1.8% per year during 1985-1995, and stabilized in the last 18 years. This decline is probably due to increased screening and polyp removal, which prevents progression of polyps to invasive cancers [1]. In Brazil, on the other hand, these figures are different [6]. As suggested by a recent report from the Brazilian National Cancer Institute (INCA), colorectal carcinoma affects nowadays 70% more Brazilians than in 1979. The estimate for 2003 in Brazil is approximately 10,000 new cases, and 4,000 deaths [6,7].

The development of colorectal cancer is a complex process. Among the possible causative agents are environmental and dietary factors, as well as inherited and somatic mutations [8]. The primary risk factor for colorectal cancer is age, with more than 90% of cases diagnosed in persons over the age of 50, as the consequence of environmental carcinogen exposure and genetic factors. Other risk factors include smoking, alcohol consumption, obesity and physical inactivity [9-12], but these relations are less significant and some data are contradictory. Two recent studies suggest that dietary fiber intake is inversely related to the incidence of colorectal adenomas and cancer [13,14]. Differently, in two other clinical trials, neither a high fiber dietary intervention nor fiber supplements seem to decrease the risk of adenomas [15]. Although there is controversy, it is suggested that intake of meals rich in vegetables protects against colorectal cancer, through reducing the intestinal transit time and subsequently reducing the exposure of the colon mucosa to potential carcinogens [11,12,16]. In contrast, diet rich in meat and animal fats increases its risk [4,12].

Molecular Characteristics

During the last decades some of molecular alterations in colorectal carcinoma were characterized. Based on these observations it is known that hereditary factors may predispose to colorectal carcinoma. Among these are familial adenomatous polyposis (FAP) and the hereditary non-polyposis colorectal cancer (HNPCC) syndrome (Table 1). Patients with inflammatory bowel diseases also run an increased risk for colorectal carcinoma [17,18]. FAP is characterized by the development of multiple polyps, which progress to cancer (Table 1). The disease is caused by an inherited mutation in the adenomatous polyposis coli (APC) gene, inducing polyp formation [19,20]. A number of variants of FAP have been described in which there is marked variability in the number of adenomas seen in affected individuals. Among these are Gardner's syndrome, wherein affected individuals have extensive polyposis together with epidermoid cysts and osteomas; and Turcot's syndrome, in which polyposis and brain tumors can be seen [reviewed in ref. 8]. Individuals with Gardner's syndrome are at the same risk for colorectal cancer as classic FAP [21]. Cancers in affected individuals with HNPCC (Table 1) syndromes arise from adenomas through a multistep process [22,23]. HNPCC is recognized by the early occurrence of colorectal and extracolonic cancers [24]. The adenomas found in patients with HNPCC are more often histologically advanced and have areas of high-grade dysplasia [25]. Two different variations of the HNPCC syndrome have been described: Lynch Type I, in which only colorectal cancers are seen; Lynch Type II, in addition to colorectal cancer, stomach and endometrial cancer can be seen [reviewed in ref. 8]. HNPCC involving mutations in two DNA mismatch repair (MMR) genes, hMSH2 and hMLH1, that induce microsatellite instability [22,23]. The MMR system consist in a complex of proteins that recognized and repair base pair mismatches during DNA replication [26]. The analyses of 86 families with know MMR gene mutation indicated that the *MMR* defects are involved in the early stages of development of adenomas [27].

Based on familial studies, it is estimated that 20%-30% of colorectal cancers have a potentially genetic cause [28]. Indeed, persons who have first-degree relatives with colorectal cancers increased, at least, 2-fold the risk of developing colorectal cancer compared with the general population [28]. There is strong evidence that the majority of colorectal carcinoma arose from pre-neoplastic lesions called adenomas. The transformation of adenoma in carcinoma is a result from a series of pathologic changes from normal colonic mucosa to invasive carcinoma (Figure 1) [17,29]. The sequence of genetic alterations leading to colorectal cancer usually begins with the inactivation of the pathway involving the *APC* tumor suppressor gene [reviewed in ref. 20,30]. Other important alteration is *ras*-gene mutation, which occurs in approximately 50% of malignant colorectal tumors in the initial steps of colon carcinogenesis [29]. The following events include deletion in chromosome 18q that encodes for the tumor suppressor genes *DCC*, and deletion in chromosome 17p in which is the tumor suppressor gene *p53* [8].

Table 1: Features of familial adenomatous polyposis and hereditary nonpolyposis colorectal cancer syndromes.

Features	FAP	HNPCC
Inheritance pattern	Autossomal dominant	Autossomal dominant
Incidence	*1:10,000*	*1: 2,000*
Genes[a]	APC *(>90%)*	MLH1 *(59%)* *MSH2* (38%) *MSH6* (1.3%) *PMS2* (0.8%) *PMS1* (0.4%)
Colon cancer[b]	*39*	*44*
Extracolonic cancers[c]	Duodenal (5%-10%) Pancreatic (2%) Thyroid (2%) Gastric (0.5%) Hepatoblastoma (1.6%) CNS (<1%)	Endometrial (43-60%) Ovarian (9-12%) Gastric (13-19%) Urinary tract (4-10%) Renal (3.3%) CNS (3.7%) Small bowel (1-4%)
Colon polyps	> 100 polyps in teens	Few colon polyps detected by endoscopy
Variant syndromes	Gardner's (extensive polyposis, epidermoid cysts, osteomas) Turcot's (polyposis and brain tumor)	Lynch Type I (colorectal cancer without extensive polyps) Lynch Type II (colorectal cancer without extensive polyps, and stomach cancer, endometrial cancer, urothelial cancer)

FAP = Familial adenomatous polyposis; HNPCC = Hereditary nonpolyposis colorectal cancer; CNS = Central nervous system. [a] Percentage of cases with gene mutation; [b] Average age (year); [c] Lifetime risk.

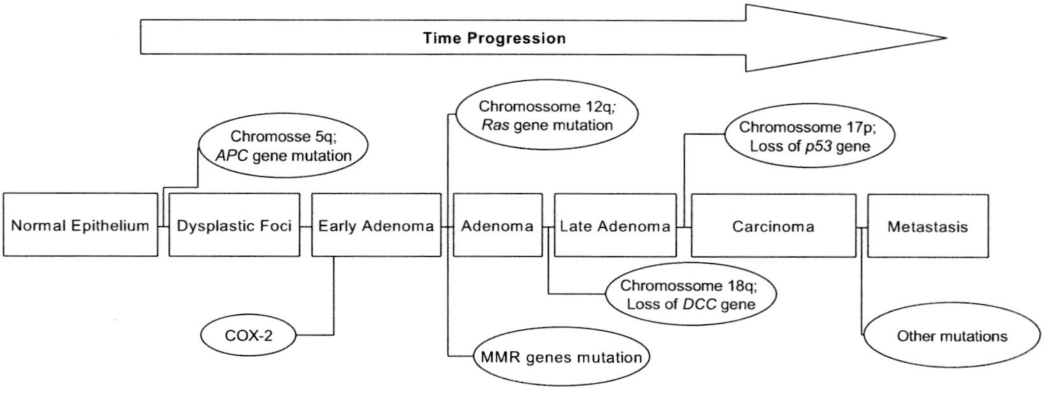

Figure 1: Genetic model of colorectal cancer progression.

About 15% percent of sporadic colorectal cancers have insertions and deletions of nucleotides with repeated sequences of DNA, termed microsatellite instability (MSI), due to defective repair of mismatched nucleotides [17,22,23,30,31]. Some of these genetic alterations are prognostic markers in colorectal cancer and will be discussed further in this chapter. [32]. Loss of heterozygosity at chromosome 18q indicates a poor prognosis [17,18,32]. Other alterations interfere with prognosis are mutations in chromosome 17p, 5q, [30]; and increased expression of genes involved in fluoropyrimidine metabolism [32,33]. Several results of pre-clinical and clinical studies indicated that the pattern of the enzymes involved in the metabolism of 5-fluorouracil (5-FU) might predict response to 5-FU [34].

Many other mechanisms have been suggested to be involved in the adenoma- carcinoma transformation; among these the participation of the enzyme cyclooxygenase (Cox) The involvement of Cox in the carcinogenic sequence of colorectal carcinoma has been derived from studies on prostaglandins [35]. High levels of prostaglandins especially PGE_2 have been founded in human colonic and rectal tumors [36]. Consistent with these observations, several studies demonstrated that *Cox-2* gene and protein expression are associated with colonic neoplasia [37-41]. The expression of *Cox-2* in colorectal tumors seems to occur in early stage (Figure 1) of carcinogenesis [38], and has been associated with tumor invasiveness [39,40].

In this chapter we examined the current status of the treatment for advanced colorectal carcinoma, as well as the new modalities of therapy and potential prognostic markers for this disease.

Treatment Modalities

Approximately 80% of colorectal cancer patients present with localized disease, for which surgery is the primary treatment modality, resulting in complete remission in approximately 50% of patients [17,18]. The prognosis of patients following surgery depends on the tumor stage [17]. The majority of patients with stage I or II disease are cured by surgery alone [42]. In those patients with lymph node involvement, approximately 50% will eventually experience metastatic disease progression following surgery [17]. Systemic chemotherapy, therefore, plays an important role in such patients. Unfortunately, cytotoxic drug therapy generally produces partial clinical responses of short duration, making this form of treatment only of palliative value [2,17].

The standard treatment for stage III colon cancer is surgery followed by six months of adjuvant 5-FU and leucovorin. The 5-year survival of patients with stage I colon cancer is approximately 85%, stage II colon cancer 70 to 80% and stage III colon cancer 25 to 60% [2,42].

Conventional Chemotherapy

5-Fluorouracil

In the absence of any more effective agent, 5-FU served as the mainstay of treatment for patients with advanced colorectal cancer for nearly 50 years [43]. A fluorinated pyrimidine, 5-FU acts by inhibiting thymidylate synthase (TS), an enzyme necessary for the production of thymidine nucleotides required for DNA synthesis. TS is a cytosolic enzyme that catalyzes the methylation of deoxyuridine-5'-monophosphate (dUMP) to give deoxythymidine-5'-monophosphate (dTMP), a precursor of deoxythymidine triphosphate (dTTP), one of the deoxyribonucleotides required for DNA synthesis [44,45]. Intracellularly generated, the active phosphate 5-fluorodeoxyuridine monophosphate (FdUMP) associates covalently with TS and 5,10-methylene-tetrahydrofolate to form a stabilized ternary complex (Figure 2), leading to the inhibition of dTMP production and thus DNA synthesis [46].

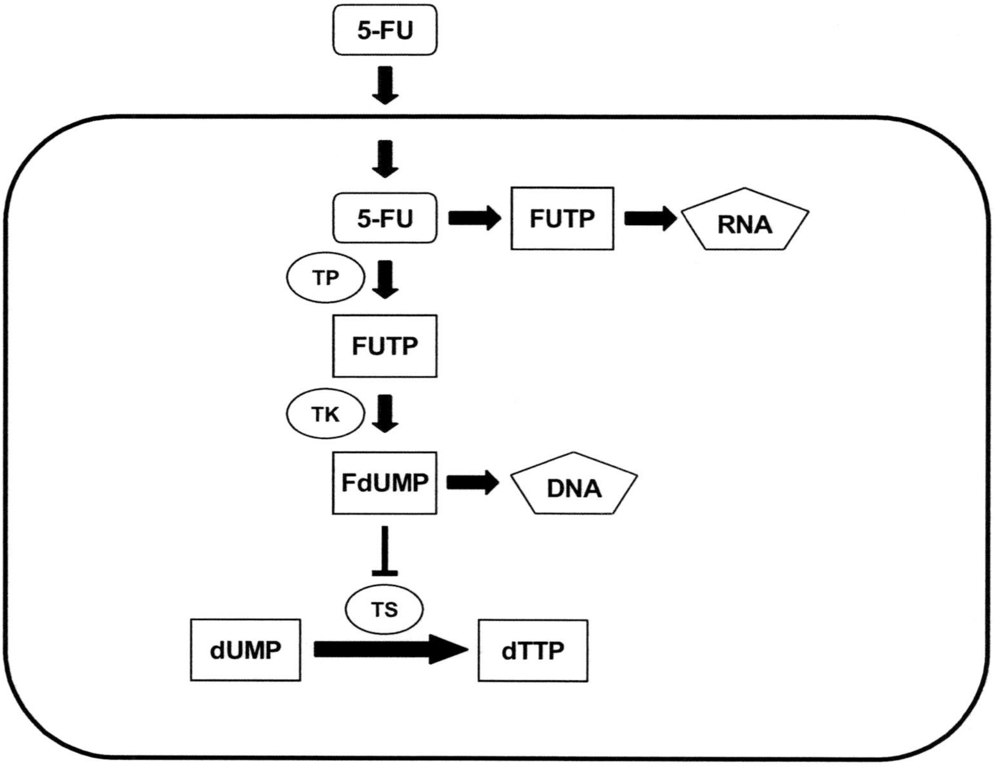

Figure 2: Metabolic pathway of 5-Fluorouracil. (thymidine phosphorylase; TK=thymidine kinase; TS=thymidylate synthase).

Although these data support that inhibition of TS is the principal mechanism of 5-FU cytotoxicity, abnormal RNA and protein processing after incorporation of fluorouridine-5'-triphosphate (FUTP) into various RNA species [47], and premature chain termination and/or DNA strand breakage upon incorporation of fluorodeoxyuridine-5'-triphosphate (FdUTP) into DNA [48], may also contribute to varying degrees to 5-FU cytotoxicity (Figure 2).

5-FU is administered either as a bolus or a continuous infusion. It has been suggested that the RNA pathway dominates the mechanism of action of 5-FU following bolus administration while the TS pathway is central with continuous infusion [49]. Bolus administration is associated with myelosuppression, oral mucositis and gastrointestinal toxicity, while continuous infusion can result hand-foot syndrome [50]. 5-FU, as a single agent given as an intravenous bolus, is only modestly active against advanced colorectal cancer, producing typical response rates of 10 to 15%, which in general last less than one year [17,44].

The failure of better responses of 5-FU as a single agent against advanced colorectal cancer has prompted investigators to look for more effective strategies. These included its administration by continuous infusion instead of by bolus injection in order to increase dose-intensity [50], and its local or regional administration, such as by direct hepatic arterial infusion for patients with liver metastases [51]. Also, several combinations of 5-FU with other cytotoxic drugs have been evaluated, such as with methyl CCNU, mitomycin C, cisplatin, irinotecan or oxaliplatin [18,45,52].

Furthermore, many attempts have been undertaken to pharmacologically manipulate intracellular metabolizing pathways of 5-FU, with the aim to selectively increase its antitumor efficacy and/or to decrease its toxicity [52]. Examples are the use of methotrexate or *N*-phosphon-acetyl-*L*-aspartate (PALA) to increase 5-phosphoribosyl-1-pyrophosphate and thus the conversion of 5-FU into FUMP; interferons, to reduce 5-FU plasma clearance, thus increasing drug tissue exposure and 5-FU-mediated DNA damage; uridine to prevent 5-FU incorporation into RNA and reduce toxic side effects; thymidine, to prevent 5-FU degradation, prolonging 5-FU exposure; allopurinol, to inhibit orotic acid accumulation, improving 5-FU activation; dipyridamol, to inhibit 5-fluorodeoxyuridine efflux, thus increasing FdUMP retention; levamisole as an immunomodulator of 5-FU cytotoxicity; and leucovorin (5-formyltetrahydrofolate), to increase TS inhibition and retention [18,52]. Of these, only the combination with leucovorin improves of the treatment results [52,53].

5-FU and Leucovorin

5-FU and leucovorin (LV) have been used in various doses and schedules in advanced colorectal cancer. This combination produced significantly superior response rate over 5-FU monotherapy although without any marked survival difference [54]. The efficacy of 5-FU/LV as adjuvant therapy has been confirmed in Intergroup-0085 [54], NSABPC-03 [55] and IMPACT-1 [56] studies. This combination can increase response rates of colorectal carcinoma to 5-FU approximately two-fold when compared to 5-FU alone. This is because of an enhanced inhibition of TS in the presence of an excess of LV.

LV is a tetrahydrofolate derivative and an intracellular source of reduced folates, which prolonged stabilization of the FdUMP - TS - folate ternary complex [45,52]. The dose-limiting toxicity of 5-FU/LV is stomatitis [57]. This finding provided the rationale for the current use of 5-FU/LV as first-line therapy in advanced colorectal carcinoma.

Irinotecan

Irinotecan (Camptosar®; 7-ethyl-10-(4-(1-piperidino)-1-piperidino) carbonyloxy-camptothecin; CPT-11), a semi-synthetic derivative of the natural alkaloid camptothecin [58], displays meaningful activity against colorectal carcinoma, both single and in certain combinations, in first- as well as in second-line therapy [59]. Irinotecan has a piperino side chain at the C-10 position, which can be cleaved by carboxyl esterases that are abundantly present in the liver, but can also be found in other tissues and cells. This reaction yields the 100- to 1000-fold biologically more active metabolite, 7-ethyl-10-hydroxycamptothecin or SN-38 [60].

Like camptothecin, both irinotecan and SN-38 act by introducing single-strand DNA breaks upon the stabilization of DNA-topoisomerase I complexes [59,61]. The single-strand breaks themselves are not cytotoxic, because they are highly reversible and are rapidly repaired when the drug is removed (Figure 3). According to the 'fork collision model', lethal, irreversible DNA damage only occurs with ongoing DNA synthesis, *i.e.* when a replication fork encounters a cleavable complex, resulting in the formation of a complete double-strand DNA break (Figure 3) [59,61].

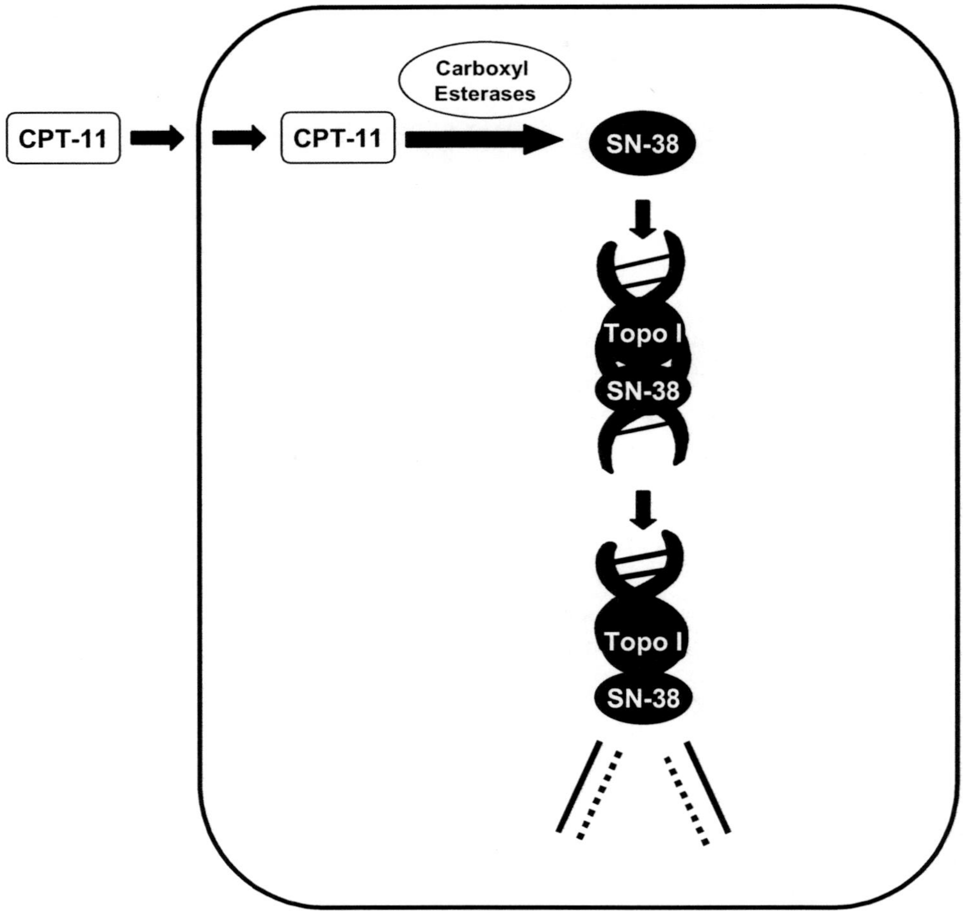

Figure 3: Mechanism of action of irinotecan.

Irinotecan displays meaningful activity against colorectal carcinoma, both singly and in certain combinations, in first- as well as in second-line [reviewed in Ref. 59]. These and other observations encouraged the hope for an alternative option for patients with advanced colorectal carcinoma who relapsed after a 5-fluorouracil-based treatment. This hope was confirmed in a randomized phase III clinical trials [62]. Comparing irinotecan with best supportive care, or with best high-dose 5-fluorouracil given by infusion, irinotecan was demonstrated to provide significant quality of life and survival advantages (8-10 months) for patients who had failed a prior 5-fluorouracil-based therapy, producing response rates of 14-

22%. An added benefit of irinotecan was its cost-effectiveness when compared to 5-fluorouracil or 5-fluorouracil plus leucovorin [62]. In a recent phase II study, the efficacy and toxicity of irinotecan (350 mg/m2, i.v., once every 3 weeks) was evaluated in 60 patients with advanced colorectal cancer showing failure to 5-FU treatment. The overall objective response rates was 13.6%, 42.4% of patients showed stable disease, the median time to disease progression was 4.4 months and the median survival was 10.5 months. These data confirm the use of CPT-11 as second-line treatment for colorectal cancer in 5-FU resistant patients [63].

Irinotecan/5-FU/Leucovorin

Many studies have been carried out to evaluate the combination of irinotecan/5-FU/LV for its therapeutic efficacy against advanced colorectal carcinoma. *In vitro* and *in vivo* evidence suggested schedule-dependent cytotoxic interactions for the combination of TS inhibitors and irinotecan or its active metabolite SN-38 [18,64]. Different schedules and sequences combining irinotecan and 5-FU have been investigated in phase I trials in Europe, United States, and Japan [65-67].

In subsequent phase II studies, this combination was evaluated as second- or first-line treatment of colorectal carcinoma. In one of these studies [68], bimonthly irinotecan 180 mg/m^2 and LV 400 mg/m^2 were given on day 1 as a 90-minute and a 2-hour infusion, respectively, immediately followed by a 5-FU bolus of 400 mg/m^2 and a 46-hour continuous infusion of 5-FU 2.4-3 g/m^2. Of the 33 pretreated patients, 2 experienced a partial response (6%), 20 had stabilization of their disease (61%), and 11 progressed (33%). Grade 3-4 toxicities occurred in 10 patients (33%), but were manageable. Thus, this so-called FOLFIRI regimen (FOLinic acid, 5-Fluorouracil, IRInotecan) was efficacious as second-line therapy against metastatic colorectal carcinoma, producing acceptable toxicity.

Another trial [69] included 683 patients who where assigned randomly to 1 of 3 arms. Patients on one of the arms received 5-FU 452 mg/m^2 as an intravenous bolus and LV 20 mg/m^2 as an intravenous bolus daily for 5 consecutive days, every 4 weeks; irinotecan alone at 125 mg/m^2 intravenously, weekly for 4 weeks, every 6 weeks; irinotecan 125 mg/m^2 intravenously, 5-FU 500 mg/m^2 intravenous bolus, and LV 20 mg/m^2 intravenous bolus, weekly for 4 weeks, every 6 weeks. Irinotecan alone did not show any benefit to 5-FU/LV, but the three-drug combination compared to the standard therapy increased tumor response rate (39 % *vs* 21 %), the time to disease progression (7 months *vs* 4.3 months), and the median survival time (14.8 months *vs* 12.6 months).

Two randomized, controlled, clinical trials [69,70] led to the approval of the irinotecan/5-FU/LV regimen by the FDA in April 2000, in USA. In these studies (Table 2), the combination of irinotecan and 5-FU/LV resulted in a significant delay in the time at which tumors progressed and significant improvement in survival compared with 5-FU/LV alone [Reviewed in Ref.18]. For this reason, since 2000, the irinotecan/5-FU/LV regimen has been the most widely used front-line chemotherapy in North America for patients with metastatic colorectal cancer [61].

Table 2: Current recommended combinations regiments in the treatment of advanced colon cancer.

Treatment arms	Patients (n)	Response rates (%)	Median survival (months)	Ref.
CPT-11/5-FU/LV	231	39	14.8	
5-FU/LV	226	21	12.6	[69]
CPT-11	226	18	12.0	
CPT-11/5-FU/LV	199	41	17.4	
5-FU/LV	188	23	14.1	[70]
OXA/5-FU/LV	210	50	16.2	
5-FU/LV	210	21.9	14.7	[72]
OXA/5-FU/LV	100	53	19.4	
5-FU/LV	100	16	19.9	[73]

CPT-11 = Irinotecan; 5-FU = 5-Fluorouracil; LV = Leucovorin; OXA = Oxaliplatin.

Several studies with different schedules of irinotecan/5-FU/LV are under investigation for identify a more practical and tolerable treatment option [71]. For instance, a biweekly irinotecan/5-FU/LV regimen was assessed in 28 patients with advanced colorectal cancer. One treatment cycle consisted of irinotecan (180 mg/m^2) on days 1 and 15; 5-FU (425 mg/m^2) on days 1,2, 15 and 16; and LV (20 mg/m^2) on days 1,2,15,16, every 4 weeks. The overall response rate of 21.5% was achieved, and toxicities were mild and manageable [71].

Oxaliplatin

Oxaliplatin (Eloxatin®; trans-*l*-diaminocyclohexane oxaloplatinum; L-OHP) is a third generation platinum compound that has shown promise in advanced colorectal cancers (Table 2) and is used widely in Europe [72,73]. Oxaliplatin undergoes nonenzymatic conversion of the labile oxalate ligand to several transient reactive species that covalently bind with macromolecules in physiologic solutions. This type of binding produces both inter- and intra-strand Pt-DNA cross-links (Figure 4) that result in the inhibition of DNA replication and transcription that is cell-cycle nonspecific [74].

Clinical testing of oxaliplatin more than one decade later revealed its meaningful antitumor activity and favorable toxicity profile. Indeed, oxaliplatin proved effective in colorectal cancer both as first-line and as second-line treatment of 5-FU-refractory tumors [75]. A phase II evaluation of oxaliplatin alone confirmed its therapeutic efficacy against advanced colorectal carcinoma. For instance, oxaliplatin 130 mg/m^2 every 21 days produced 9 partial responses (24.3%) among 38 previously untreated patients with metastatic colorectal carcinoma, with response duration of 216 days [75]. Disease stabilization was noted in 15 patients (40.5%), and 13 patients progressed (35.2%). The main side effect was peripheral sensory neuropathy, but hematologic and gastrointestinal toxicities were mild. The results from two other clinical trials with oxaliplatin 130 mg/m^2 q 21 days in chemotherapy-naive patients were in agreement with those from the latter study, showing 20% objective responses and 32% stable diseases among 25 patients [77], an overall response rate of 18% among 63 patients, and a median overall survival of 13-14 months [reviewed in Ref. 78]. These data suggested that oxaliplatin monotherapy might be considered as first-line treatment of advanced colorectal carcinoma.

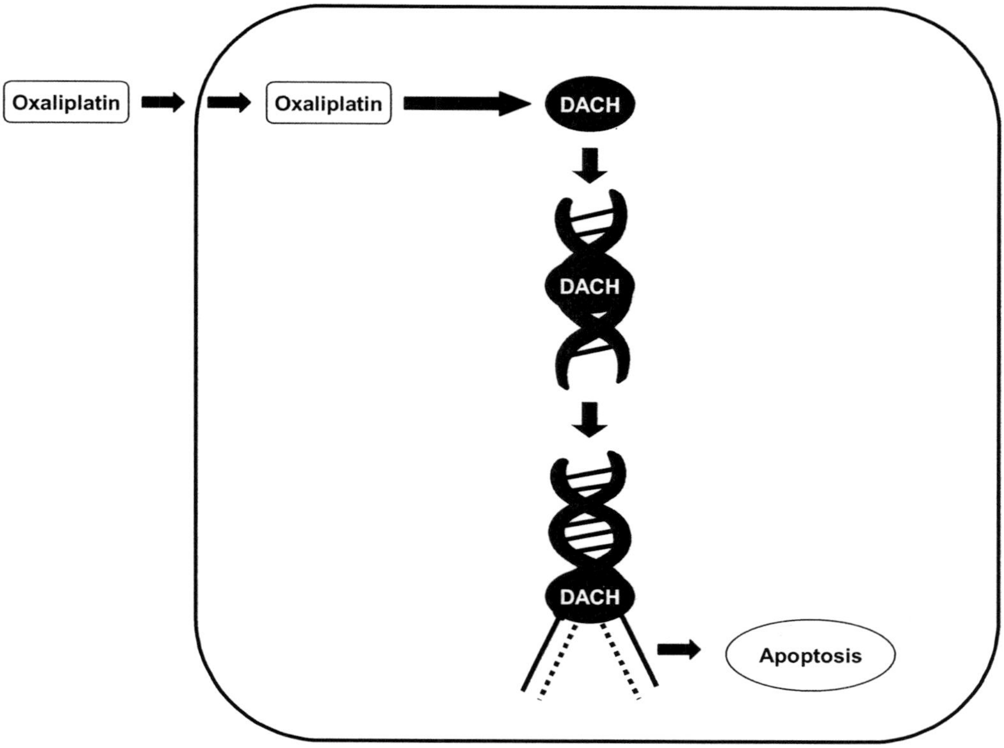

Figure 4: Mechanism of action of oxaliplatin.

Oxaliplatin/ 5-Fluorouracil/Leucovorin

Oxaliplatin is indicated for use only in combination with infusional 5-fluorouracil/LV for the treatment of patients with metastatic carcinoma of the colon or rectum whose disease has recurred or progressed during or within 6 months of completion of first-line therapy (a combination of irinotecan and bolus 5-FU/LV) [79].

Studies to assess the benefits of the addition of oxaliplatin to 5-FU/LV were initiated following the observation that this combination acted synergistically *in vitro* as well as *in vivo* murine models [80]. These studies enrolled chemotherapy-naive and 5-FU-pretreated patients, and were performed according to various trial designs, such as one-armed phase II trials, two-armed phase III trials, and compassionate-use programs.

The results from these studies were comparable with regard to the efficacy and the tolerability of the combination of oxaliplatin/5-FU/LV. Response rates, progression-free survival, and overall survival were consistently and significantly higher with oxaliplatin/5-FU/LV when compared with 5-FU/LV alone. The main problem with the addition of oxaliplatin to 5-FU/LV was diarrhea, which was probably related to a cumulative effect of both drugs, but could be managed [73,81]. Peripheral neuropathy is the dose-limiting toxicity, which could be reversible [82]. These data led to proposals to use the oxaliplatin/5-FU/LV combination as first- or second-line treatment against advanced colorectal carcinoma, as well as against liver metastases associated with the disease [73,81]. Indications for the applicability of oxaliplatin/5-FU/LV as second- or third-line treatment of colorectal carcinoma came from various studies evaluating this combination in patients with metastatic colorectal carcinoma who were refractory to 5-FU and/or irinotecan, or who progressed while on a second 5-FU-based therapy [81].

An important phase III study [72] investigated the effect of combining oxaliplatin with 5-FU/LV, with progression-free survival as the primary end point. For that purpose 420 previously untreated patients with measurable disease were randomized to receive a 2-hour infusion of LV 200 mg/m^2 daily, followed by a 5-FU bolus 400 mg/m^2 daily, and 22-hour infusion 600 mg/m^2 daily for 2 consecutive days, every 2 weeks, either alone or together with oxaliplatin 85 mg/m^2 as a 2-hour infusion on day 1. Patients allocated to oxaliplatin plus 5-FU/LV had significantly longer progression-free survival (9.0 months versus 6.2 months) and better response rate (50.7% *vs* 22.3%) when compared with the control arm. The improvement in overall survival did not reach significance (16.2 months versus 14.7 months).

In another phase III study [73] 200 patients were randomly assigned to receive a 5-day course of chronomodulated 5-FU/LV (700 and 300 mg/m^2 daily, respectively) with or without oxaliplatin (125 mg/m^2) on the first day of each course. The treatment was repeated every 21 days. Oxaliplatin improved response rates (53% *vs* 16%) and median progression-free survival (8.7 *vs* 6.1 months), with no improvement in median survival (19.9 *vs* 19.4 months).

The oxaliplatin/5-FU/LV combination seems beneficial as first-line therapy in advanced colorectal cancer. In France, oxaliplatin with infusional 5-FU/LV combinations was approved as second line treatment in 1996 and first line in 1998. European Union approval first line was obtained in 1999, while in USA this combination was approved as second line in 2002 [72,73]. In a randomized controlled trial comparing oxaliplatin/5-FU/LV combination with irinotecan/5-FU/LV combination in 795 patients with metastatic colorectal cancer who had not been treated previously, oxaliplatin/5-FU/LV regimen showed superior response rates (45% *vs* 31%) and median survival time (19.5 *vs* 15.0 months) than irinotecan/5-FU/LV combination [83].

New Agents in Advanced Colorectal Carcinoma

Despite the greater clinical efficacy of 5-FU plus LV over 5-FU alone, it did not lead to significant improvements in survival rates, and relapses continued to be the rule. The same held true for combinations of 5-FU/LV with irinotecan or oxaliplatin [18,52]. Therefore, in the last few decades, much interest was put in the search for alternative ways of administration, e.g. as a prodrug and for more efficacious agents for the treatment of advanced, 5-FU-refractory colorectal carcinoma.

Oral Fluoropyrimidines

Several studies demonstrated that oral fluoropyrimidines and intravenous fluoropyrimidines are equally active [84]. The results of these studies led to development of three active oral drugs: capecitabine, UFT and eniluracil. These three drugs have been completed phase III clinical trials as first line treatment for advanced colorectal carcinoma (Table 3).

Table 3: New agents in advanced colon carcinoma in phase III studies.

Treatment arms	Patients (n)	Response rates (%)	Median overall survival (months)	Ref.
Capecitabine	302	25.8	12.5	[86]
Bolus 5-FU/LV	303	11.6	13.3	
Capecitabine	301	18.9	13.2	[87]
Bolus 5-FU/LV	301	15.0	12.1	
UFT/LV	409	12.0	12.4	[93]
Bolus 5-FU/LV	407	15.0	13.4	
UFT/LV	190	11.0	12.2	[96]
Bolus 5-FU/LV	190	9.0	10.3	
Eniluracil/5-FU	485	12.2	13.3	[97]
Bolus 5-FU/LV	479	12.7	14.5	
Raltitrexed/5-FU	439	19.0	10.1	[101]
Bolus 5-FU/LV	439	17.0	12.2	

5-FU = 5-Fluorouracil; LV = Leucovorin.

Capecitabine (Xeloda®; N^4-pentoxycarbonyl-5'-deoxy-5-fluorocytidine) is an oral fluoropyrimidine carbamate that was approved for the treatment of metastatic colorectal cancer in April 2001. It was designed as an inactive precursor that passes intact through the intestinal mucosa and is sequentially converted to 5'-deoxy-5-fluorocytidine (5'-DFCR), 5'-deoxy-5-fluorouridine (5'-DFUR) and finally 5-FU in the liver and tumor tissues selectively [85]. In two-phase III studies this agent has been shown to have equivalent survival to bolus 5-FU/LV in advanced colorectal cancer [86,87]. In addition, the oral regimen was associated with significantly less toxicity [88]. The moderate toxicity of capecitabine (above all its low incidence of neutropenia) makes it a suitable candidate for novel combination therapies involving other agents that are active in colorectal cancer, including irinotecan and oxaliplatin [89]. Capecitabine seems to be synergistic with irinotecan in a recent phase I study of patients with metastatic colorectal cancer [90]. A randomized multicenter phase II trial of irinotecan with capecitabine demonstrated that this combination was a highly active first-line treatment in advanced colorectal cancer [91]. In a randomized phase II trial capecitabine plus oxaliplatin showed substantial antitumor activity in patients with previously untreated advanced colorectal cancer [82].

UFT (Orzel®), another oral fluoropyrimidine, is a combination of uracil and tegafur (1-[2-tetrahydrofuranyl]-5-FU, ftorafur) in a fixed molar ratio of 4:1 [92]. Tegafur is a prodrug of 5-FU and is completely and rapidly absorbed after oral administration. After the absorption it is hydroxylated and converted to 5-FU by the hepatic microsomal P450 enzymes. Uracil inhibits the dihydropyrimidine dehydrogenase (DPD) the main catabolic enzyme of 5-FU. This prevents degradation of 5-FU, ensuring elevated concentrations of 5-FU in the body [93]. The inhibition of DPD, allows tegafur absorption and to increase the plasma concentrations of 5-FU [88]. Two-phase III trials in patients with advanced colorectal cancer have been reported that UFT/LV demonstrated equivalence in activity and in survival compared with intravenous 5-FU/LV [92,93]. Aside the efficacy, UFT/LV resulted in significantly less grade 3/4 stomatitis, neutropenia, and infections compared with bolus 5-FU/LV [93]. The most common reported factor for patient preference was the possibility of the UFT to be taken at home. Despite this UFT/LV has not gained approval in USA yet [94]. UFT/LV has also been investigated in combination with both irinotecan and oxaliplatin, and recently presented data suggest that both of these combinations are feasible. In a phase I/II trial of irinotecan plus UFT/leucovorin as first-line therapy in 33 patients with advanced or metastatic colorectal cancer, the dose-limiting toxicities included diarrhea and febrile neutropenia [95]. Preliminary efficacy results were promising.

Eniluracil (5-Ethynyluracil; GW776), a uracil analogue, is a highly irreversibly inhibitor of DPD. Administration of eniluracil with 5-FU significantly increases the oral bioavailability of 5-FU to 100%, promoting a uniform absorption and predictable toxicity. Although eniluracil is neither toxic nor active as a single agent in animals, it improves the antitumor efficacy and therapeutic index of 5-FU [92]. One phase III trial with eniluracil/5-FU has been demonstrated similar survival rates when compared with bolus 5-FU/LV [96]. However in another study patients treated with eniluracil/5-FU showed inferior overall survival than 5-FU/LV [97]. Eniluracil is a promising drug, which has the potential to overcome 5-FU resistance mediated by overexpression of DPD; the clinical development of eniluracil/5-FU needs more investigation.

Phase I and II trials combining Capecitabine or UFT with irinotecan or oxaliplatin are now ongoing. However, it is too early to know whether the oral fluoropyrimidines will be able to replace 5-FU/LV in combination with irinotecan or oxaliplatin [94].

TS Inhibitors

Raltitrexed (Tomudex®; ZD1694), a water-soluble quinazoline antifolate, is a direct and specific TS inhibitor, without secondary effects on RNA or protein synthesis. Prolonged TS inhibition is reached by rapid polyglutamylation of folates and its subsequent retention in cells [98]. In three phase III trials, patients with advanced colorectal cancer were randomized between Raltitrexed and a bolus 5-FU/LV [99-101]. These studies demonstrated similar median survival for Raltitrexed and bolus 5-FU/LV in two studies, but inferior survival was found for Raltitrexed and 5-FU/LV in another. The major side effects from Raltitrexed are gastrointestinal, hematological and asthenia [101]. Raltitrexed is approval as monotherapy, at a dose of 3.0 mg/m^2 every 3 weeks, for the first-line treatment of advanced colorectal cancer. A number of phase I and phase II trials have been performed with the combination of Raltitrexed and 5-FU or irinotecan or oxaliplatin. Phase II studies have shown a remarkable activity of some of these combinations [102]. Phase III studies (Table 3) comparing 5-FU/LV with Raltitrexed /5-FU showed similar dose response rates as well as overall survival [98]. For current use of these combinations in clinical practice, randomized phase III studies are necessary.

Thymitaq (Nolatrexed®; AG337); is a lipophilic antifolate that does not require activation by folylpolyglutamate synthetase (FPGS), and does not require transport into cells by the reduced folate carrier (RFC) [98]. This would yield the theoretical advantage of circumvention of resistance mechanisms involving low FPGS and/or low RCF expression. Thymitaq has a greater potency in terms of TS inhibition. In phase II studies, AG337 displayed modest activity in untreated head and neck cancer patients [103].

ALIMTA (Pemetrexed®; LY231514) is a potent novel antifolate, which inhibits three folate-dependent reactions that are essential for cell proliferation. Its primary target is TS but it also inhibits dihydrofolate reductase and glycinamide ribonucleotide formyltransferase [104]. In a phase II trial, ALIMTA has shown about 16% overall response rate in untreated patients with colorectal carcinoma, and the dose-limiting toxic effect is neutropenia [98]. The response rates with single-agent ALIMTA in patients with colorectal carcinoma are comparable to those with bolus 5-FU/LV [105].

Novel Agents and Targets

Various new agents acting in different targets are in pre-clinical and early clinical investigation in colorectal carcinoma. These agents include the vascular endothelial cell growth factor inhibitors, the epidermal growth factor inhibitors, and the Cox-2 inhibitors

Vascular Endothelial Cell Growth Factor and Vascular Endothelial Cell Growth Factor Receptor Inhibitors

Tumor angiogenesis is the process leading to the formation of blood vessels within a tumor and plays a key role in the growth and metastases of many cancers. New blood vessels are required to provide a sufficient oxygen and nutrient supply to the growing tumor as well as initiating invasion and metastasis. Growth factors and growth inhibitors are known to regulate angiogenesis. The vascular endothelial growth factor (VEGF) plays a crucial role in promoting angiogenesis (Figure 5), and it is the target of innovative anti-cancer therapies [106]. Inhibition of angiogenesis may stop tumor growth and decrease metastatic potential [107].

Colorectal cancer has been shown to express elevated level of VEGF. In this type of tumor, an increase in the VEGF expression has been correlated with metastasis and poor prognosis [106]. It was demonstrated that patients with low VEGF expression had a significantly better survival than patients with high VEGF expression [107]. VEGF binds to two distinct receptors on endothelial VEGFR-1 (Flt-1) and VEGFR-2 (Flk-1/KDR) [108]. Disruption of cellular signaling through the VEGF/VEGFR pathway represents an attractive target for therapy. A series of studies have attempted to determine the role of VEGF in angiogenesis, metastasis, and proliferation of human colon cancer [107]. A variety of small molecules tyrosine kinase inhibitors with antiangiogenic activity are in preclinica and clinical investigation [109]. SU5416 Z-3- [(2,4-dimethylpyrrol-5-yl)methylidenyl]-2-indolinone) is a small molecule inhibitor of the VEGFR-2 signaling pathway, which demonstrated potent activity in preclinical studies [107,110]. ZD6474, is an anilinoquinazoline derivative with an inhibitory activity on VEGFR-2, which significantly inhibits tumor growth in a wide range of established human cancer xenografts in nude mice and is currently in Phase I clinical trials [111,112].

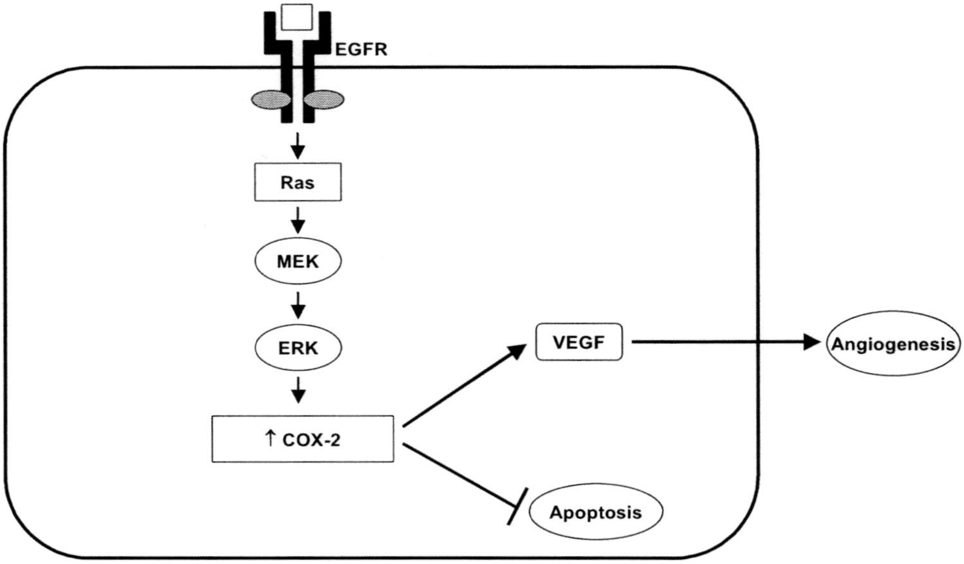

Figure 5: Role of epidermal growth factor receptor (EGFR), vascular endothelial growth factor (VEGF) and cyclooxygenase-2 (Cox-2) in tumor progression.

In addition, antibodies targeting VEGF have been tested alone and combined with chemotherapy. Among these, Bevacizumab (Avastin®; beh-vah-SIH-zoo-mab), a recombinant humanized monoclonal antibody to VEGF is under investigation in non-small cell lung, breast, prostate, renal, and colorectal tumors. In phase I trials, Avastin was in general, well tolerated and did not display dose-limiting toxicity [113,114]. In a randomized phase II trial the safety and efficacy of Avastin plus 5-FU/LV *vs* 5-FU/LV alone as first-line treatment for metastatic colorectal cancer was investigated [115]. This study demonstrated that Avastin combined with 5-FU/LV, increases response rate (24% to 40% *vs* 17%), prolongs time to disease progression (7.2 to 9.0 months *vs* 5.2 months), and prolongs median survival (16.1 to 21.5 months *vs* 13.8 months) compared to 5-FU/LV alone [115]. There are two phase III trials ongoing comparing 5-FU/LV/irinotecan with either 5-FU/LV/irinotecan/Avastin or 5-FU/LV/Avastin.

Epidermal Growth Factor Receptor Inhibitors

Tumor growth depends on the activation of cell membrane receptors that control the intracellular signal transduction pathways for proliferation, adhesion and motility [116]. Epidermal growth factor receptor (EGFR) overexpression (Figure 5) has frequently been correlated with poor response to treatment, disease progression and poor survival [116,117]. Approximately 70% of colorectal carcinomas have been shown to express the EGFR [118], and this expression was shown to be higher in tumors of more advanced stage [119,120]. Despite conflicting results, it has been shown that expression of EGFR correlates with a reduction in disease-free survival, increase in risk of recurrence and metastases, and advanced tumor stage [17,121]. EGFR expression correlates with the ability of colorectal cancer cells to produce hepatic metastases [121]. Inhibition of EGFR signaling with an EGF antibody is accompanied by a reduction in the level and activity of DNA-dependent protein kinase in the nucleous, resulting in a tumor regression [122]. EGF-inhibitors under development are the monoclonal antibody Cetuximab [123,124] and the EGF receptor-tyrosine kinase inhibitor ZD1839 [123,124].

Cetuximab (Erbitux®; IMC-C225) is an IgG1 monoclonal antibody that targets EGFR with a high affinity, preventing the ligand from interacting with the receptor [116,123,124]. It has a higher affinity for the EGFR than either TGF-α or EGF and effectively blocks ligand-induced EGFR phosphorylation. The binding of Cetuximab to EGFR blocks ligand-induced EGFR signaling and results in the inhibition of proliferation, angiogenesis and stimulation of apoptosis [116]. Cetuximab has been shown to inhibit the growth of human colon carcinoma by disrupting the EGFR- mediated signal transduction [126]. Preclinical studies have shown that cetuximab has remarkable activity in colorectal tumor model systems *in vitro* and *in vivo* [124,126]. Both animal studies and human xenografts have shown that Cetuximab enhances the antitumor effects of cytotoxic agents including cisplatin and topotecan when given in combination [121,127]. In a colorectal tumor models in nude mice combining Cetuximab with irinotecan, it was demonstrated an enhanced antitumor activity with the combination of Cetuximab with irinotecan therapy compared with irinotecan or Cetuximab treatment alone [126]. Initial clinical trials demonstrated that Cetuximab showed complete and partial responses in patients who had relapsed to chemotherapy. In addition, this antibody appears to enhance the activity of chemotherapeutic agents [127]. Cetuximab is currently in Phases II and III clinical testing in a number of malignancies overexpressing EGFR [128]. In a randomized phase II trial in 329 patients with EGFR-expressing metastatic colorectal cancer, Cetuximab was evaluated combined with irinotecan. In this study 218 patients received Cetuximab plus irinotecan and 111 patients Cetuximab alone. The response rates (23% *vs* 11%) and median survival time (8.6 *vs* 6.0 months) was higher with Cetuximab plus irinotecan than Cetuximab alone [129]. This antibody is well tolerated, lacks the hematological toxicity [130] commonly associated with the most anticancer agents, and does not intensify the toxicity of the common chemotherapeutic drugs [123].

ZD1839 (Iressa®, Gefitinib), an anilinoquinazoline orally active, selective inhibitor of EGFR, that block signaling pathways responsible for proliferation, invasion, and survival of cancer cells [125]. Several studies have correlated EGFR activation with the ability to stimulate normal endothelial cell growth through paracrine mechanisms and to up-regulate VEGF production in human cancer cells at the transcription levels [131,132]. In this regard, it was demonstrated that ZD1839 is also able to inhibit VEGF expression and neoangiogenesis *in vitro* an in nude mice xenografts [133]. In addition to have activity against several human xenograft models, including colorectal carcinoma, ZD1839 exhibited an additive effect when combined with a variety of cytotoxic drugs *in vitro* [134,135]. For instance, ZD1839 in combination with irinotecan generated supra-additive inhibitory effect in COLO320DM, WiDr and Lovo human colorectal cancer cell lines [136]. In a phase I trial, ZD1839 has shown promising clinical activity in patients with a variety of tumors types [137]. A phase I/II trial of ZD1839 with 5-FU/LV has been performed [138], and shown that this combination can be safely administered with promising antitumor efficacy.

Cyclooxygenase-2 Inhibitors

Cyclooxygenase is an enzyme that is responsible for the conversion of arachidonic acid into prostaglandins. There are two isoforms: Cox-1 and Cox-2. Cox-1 is a constitutive form, while Cox-2 is expressed only after stimulation via numerous growth factors, cytokines and mitogens [35,139]. Recent studies have demonstrated that activation of receptor tyrosine kinase such as EGFR may induce Cox-2 expression [140]. Overexpression of Cox-2 is also involved in cancer cell proliferation, induction of neoangiogenesis, increased invasiveness and metastases [36,37,41,141-143]. These events may be responsible for the worse prognostic observed in patients with different types of cancer overexpressing Cox-2 [37,140]. Studies with this enzyme led to development of drugs known as non-steroidal anti-inflammatory drugs (NSAIDs). In addition to the anti-inflammatory properties of NSAIDs, anticancer activity has been observed [reviewed in ref. 36]. Various NSAIDs, such aspirin, sulindac, have shown anticancer properties in animal models [144].

Recently celecoxib (Celebrex®) has been tested in a xenograft models and shown to have a dose-dependent effect on growth inhibition [145]. Combination chemotherapy is known to be a beneficial strategy in cancer treatment. The addition of Cox-2 inhibitor may enhance the effects of current chemotherapeutic regimens [144]. A phase I trial using sulindac and 5-FU in 15 patients with advanced colorectal cancer, which had been refractory to 5-FU treatment, demonstrated a potential benefit [146]. These results suggest that celecoxib may add to responses obtained from chemotherapy and decrease some of its drug toxicities. Celecoxib was evaluated combined with capecitabine and demonstrated an increased tumor response, proportion of stable disease (62.5% *vs* 22.8%), and increase in median time to tumor progression (6 *vs* 3 months) compared with capecitabine alone. It is also observed that celecoxib appeared to attenuate capecitabine-induced hand-foot syndrome [147]. More recently a second generation of Cox-2 inhibitors has been developed. Among these, Valdecoxib (Bextra®), Parecoxib (Dynastat®), have been made available [148]. The specific mechanism of action as anticancer agents for Cox-2 remains unclear [36]. However an impact of these agents in apoptosis [149,150] and angiogenesis [151] has been observed (Figure 5). Additionally, there is evidence that Cox-2 inhibitors have effects on cellular proliferation and adhesion [150,152]. The combination of a selective Cox-2 inhibitor SC-236 with the selective EGFR tyrosine kinase inhibitor ZD1839 in human colon and breast cancer cells, demonstrated an antitumor activity as well as a down regulation of the Cox-2 and VEGF expression [153].

Chemoprevention of colorectal cancer requires the administration of agents to prevent either the development of precancerous polyps or the progression of polyps to invasive disease [154]. Aspirin and sulindac showed the ability to suppress the development of intestinal polyps in a mouse model, with defective *APC* gene, similar to that found in FAP patients [155,156]. In another murine model of FAP, sulindac in combination with a inhibitor of EGFR, conferred protection from development of intestinal neoplasia [157]. A large number of epidemiological studies have shown that regular use of aspirin results in a 40-50% decreased risk of colorectal cancer [141,158]. Celecoxib inhibited the incidence of colon tumors by 93% in rat colon tumor [159]. A recent study with 77 individuals with FAP, demonstrated that celecoxib reduced the mean number of colonic polyps in 28% [160]. Based on these studies the FDA has recently approved the use of celecoxib as a chemopreventive therapy in patients with FAP [161].

PROGNOSTIC MARKERS IN COLORECTAL CANCER

The efficacy of chemotherapy is limited by a number of disparities in response and toxicity by different individual. Such variations are frequently initiated by genetic alterations. A series of genetic alterations (Table 4) are prognostic markers in colorectal cancer [32], and can predict survival after chemotherapy [30,162]. Predictive markers that direct the selection of the accurate chemotherapy regimen would benefit the responses for adjuvant therapy.

Table 4: Promising molecular markers for colorectal carcinoma.

Marker	Gene alteration	Function of wild-type gene	Prognostic in colorectal cancer with gene mutation
Loss of heterozigosity at chromossome 18q	*DCC*	Caspase substrate in apoptosis; cell adhesion molecule; tumor suppressor	Adverse prognostic
Loss of heterozigosity at chromossome 17q	*p53*	Transcription factor; regulator of cell cycle progression, apoptosis, gene expression and DNA repair; tumor suppressor	Adverse prognostic
Microsatellite instability	*MMR*	Repair of nucleotide mismatches	Favorable prognostic
Mutation in bax gene	*BAX*	Proapoptosis	Adverse prognostic

MMR = mismatch repair genes, DCC=deleted in colon cancer gene.

In several studies loss of heterozygosity at 18q was an indicator of a poor prognosis in patients with stage II and III cancer [32,163]. In colorectal cancer, loss of *DCC* is associated with metastasis and inhibition of apoptosis led to an adverse prognosis [164-166]. Loss of *DCC* as a result of loss of 18q could impair apoptosis, thereby conferring resistance to chemotherapy. Based on these observations it has been suggested that loss of heterozygosity at 18q may be a specific marker for survival [30]. Although alterations of *p53* are a plausible predictive marker [167-169] there are studies in which no significant relation between survival and *p53* status were observed [170]. It is believed that all cases of FAP or its variants are a result from germline alterations in the *APC* gene [171]. Based on this a number of investigations have been done in attempt to correlate the mutations in *APC* gene with risk and prognostic for colorectal carcinoma. Polymorphisms in the *APC* (I1307K and E1317Q) are associated with an increased risk for colorectal cancer. For instance, I1307K polymorphism occurs exclusively in Ashkenazi Jewish descendents and result in a 2-fold increased risk for adenocarcinomas compared with general population [172,173].

Microsatellite instability (MSI) in tumors from patients with hereditary non-polyposis colorectal cancer (HNPCC) is caused by germline mutations in mismatch repair (MMR) genes, principally hMSH2 and hMLH1, as mentioned in the beginning of this chapter. Tumors with high MSI are associated with a less aggressive clinical course and better prognosis [174]. MSI may impart a favorable prognosis in colorectal cancer. In clinical studies colorectal cancers demonstrating MSI respond better to chemotherapy while in vitro studies using MSI positive cell lines show resistance to chemotherapy. Based on these findings, MSI may be a useful genetic marker in prognosis and could be an influential factor in deciding treatment options [175].

Furthermore, the identification of critical roles of various factors related to drug activity, cell death or cell growth inhibition in resistance and sensitivity of anticancer agents will modify the response for chemotherapy. For instance, oncogenes, tumor suppressor genes, as well as activity and expression of TS and DPD can play a role in increase response rates to chemotherapeutic agents by better section of patient [34].

A number of studies postulated that high TS levels are responsible for the resistance to TS inhibitors, either fluoropyrimidines or antifolates. However, contradictory data were observed in studies on metastatic disease and adjuvant treatment [176]. Early data with patient material suggested a relation between TS inhibition and response to 5-FU therapy. Spears *et al.* [177] reported that the ratio between FdUMP and dUMP (as a measured for TS inhibition) was higher in patients with gastrointestinal cancer who responded to 5-FU therapy than those who did not. In patients not responding to hepatic artery infusion of 5-FU, total TS activity was significantly higher than in responding patients [178,179]. In the same study incorporation of 5-FU into RNA was not related to response [179]. Besides enzymatic TS levels, TS-mRNA levels are predictive indicators for response to 5-FU therapy. In 46 patients with metastatic colorectal cancer treated with protracted-5-FU infusion, a high TS-mRNA level was significantly correlated with poor response [180]. Patients with low TS-mRNA level responded to 5-FU-based chemotherapy and survival in these patients was significant longer [181]. In patients with liver metastasis from colorectal cancer the TS-mRNA level was measured with RT-PCR. In 29 patients a low TS level was significantly related to response to 5-FU-based hepatic artery infusion [176].

It was also observed that TS may function as a biomarker for the malignant potential of each tumor independent of 5-FU treatment [182]. In a study of 86 patients with colorectal carcinoma, high TS levels measured by immunostaining with an anti-TS polyclonal AB, were correlated with shorter survival [183]. Subgroup analysis to correlate chemotherapy response to TS levels was not significant because the groups were too small [183].

Besides the above mentioned studies reporting correlation between TS levels and response to 5-FU-based chemotherapy regimens, negative studies have also been reported (Table 5). In another study TS levels were measured with polyclonal TS antibody in biopsies of primary colon tumors of 134 patients who were treated with 5-FU or a folate-based TS inhibitor ZD1694 for advanced metastatic disease. In this very heterogeneous patient group, no significant relationship between TS levels and response to therapy could be observed. This result was possibly related to the observation that primary tumors are different from their metastasis [185].

Table 5. Thymidylate Synthase as a prognostic parameter for survival and as a predictive marker of response to chemotherapy in clinical studies.

Tumor Type	Patients (n)	Chemo-therapy	Methods[1]	Correlation with Survival[2]	Correlation with Response	Ref.
mCRC	40	5FU intrahepatic	Biochemical	yes	high TS worse	[178, 179]
mCRC	46	protracted-5FU infusion	RT-PCR	yes	high TS worse	[181]
mCRC	29	5FU intrahepatic	RT-PCR	no	high TS worse	[176]
mCRC	86	mitomycin C + 5FU	Polyclonal-TS AB	yes	no	[183]
colon cancer	134	5FU or ZD1694	Polyclonal TS AB	no	no	[184]

[1]Methods for TS level detection: biochemical measurement of TS activity, TS mRNA level detected by RT-PCR, TS expression by immunostaining. mCRC = metastatic colorectal cancer; AB = antibody.
[2] Yes = High TS expression significantly related to worse survival.

Recent studies [183,186,187] showed that, patients with tumors expressing low TS had no or only marginal benefits of adjuvant 5-FU-based chemotherapy both with respect to overall and recurrence-free survival. Compared with surgery alone, adjuvant chemotherapy prolonged the survival of patients with high TS levels, whereas there was no such survival prolongation by adjuvant chemotherapy for patients with low TS levels. There was also an increase in the 5-year survival rate in patients with chemotherapy and high TS expression level compared with patients with chemotherapy and low TS [186]. These results indicate that patients with high TS levels may profit from the presently used adjuvant chemotherapy regimens.

The above mentioned studies focused on TS as a target for chemotherapy and its relationship with prognosis and clinical outcome. More recently several groups tried to elucidate the molecular events leading to cell death and whether or not these are determinants of prognosis and response to chemotherapy. One of the most studied tumor suppressor gene is p53 and the activation of wild-type p53 is of importance for drug (e.g. 5-FU) induced cell death. p53 is inducible by DNA damage resulting in activated wild-type p53, which can arrest the cell cycle so DNA repair can occur [188,189]. Activated wild-type p53 induces various targets including cyclin G, damage response genes Gadd45 and ERCC3, the cell cycle kinase inhibitor $p21^{cip1/waf1}$ and bax, a cell death promoting gene. p53 is mutated in a high number of cancers with disruption of the protection mechanism to DNA damage as a result [190]. In 36 patients with advanced colorectal cancer a high incidence of p53 mutations detected by sequencing was related to poor response to 5-FU based chemotherapy. 19% of the patients with mutant p53 responded compared to 50% of the patients with wild type p53. When TS mRNA expression was included high TS mRNA and mutant p53 were poor prognostic factors for response; none of the patients with these characteristics responded to 5-FU based chemotherapy. Besides predicting for response for 5-FU based therapy the combination of high TS levels and mutant p53 also predicted recurrence in this patient group [191,192]. Another study reported on the relationship between p53, p21 and TS in patients with rectal cancer. Thirty-four patients with stage II and III rectal cancer were retrospectively analyzed for their level of p53, p21 and TS as measured with immunostaining. The authors hypothesized that patients with tumors with wild-type p53 (= no p53 overexpression) with subsequent p21 upregulation and low TS expression should benefit from the adjuvant chemoirradiation regimen. In this small study 32% of the patients with p53 overexpression recurred, 40% of the patients without p21 expression recurred and 31% of the patients with high TS expression recurred [193]. Another study in 30 patients with rectal cancer related TS and p53 protein expression to response. No relationship between TS expression and response was observed, whereas wild-type p53 protein expression was related to response to 5-FU-based chemo-radiotherapy [194]. In patients with colon cancer stage II or III p53 (n=164) and TS (n=141) levels were determined by immunohistochemical staining. These patients were randomized according to two arms one with surgery alone and the other arm with surgery combined with adjuvant 5-FU/LV. TS and p53 expression predicted for disease free survival but not for efficacy of 5-FU/LV adjuvant therapy in these patients [195]. In patients with advanced colorectal cancer treated with a regimen of alternating bolus 5-FU, modulated by methotrexate and continuous 5-FU modulated with LV no association between p53 expression in tumor samples and response to 5-FU-based chemotherapy could be measured [196].

In addition to TS protein expression, TS gene polymorphisms have been found to potentially predict clinical effect, toxicity or risk to develop cancer. Large groups of patients have been evaluated for the prognostic and predictive value of genetic polymorphisms. TS mRNA has a unique tandemly repeated sequence in the 5'UTR, which is polymorphic [197]. A triple repeat has been postulated to be associated with a higher TS expression than a double repeat. This tandem repeat possibly controls the expression of TS protein, since in 52 patients with a 3R/3R (triple tandem repeat) the TS mRNA/TS protein (FdUMP binding assay) ratio was about 2 times higher than in 5 patients with a 2R/2R (homogenous double repeat) or 35 patients with a 2R/3R genotype. However, TS mRNA expression was comparable. In an in vitro transcription system with a luciferase reporter construct it was demonstrated that RNA with the three-repeat sequence was translated three to four times more efficiently than that with the two-repeat sequence. However, in a panel of 16 cell lines, cells with a triple repeat sequence did not have a higher TS mRNA expression, TS protein or TS activity than cells with a double repeat, while induction of resistance did not change the polymorphisms from a double to a triple repeat [198].

These data indicate that this TS polymorphism is a somatic property, which can however be influenced by allelic loss [199]. TS polymorphisms have now been evaluated as a risk factor in developing cancer or leukemia, as a risk factor in developing toxicity in antifolate therapy, and as a prognostic factor for outcome of treatment. In addition, ethnic differences have been described for the presence of triple repeats. In Asians (both Japanese and Chinese) the occurrence of the 2R/3R and 3R/3R genotype is much higher (60%), while higher repeats (4R and 5R) are not uncommon [197,200,201]. In Caucasians this occurrence is about 29% [202]. Next to the triple repeat in the 5'UTR, an additional 6-bp deletion (TS1494del6) in the 3'UTR region may affect RNA stability.

Ulrich *et al.* [203] investigated the occurrence of TS polymorphisms, folate intake and the risk of colorectal carcinoma in a case control study of 510 patients with adenomatomous polyps and 604 polyp-free individuals, but the incidence was comparable. However, persons with a 3R/3R polymorphism and a high folate intake (>440 μg/day) showed a decreased risk compared to those with a lower intake (odds ratio 1.0 vs 0.5), while in the 2R/2R group high folate intake was associated with an increased risk (odds ratio 0.6 vs. 0.9; p=0.03). For another polymorphism, a 6-bp deletion no clear pattern was found. Skibola *et al.* [204] observed that the occurrence of a 2R/3R or 2R/2R was associated with a higher chance to get adult acute lymphoblastic leukemia (ALL) than 3R/3R. The risk was even further reduced (13.9-fold) when the 3R/3R genotype was associated with a CT/TT genotype for serine hydroxymethyltransferase. It was hypothesized that uracil misincorporation resulting in chromosomal damage may play a role in the pathogenesis of ALL, and that genetic interactions involving low penetrance polymorphisms in folate-metabolizing genes may increase ALL risk.

A number of studies have been published examining the relation between polymorphisms and outcome of treatment. In colon cancer it was demonstrated in a small group of patients that ¾ patients with a 2R/2R genotype responded to capecitabine, compared to 1/12 and 2/8 with a 2R/3R and 3R/3R genotype [205]. Interesting data were also observed in ALL, which is frequently been treated with methotrexate. Krajinovic *et al.* [206] observed that in a group of 205 patients those with a 3R/3R genotype had a shorter event-free median survival than patients with a 2R/2R genotype (odd ratio 0.2, p<0.005). Genetic polymorphisms for folate-metabolizing enzymes may also play a role in other diseases such as rheumatoid arthritis [203]. Pretreatment analysis of genetic polymorphisms may become an essential part in the future planning of treatment, especially in combinations with drugs, with known but different genetic polymorphisms. In addition several polymorphisms, either within one gene or targeting for another drug, should be considered when designing combination chemotherapy, such as irinotecan combined with a fluoropyrimidine [207,208].

Next to the role of DPD in 5-FU pharmacokinetics, the current data also clearly demonstrate that DPD plays a crucial role in the efficacy of fluoropyrimidines, not only by influencing the systemic bioavailability (and toxic side effects) but also at the cellular tumoral level (antitumor activity). DPD levels in normal tissues (especially liver) will predominantly affect 5-FU's metabolic clearance. Hence, deficiency will dramatically increase 5-FU plasma and tissue concentration. Mutations in DPD are likely to affect DPD activity. In addition to the studies on TS polymorphisms, similar studies on DPD, revealed the presence of a number of mutations in the DPD gene [209,210]. Some of these mutations are relatively frequent (e.g. resulting in exon 14 skipping) and affect enzyme levels markedly. The prevalence of a common point mutation, leading to exon 14 skipping, was also associated with an increase in 5-FU plasma concentration in patients receiving 5-FU treatment. This mutation leads to the absence of DPD protein and was associated with more toxicity upon 5-FU treatment. Also Haring *et al.* [211] observed an association between 5-FU toxicity and DPD deficiency. Also the bioavailability was related to DPD mutations. Therefore research on the role of DPD and DPD genomic alterations, received quite some attention. At least 21 mutations have been observed, some of them encoding for a deficient enzyme [212]. At least 16 mutations occur in the open reading frame [213]. Improved technology has enabled to characterize the molecular defect in DPD deficient patients which were diagnosed more than 10 years ago and it was confirmed that this patient was heterozygote for two different mutations [214] one in each allele. It seems worthwhile to include characterization of DPD polymorphisms together with that of TS in patients receiving 5-FU based therapy.

Next to the role of DPD in toxicity it has also been demonstrated that DPD expression is related to response to 5-FU based treated [33]. However, the most striking effect was found when DPD and TS expression were combined; almost all patients with a low TS and DPD expression response to 5-FU based treatment, but none of the patients with both high TS and DPD. These studies form an excellent basis to use TS and DPD expression to select patients for a 5-FU based combination, while those with a high expression should receive another type of treatment, e.g. with oxaliplatin and/or irinotecan [215].

CONCLUSIONS

Colorectal cancer remains a significant health problem in the world. Advances in early detection and surgical therapy have contributed to decreasing death rates. Although successful surgery is possible in selected patients, current treatment modalities are still insufficiently efficacious. Adjuvant therapies have shown some promising results, with enhanced antitumor response and quality of life. Nevertheless, there is a continued search for improved treatment modalities, including cytotoxic chemotherapy. The availability of a number of new 5-FU analogues, new folate antagonists, effective cytotoxic agents such as irinotecan and oxaliplatin, as well as Cox-2 and growth factors inhibitors produced new options on the therapy of advanced colorectal carcinoma. Clinical trials already established the efficacy and tolerability of these agents at single therapy, which led to their recommended use as second-line treatment in 5-FU-refractory disease, or in patients in whom 5-FU is contraindicated. Other studies showed that their addition to the classical 5-FU/LV combination significantly increases response rates, time to disease progression, and survival. However, the optimal integration and sequence of use of these drugs still needs to be defined. In addition, with the improved understanding of colorectal cancer biology, novel molecular targets such as EGFR, VEGF, and Cox-2 have been identified. Combined with cytotoxic drugs, the inhibition of these new targets may have an impact on the survival of these patients. The same holds true for the use of genetic testing. Through understanding the gene functions, we come closer to understanding precisely how tumors develop, and then offer a more efficacious treatment.

REFERENCES

[1] Jemal A, Murray T, Samuels A, Ghafoor A, Ward E, Thun MJ. Cancer statistics, 2003. *CA Cancer J Clin*. 2003;53:5-26.

[2] Van Cutsen E, Verslpe C. Integration of new cytotoxic agents in the management of advanced colorectal cancer: where are we now and where do we go? *Educational Book 38th Annual Meeting of the American Society of Clinical Oncology*; 2002:240-247.

[3] Parker SL, Tong T, Bolden S, Wingo PA. Cancer statistics, 1996. *CA Cancer J Clin.* 1996;46:5-27.

[4] Potter JD. Colorectal cancer: molecules and populations. *J Natl Cancer Inst.* 1999; 91:916-932.

[5] McMichael AJ, Giles GG. Cancer in migrants to Australia; extending the descriptive epidemiological data. *Cancer Res.* 1988; 48:751-756.

[6] Ministério da Saúde. Instituto Nacional de Câncer (INCA). Coordenação de programas de controle de câncer - pro-onco. O problema do câncer no Brasil. Rio de Janeiro, 2003. Available at: http://www.inca.org.br. Accessed at 7 October 2003.

[7] Parkin DM, Bray FI, Devesa SS. Cancer burden in the year 2000. The global picture. *Eur J Cancer.* 2001; 37(Suppl 8):S4-S66.

[8] Fearon ER, Gruber SB. Molecular abnormalities in colon and rectal cancer. In Mendelsohn J, Howley PM, Israel MA, Liotta LA, ed. *The molecular basis of cancer.* Philadelphia: WB Sauders Company; 2001: 289-312.

[9] Shields PG, Harris CC. Cancer risk and low-penetrance susceptibility genes in gene-environment interactions. *J Clin Oncol.* 2000; 18:2309-2315.

[10] Willer A. Reduction of the individual cancer risk by physical exercise. *Onkologie.* 2003; 26:283-289.

[11] Sanjoaquin MA, Appleby PN, Thr命rogood M, Mann JL, Key TJ. Nutrition, lifestyle and colorectal cancer incidence: a prospective investigation of 10998 vegetarians and non-vegetarians in the United Kingdom. *J Cancer.* 2004; 90:118-121.

[12] Mathew A, Peters U, Chatterjee N, Kulldorff M, Sinha R. Fat, fiber, fruits, vegetables, and risk of colorectal adenomas. *Int J Colorectal Dis.* 2004; 19:23-42.

[13] Peters U, Sinha R, Chatterjee N, *et al.* Dietary fiber and colorectal adenoma in a colorectal cancer early detection programme. *Lancet.* 2003; 361:1491-1495.

[14] Bingham SA, Day NE, Luben R, *et al.* Dietary fiber in food and protection against colorectal cancer in the European Prospective Investigation into Cancer and Nutrition (EPIC): an observational study. *Lancet.* 2003; 361: 1496-1501.

[15] Two studies find high-fiber diet lowers colon cancer risk. *CA Cancer J Clin.* 2003; 53:201-202.

[16] Dashwood RH. Early detection and prevention of colorectal cancer. *Oncol Rep.* 1999; 6:277-281.

[17] Skibber JM, Minsky BD, Hoff P. Cancer of the colon. In DeVita VT, Hellman S, Rosenberg AS, eds. *Cancer: principles and practice of oncology.* Philadelphia, PA: Lippincott Williams & Wilkins, 2001.

[18] Grivicich I, Mans DRA, Peters GJ, Schwartsmann G. Irinotecan and Oxaliplatin: an overview of the novel chemotherapeutic options for the treatment of advanced colorectal cancer. *Braz J Med Biol Res.* 2001; 34:1087-1103.

[19] Nishisho I, Nakamura Y, Miyoshi Y, *et al.* Mutations of chromosome 5q21 genes in FAP and colorectal cancer patients. *Science.* 1991; 253:665-669.

[20] Groden J, Thliveris A, Samowitz W, *et al.* Identification and characterization of the familial adenomatous polyposis coli gene. *Cell.* 1991; 66:589-600.

[21] Burt RW. Colon cancer screening. *Gastroenterology.* 2000; 119:837-853.

[22] Peltomaki P, De la Chapelle A. Mutations predisposing to hereditary non-polyposis colorectal cancer. *Adv Cancer Res*. 1997; 71:93-119.

[23] Thibodeau SN, Bren G, Schaid D. Microsatellite instability in cancer of the proximal colon. *Science*. 1993; 260:816-819.

[24] Lynch H, Smyrk T. Hereditary nonpolyposis colorectal cancer (Lynch syndrome): an update review. *Cancer*. 1996; 78:1149-1167.

[25] Jass JR, Stewart SM. Evolution of hereditary non-polyposis colorectal cancer. *Gut*. 1992; 33:780-783.

[26] Wu Y, Berends MJ, Post JG, *et al*. Germline mutations of EXO1 gene in patients with hereditary nonpolyposis colorectal cancer (HNPCC) and atypical HNPCC forms. *Gastroenterology*. 2001; 120:1580-1877.

[27] De Jong AE, Morreau H, Van Puijenbrock M, et al. The role of mismatch repair gene defects in the development of adenomas in patients with HNPCC. *Gastroenterology*. 2004; 126:42-48.

[28] Johns LE, Houlston RS. A systematic review and meta-analysis of familial colorectal cancer risk. *Am J Gastroenterol*. 2001; 96:2992-3003.

[29] Vogelstein B, Fearon ER, *et al*. Genetic alterations during colorectal-tumor development. *N Engl J Med*. 1988; 319:525-532.

[30] Watanabe T, Wu TT, Catalano PJ, *et al*. Molecular predictors of survival after adjuvant chemotherapy for colon cancer. *N Engl J Med*. 2001; 344:1196-1206.

[31] Prolla TA. DNA mismatch repair and cancer. *Curr Opin Cell Biol*. 1998; 10:311-316.

[32] McLeod HL, Murray GI. Tumour markers of prognosis in colorectal cancer. *Br J Cancer*. 1999; 79:191-203.

[33] Salonga D, Danenberg KD, Johnson M, *et al*. Colorectal tumors responding to 5-fluorouracil have low gene expression levels of dihydropyrimidine dehydrogenase, thymidylate synthase, and thymidine phosphorylase. *Clin Cancer Res*. 2000; 6:1322-1327.

[34] Backus HHJ, Rustum YM, van Groeningen CJ, Peters GJ. Chemotherapeutic strategies for treatment of colorectal cancer: present and future developments. *Clin Colorectal Cancer*. 2001; 1:121-127.

[35] Ferrandez A, Prescott S, Burt RW. COX-2 and colorectal cancer. *Curr Pharm Des*. 2003; 9:2229-2251.

[36] Church RD, Fleshman JW, McLeod HL. Cyclo-oxygenase 2 inhibition in colorectal cancer therapy. *Br J Surg*. 2003; 90:1055-1067.

[37] Eberhart CE, Coffey RJ, Radhika A, Giardiello FM, Ferrenbach S, DuBois RN. Up-regulation of cyclooxygenase 2 gene expression in human colorectal adenomas and adenocarcinomas. *Gastroenterology*. 1994; 107:1183-1188.

[38] Hao X, Bishop AE, Wallace M, *et al*. Early expression of cyclo-oxygenase-2 during sporadic colorectal carcinogenesis. *J Pathol*. 1999; 187:295-301.

[39] Fujita T, Matsui M, Takaku K, *et al*. Size- and invasion-dependent increase in cyclooxygenase 2 levels in human colorectal carcinomas. *Cancer Res*. 1998; 58:4823-4826.

[40] Tomozawa S, Tsuno NH, Sunami E, *et al.* Cyclooxygenase-2 overexpression correlates with tumour recurrence, especially haematogenous metastasis, of colorectal cancer. *Br J Cancer.* 2000; 83:324-328.

[41] Chen WS, Wei SJ, Liu JM, Hsiao M, Kou-Lin J, Yang WK. Tumor invasiveness and liver metastasis of colon cancer cells correlated with cyclooxygenase-2 (COX-2) expression and inhibited by a COX-2-selective inhibitor, etodolac. *Int J Cancer.* 2001; 91:894-899.

[42] Plate S. ESMO minimum clinical recommendations for diagnosis, adjuvant treatment and follow-up of colon cancer. *Ann Oncol.* 2001; 12:1053-1054.

[43] Mayer, RJ. Moving beyond fluorouracil for colorectal cancer. *N Engl J Med.* 2000; 343:963-964.

[44] Grem, JL. Fluoropyrimidines. In Chabner BA, Longo DL, eds. Cancer chemotherapy and biotherapy: principles and practice. Philadelphia (USA): Lippincott-Raven, 1996.

[45] Pinedo HM, Peters GJ. Fluorouracil: biochemistry and pharmacology. *J Clin Oncol.* 1998; 10:1653-1664.

[46] Santi DV, McHenry CS, Sommer H. Mechanism of interaction of thymidylate synthase with 5-fluorodeoxyuridylate. *Biochemistry.* 1974; 13:471-481.

[47] Mandel HG. The target cell determinants of the antitumor actions of 5-FU: does 5-FU incorporation into RNA play a role. *Cancer Treat Rep.* 1981; 65(suppl 3):63-71.

[48] Schuetz JD, Diasio RB. The effect of 5-fluorouracil on DNA chain elongation in intact bone marrow cells. *Biochem Biophys Res Commun.* 1985; 133:161-167.

[49] Sobrero A, Zaniboni A, Frassineti GL, *et al.* Schedule specific biochemical modulation of 5-fluorouracil in advanced colorectal cancer: a randomized study. GISCAD, IOR and collaborating centers. *Ann Oncol.* 2000;11:1413-1420.

[50] Meta-analysis Group in Cancer. Efficacy of intravenous continuous infusion of fluorouracil compared with bolus administration in advanced colorectal cancer. *J Clin Oncol.* 1998; 16:301-308.

[51] Kemeny N, Huang Y, Cohen AM, *et al.* Hepatic arterial infusion of chemotherapy after resection of hepatic metastases from colorectal cancer. *N Engl J Med.* 1999; 341:2039-2048.

[52] Peters GJ, Van Groeningen CJ. Clinical relevance of biochemical modulation of 5-fluorouracil. *Ann Oncol.* 1991; 2:469-480.

[53] Advanced Colorectal Cancer Meta-analysis Project. Modulation of fluorouracil by leucovorin in patients with advanced colorectal cancer: evidence in terms of response rate. *J Clin Oncol.* 1992; 10:896-903.

[54] O'Connell MJ, Mailliard JA, Kahn MJ, *et al.* Controlled trial of fluorouracil and low-dose leucovorin given for 6 months as postoperative adjuvant therapy for colon cancer. *J Clin Oncol.* 1997; 15:246-250.

[55] Wolmark N, Rockette H, Fisher B, *et al.* The benefit of leucovorin-modulated fluorouracil as postoperative adjuvant therapy for primary colon cancer: results from National Surgical Adjuvant Breast and Bowel Project protocol C-03. *J. Clin Oncol.* 1993; 11:1879-1887.

[56] NIH consensus conference. Adjuvant therapy for patients with colon and rectal cancer. *JAMA.* 1990; 264:1444-1450.

[57] Hejna M, Kornek GV, Raderer, *et al.* M 5-methyltetrahydrofolate for biochemical modulation of fluorouracil (FU) in patients with advanced colorectal cancer: a randomized phase I-II study of two different FU administration schedules. *Ann Oncol.* 1998; 9:1309-1314.

[58] Wall M, Wani MC, Cook CE, *et al.* Plant antitumor agents: I. The isolation and structure of camptothecin, a novel alkaloidal leukemia and tumor inhibitor from *Camptotheca acuminata. J Am Chem Soc.* 1966; 88:3888-3890.

[59] Takimoto CH, Kieffer LV, Arbuck SG. DNA topoisomerase I inhibitors. In Pinedo H, Longo DL, Chabner BA, eds. Cancer Chemotherapy and Biological Response Modifiers Annual 17. Elsevier Science, 1997.

[60] Rivory LP, Bowles R, Robert J, Pond SM. Conversion of Irinotecan (CPT-11) to its active metabolite, 7-ethyl-10-hydroxycamptothecin (SN-38), by human liver carboxylesterase. *Biochem Pharmacol.* 1996; 52:1103-1111.

[61] Hsiang YH, Liu LF. Identification of mammalian topoisomerase I as an intracellular target of the anticancer drug camptothecin. *Cancer Res.* 1988; 48:1722-1726.

[62] Vanhoefer U, Harstrick A, Achterrath W, Cao S, Seeber S, Rustum YM. Irinotecan in the treatment of colorectal cancer: clinical overview. *J Clin Oncol.* 2001; 19:1501-1518.

[63] Anton A, Aranda E, Carrato A, *et al.* Irinotecan (CPT-11) in metastatic colorectal cancer patients resistant to 5-fluorouracil (5FU): a phase II study. *Methods Find Exp Clin Pharmacol.* 2003; 25:639-643.

[64] Mans DR, Grivicich I, Peters GJ, Schwartsmann G. Sequence-dependent growth inhibition and DNA damage formation by the Irinotecan-5-fluorouracil combination in human colon carcinoma cell lines. *Eur J Cancer.* 1999; 35:1851-1861.

[65] Comella P, Casaretti R, De Vita F, *et al.* Concurrent Irinotecan and 5-fluorouracil plus leuvo-folinic acid given every other week in the first-line management of advanced colorectal carcinoma: a phase I study of the southern Italy cooperative oncology group. *Ann Oncol.* 1999; 10:915-921.

[66] Ducreux M, Ychou M, Seitz JF, *et al.* Irinotecan combined with bolus fluorouracil, continuous infusion fluorouracil, and high-dose leucovorin every two weeks (LV5FU2 regimen): a clinical dose-finding and pharmacokinetic study in patients with pretreated metastatic colorectal cancer. *J Clin Oncol.* 1999; 17:2901-2908.

[67] Vanhoefer U, Harstrick A, Kohne C-H, *et al.* Phase I study of a weekly schedule of Irinotecan, high-dose leucovorin, and infusional fluorouracil as first-line chemotherapy in patients with advanced colorectal cancer. *J Clin Oncol.* 1999; 17:907-913.

[68] Andre T, Louvet C, Maindrault-Goebel F, *et al.* CPT-11 (Irinotecan) addition to bimonthly, high-dose leucovorin and bolus and continuous-infusion 5-fluorouracil (FOLFIRI) for pretreated metastatic colorectal cancer. *Eur J Cancer.* 1999; 35:343-1347.

[69] Saltz LB, Cox JV, Blanke C, *et al.* Irinotecan plus fluorouracil and leucovorin for metastatic colorectal cancer. Irinotecan Study Group. *N Engl J Med.* 2000; 343:905-914.

[70] Douillard JY, Cunningham D, Roth AD, *et al.* Irinotecan combined with fluorouracil compared with fluorouracil alone as first-line treatment for metastatic colorectal cancer: a multicentre randomised trial. *Lancet.* 2000; 355:1041-1047.

[71] Yalcin S, Oksuzoglu B, Tekuzman G, *et al.* Biweekly irinotecan plus bolus 5-Fluorouracil and folinic acid in patients with advanced stage colorectal cancer. *Jpn J Clin Oncol.* 2003; 33:580-583.

[72] de Gramont A, Figer A, Seymour M, *et al.* Leucovorin and fluorouracil with or without Oxaliplatin as first-line treatment in advanced colorectal cancer. *J Clin Oncol.* 2000; 18:2938-2947.

[73] Giacchetti S, Perpoint B, Zidani R, *et al.* Phase III multicenter randomized trial of Oxaliplatin added to chronomodulated fluorouracil-leucovorin as first-line treatment of metastatic colorectal cancer. *J Clin Oncol.* 2000; 18(1):136-147.

[74] Raymond E, Faivre S, Woynarowski JM, Chaney SG. Oxaliplatin: mechanism of action and antineoplastic activity. *Semin Oncol.* 1998; 25(2 suppl 5):4-12.

[75] Machover D, Diaz-Rubio E, de Gramont A, *et al.* Two consecutive phase II studies of oxaliplatin (L-OHP) for treatment of patients with advanced colorectal carcinoma who were resistant to previous treatment with fluoropyrimidines. *Ann Oncol.* 1996; 7:95-98.

[76] Becouarn Y, Ychou M, *et al.* Phase II trial of oxaliplatin as first-line chemotherapy in metastatic colorectal cancer patients. *J Clin Oncol.* 1998; 16:2739-2744.

[77] Diaz-Rubio E, Sastre J, Zaniboni A, *et al.* Oxaliplatin as single agent in previously untreated colorectal carcinoma patients: a phase II multicentric study. *Ann Oncol.* 1998; 9:105-108.

[78] Becouarn Y, Rougier P. Clinical efficacy of oxaliplatin monotherapy: phase II trials in advanced colorectal cancer. *Semin Oncol.* 1998; 25(Suppl 5):23-31.

[79] Rothenberg ML, Oza AM, Bigelow RH, *et al.* Superiority of Oxaliplatin and fluorouracil-leucovorin compared with either therapy alone in patients with progressive colorectal cancer after Irinotecan and fluorouracil-leucovorin: Interim results of a phase III trial. *J Clin Oncol.* 2003; 21:2059-2069.

[80] Raymond E, Chaney SG, Taamma A, Cvitkovic E. Oxaliplatin: A review of preclinical and clinical studies. *Ann Oncol.* 1998; 9:1053-1071.

[81] Janinis J, Papakostas P, Samelis G, Skarlos D, Papagianopoulos P, Fountzilas G. Second-line chemotherapy with weekly Oxaliplatin and high-dose 5-fluorouracil with folinic acid in metastatic colorectal carcinoma: a Hellenic Cooperative Oncology Group (HeCOG) phase II feasibility study. *Ann Oncol.* 2000; 11:163-167.

[82] Scheithauer W, Kornek GV, Raderer M, *et al.* Randomized multicenter phase II trial of two different schedules of Capecitabine plus Oxaliplatin as first-line treatment in advanced colorectal cancer. *J Clin Oncol.* 2003; 21:1307-1312.

[83] Goldberg RM, Sargent DJ, Morton RF, *et al.* A randomized controlled trial of fluorouracil plus leucovorin, irinotecan, and oxaliplatin combinations in patients with previously untreated metastatic colorectal cancer. *J Clin Oncol.* 2004; 22:23-30.

[84] Mayer RJ. Oral versus intravenous fluoropyrimidines for advanced colorectal cancer: by either route, it's all the same. *J Clin Oncol.* 2001; 19:4093-4096.

[85] Pentheroudakis G, Twelves C. Capecitabine (Xeloda): from the laboratory to the patient's home. *Clin Colorectal Cancer.* 2002; 2:16-23.

[86] Van Cutsem E, Twelves C, Cassidy J, *et al.* Oral Capecitabine compared with intravenous fluorouracil plus leucovorin in patients with metastatic colorectal cancer: results of a large phase III study. *J Clin Oncol.* 2001; 19:4097-4106.

[87] Van Cutsem E, Verslype C, Demedts I. The treatment of advanced colorectal cancer: where are we now and where do we go? *Best Pract Res Clin Gastroenterol.* 2002; 16:319-330.

[88] Cassidy J. Potential of Xeloda® in colorectal cancer and other solid tumors. *Oncology.* 1999; 57(Suppl 1):27-32.

[89] Cassidy J. Xeloda in colorectal cancer. *Int J Clin Pract.* 2001; 55(5):326-328.

[90] Fuchs CS. Current and ongoing trials with Irinotecan in the United States. *Semin Oncol.* 2003; 30(4 Suppl 12):9-17.

[91] Bajetta E, Di Bortolomeo M, Mariani L, *et al.* Randomized multicenter phase II trial of two different schedules of irinotecan combined with capecitabine as first-line treatment in metastatic colorectal carcinoma. *Cancer.* 2004; 15:279-287.

[92] Hoff PM, Royce M, Medgyesy D, Brito R, Pazdur R. Oral Fluoropyrimidines. *Semin Oncol.* 1999; 26:640-646.

[93] Douillard JY, Hoff PM, Skillings JR, *et al.* Multicenter phase III study of uracil/tegafur and oral leucovorin versus fluorouracil and leucovorin in patients with previously untreated metastatic colorectal cancer. *J Clin Oncol.* 2002; 20:3605-3616.

[94] Chau I, Cunningham D. Adjuvant therapy in colon cancer: current status and future directions. *Cancer Treat Rev.* 2002; 28:223-236.

[95] Hill M, Mackay H, Cunningham D. Phase I/II study of oral uracil/tegafur (UFT), leucovorin and Irinotecan in patients with advanced colorectal cancer. *Ann Oncol.* 2000; 11(Suppl 4), 45 (abstr 193).

[96] Carmichael J, Popiela T, Radstone D, *et al* Randomized comparative study of tegafur/uracil and oral leucovorin versus parenteral fluorouracil and leucovorin in patients with previously untreated metastatic colorectal cancer. *J Clin Oncol.* 2002; 20:3617-3627.

[97] Schilsky RL, Levin J, West WH, *et al.* Randomized, open-label, phase III study of a 28-day oral regimen of eniluracil plus fluorouracil versus intravenous fluorouracil plus leucovorin as first-line therapy in patients with metastatic/advanced colorectal cancer. *J Clin Oncol.* 2000; 20:1519-1526.

[98] Danenberg PV, Malli H, Swenson S. Thymidylate synthase inhibitors. *Semin Oncol.* 1999; 26:621-631.

[99] Cunningham D, Zalcberg J, Smith I, *et al.* 'Tomudex' (ZD1694): a novel thymidylate synthase inhibitor with clinical antitumour activity in a range of solid tumours. 'Tomudex' International Study Group. *Ann Oncol.* 1996; 7:179-182.

[100] Vincent M, Ho C, Tomiak A, *et al.* Toxicity analysis of the 5-day bolus 5-fluorouracil/folinic acid regimen for the treatment of colorectal carcinoma from 2 randomized controlled trials: a concern about dose. *Clin Colorectal Cancer.* 2002; 2:111-118.

[101] Cunningham D, Zalcberg J, Maroun J, *et al.* Efficacy, tolerability and management of Raltitrexed (Tomudex) monotherapy in patients with advanced colorectal cancer. a review of phase II/III trials. *Eur J Cancer.* 2002; 38:478-486.

[102] Van Cutsem E, Cunningham D, Maroun J, Cervantes A, Glimelius B. Raltitrexed: current clinical status and future directions. *Ann Oncol*. 2002; 13:513-522.

[103] Niculescu-Duvaz I. Thymitaq (Zarix). *Curr Opin Investig Drugs*. 2001; 2:693-705.

[104] Curtin NJ, Hughes AN. Pemetrexed dissodium, a novel antifolate with multiple targets. *Lancet Oncol*. 2001; 2:298-306.

[105] Grothey A, Schmoll HJ. New chemotherapy approaches in colorectal cancer. *Curr Opin Oncol*. 2001; 13: 275-286.

[106] Cascinu S, Graziano F, Catalano V, *et al*. Differences of vascular endothelial growth factor (VEGF) expression between liver and abdominal metastases from colon cancer. Implications for the treatment with VEGF inhibitors. *Clin Exp Metastasis*. 2000; 18:651-655.

[107] Ellis LM, Takahashi Y, Liu W, Shaheen RM. Vascular endothelial growth factor in human colon cancer: biology and therapeutic implications. Oncologist. 2000; 5(Suppl 1): 11-15.

[108] Ferrara N. Role of vascular endothelial growth factor in physiologic and pathologic angiogenesis: therapeutic implications. *Semin Oncol*. 2002; 29(6 Suppl 16):10-4.

[109] Ciardiello F, Caputo R, Damiano V, *et al*. Antitumor effects of ZD6474, a small molecule vascular endothelial growth factor receptor tyrosine kinase inhibitor, with additional activity against epidermal growth factor receptor tyrosine kinase. *Clin Cancer Res*. 2003; 9:1546-1556.

[110] Fong TA, Shawver LK, Sun L, *et al*. SU5416 is a potent and selective inhibitor of the vascular endothelial growth factor receptor (Flk-1/KDR) that inhibits tyrosine kinase catalysis, tumor vascularization, and growth of multiple tumor types. *Cancer Res*. 1999; 59:99-106.

[111] Levitt ML, Koty PP. Tyrosine kinase inhibitors in preclinical development. *Invest New Drugs*. 1999; 17:213-226.

[112] Wedge SR, Ogilvie DJ, Dukes M, *et al*. ZD6474 inhibits vascular endothelial growth factor signaling, angiogenesis, and tumor growth following oral administration. Cancer Res. 2002; 62:4645-4655.

[113] Gordon MS, Margolin K, Talpaz M, *et al*. Phase I safety and pharmacokinetic study of recombinant human anti-vascular endothelial growth factor in patients with advanced cancer. *J Clin Oncol*. 2001; 19:843-850.

[114] Margolin K, Gordon MS, Holmgren E, *et al*. Phase Ib trial of intravenous recombinant humanized monoclonal antibody to vascular endothelial growth factor in combination with chemotherapy in patients with advanced cancer: pharmacologic and long-term safety data. *J Clin Oncol*. 2001; 19:851-856.

[115] Kabbinavar F, Hurwitz HI, Fehrenbacher L, *et al*. Phase II, randomized trial comparing bevacizumab plus fluorouracil (FU)/leucovorin (LV) with FU/LV alone in patients with metastatic colorectal cancer. *J Clin Oncol*. 2003; 21:60-65.

[116] Baselga J. The EGFR as a target for anticancer therapy-focus on cetuximab. *Eur J Cancer*. 2001;37(Suppl 4):S16-S22.

[117] Baselga J Why the epidermal growth factor receptor? The rationale for cancer therapy. *Oncologist*. 2002;7(Suppl 4):2-8.

[118] Messa C, Russo F, Caruso MG, Di Leo A. EGF, TGF-alpha, and EGF-R in human colorectal adenocarcinoma. *Acta Oncol.* 1998; 37:285-289.

[119] Kluftinger AM, Robinson BW, Quenville NF, Finley RJ, Davis NL. Correlation of epidermal growth factor receptor and c-erbB2 oncogene product to known prognostic indicators of colorectal cancer. *Surg Oncol.* 1992;1:97-105.

[120] Steele RJ, Kelly P, Ellul B, Eremin O. Epidermal growth factor receptor expression in colorectal cancer. *Br J Surg.* 1990;77:1352-1354.

[121] Radinsky R. Modulation of tumor cell gene expression and phenotype by the organ-specific metastatic environment. *Cancer Metastasis Rev.* 1995; 14:323-338.

[122] Arteaga CL. The epidermal growth factor receptor: from mutant oncogene in non human cancers to therapeutic target in human neoplasia. *J Clin Oncol.* 2001; 19(18 Suppl):32S-40S.

[123] O`Dwyer PJ, Benson AB 3rd. Epidermal growth factor receptor-targeted therapy in colorectal cancer. *Semin Oncol.* 2002; 29(5 Suppl 14):10-17.

[124] Ciardiello F, Bianco R, Damiano V, *et al.* Antitumor activity of sequential treatment with topotecan and anti-epidermal growth factor receptor monoclonal antibody C225. *Clin Cancer Res.* 1999; 5:909-916.

[125] Sirotnak FM. Studies with ZD1839 in preclinical models. *Semin Oncol.* 2003; 30(1 Suppl 1):12-20.

[126] Prewett MC, Hooper AT, Bassi R, Ellis LM, Waksal HW, Hicklin DJ. Enhanced antitumor activity of anti-epidermal growth factor receptor monoclonal antibody IMC-C225 in combination with Irinotecan (CPT-11) against human colorectal tumor xenografts. *Clin Cancer Res.* 2002; 8:994-1003.

[127] Fan Z, Baselga J, Masui H, Mendelsohn J. Antitumor effects of anti-epidermal growth factor receptor monoclonal antibody plus cis-diamminedichloroplatinum on well established A341 cell xenografts. Cancer Res. 1993; 53:4637-4642.

[128] Mendelsohn J. The epidermal growth factor receptor as a target for cancer therapy. *Endocr Relat Cancer.* 2001; 8:3-9.

[129] Cunningham D, Humblet Y, Siena S. *et al. Proc Am Soc Clin Oncol.* 2003; 22:#1012.

[130] Mendelsohn J. Targeting the epidermal growth factor receptor for cancer therapy. *J Clin Oncol.* 2002;20(Suppl 18):1S-13S.

[131] Schmitt FC, Soares R. TGFα and angiogenesis. *Am J Surg Pathol.* 1999; 23:358-359.

[132] Gille J, Swerlick RA, Caughman SW. Transforming growth factor α-induced transcriptional activation of the vascular permeability Factor (VPF/VEGF) gene requires AP2-dependent DNA binding and transactivation. *EMBO J.* 1997; 16:750-759.

[133] Ciardiello F, Caputo R Bianco R, *et al.* Inhibition of growth factors production and angiogenesis in human cancer cells by ZD1839 (Iressa), a selective epidermal growth factor receptor tyrosine kinase inhibitor. *Clin Cancer Res.* 2001; 7:1459-1465.

[134] Ciardiello F. Epidermal growth factor receptor tyrosine kinases inhibitors as anticancer agents. *Drugs.* 2000; 60(Suppl 1):25-32.

[135] Ciardiello F, Caputo R Bianco R, *et al.* Antitumor effect and potentiation of cytotoxic drugs activity in human cancer cells by ZD-1839 (Iressa), an EGFR-selective tyrosine kinase inhibitor. *Clin Cancer Res.* 2000; 6: 2053-2063.

[136] Koizumi F, Kanzawa F, Ueda Y, *et al.* Synergist interaction between the EGFR tyrosine kinase inhibitor gefitinib ("Iressa") and the DNA topoisomerase I inhibitor CPT-11 (irinotecan) in human colorectal cancer cells. *Int J Cancer*. 2004;108:464-472.

[137] Herbst RS. ZD1839: targeting the epidermal growth factor receptor in cancer therapy. *Expert Opin Investig Drugs*. 2002; 11:837-849.

[138] de Bono JS, Hammond LA, Figeroa J, *et al.* Phase I/II trial of Iressa™ (ZD1839) in combination with 5-fluorouracil (5-FU) and leucovorin (LV) in patients with metastatic colorectal cancer. *Br J Cancer*. 2002; 87(Suppl1):abstract 56.

[139] Smith ML Hawcroft G, Hull MA. The effect of non-steroidal anti-inflammatory drugs on human colorectal cancer cells: evidence of different mechanism of action. *Eur J Cancer*.2000; 36:664-674.

[140] Kulkarni S, Rader JS, Zhang F, et al. Cyclooxygenase-2 is overexpressed in human cervical cancer. *Clin Cancer Res*. 2001; 7:429-434.

[141] Tsujii M, Kawano S, Tsujii S, Sawaoka H, Hori M, DuBois RN. Cyclooxygenase regulates angiogenesis induced by colon cancer cells. *Cell*. 1998; 93: 705-716.

[142] Gately S. The contributions of cyclooxygenase-2 to tumor angiogenesis. *Cancer Metastasis Rev*. 2000; 19:19-27.

[143] Knosel T, Yu Y, Stein U, *et al.* Overexpression of cycloxygenase-2 correlates with chromosomal gain at the cyclooxygenase-2 locus and decreased patient survival in advanced colorectal carcinomas. *Dis Colon Rectum*. 2004; 47: 70-77.

[144] Thun MJ, Henley SJ, Patrono C. Nonsteroidal anti-inflammatory drugs as anticancer agents: mechanistic, pharmacologic, and clinical issues. *J Natl Cancer Inst*. 2002; 94:252-266.

[145] Masferrer JL, Leahy KM, Koki AT, *et al.* Antiangiogenic and antitumor activities of cyclooxygenase-2 inhibitors. *Cancer Res*. 2000; 60:1306-1311.

[146] Sinicrope FA, Pazdur R, Levin B. Phase I trial of sulindac plus 5-fluorouracil and levamisole: potential adjuvant therapy for colon carcinoma. *Clin Cancer Res*. 1996; 2:37-41.

[147] Lin E, Morris JS, Ayers GD. Effect of celecoxib on Capecitabine-induced hand-foot syndrome and antitumor activity. *Oncology (Huntingt)*. 2002; 16(12Suppl 14):31-37, 2002.

[148] McMurray RW, Hardy KJ. Cox-2 inhibitors: today and tomorrow. *Am J Med Sci*. 2002; 323:181-189.

[149] Richter M, Weiss M, Weinberger I, Furstenberger G, Marian B. Growth inhibition and induction of apoptosis in colorectal tumors cells by cyclooxygenase inhibitors. *Carcinogenesis*. 2001; 22:17-25.

[150] Yamazaki R, Kusunoki N, Matsuzaki T, Hashimoto S, Kawai S. Selective cyclooxygenase-2 inhibitors show a differential ability to inhibit proliferation and induce apoptosis of colon adenocarcinoma cells. *FEBS Lett*. 2002; 531:278-284.

[151] Jones MK, Wang H, Peskar BM, *et al.* Inhibition of angiogenesis by nonsteroidal anti-inflammatory drugs: insight into mechanisms and implications for cancer growth and ulcer healing. *Nat Med*. 1999; 5:1418-1423.

[152] Pan MR, Chuang LY, Hung WC. Non-steroidal anti-inflammatory drugs inhibit matrix metalloproteinase-2 expression via repression of transcription in lung cancer cells. *FEBS Lett.* 2001; 508:365-368.

[153] Tortora G, Caputo R, Damiano V, et al. Combination of a selective cyclooxygenase-2 inhibitor with epidermal growth factor receptor tyrosine kinase inhibitor ZD1839 and protein kinase A antisense causes cooperative antitumor and antiangiogenic effect. *Clin Cancer Res.* 2003; 9:1566-1572.

[154] Sharma RA. Cancer chemoprevention: a clinical reality. *J R Soc Med.* 2000; 93:518-520.

[155] Beazer-Barclay Y, Levy DB, Moser AR, *et al.* Sulindac suppresses tumorigenesis in the Min mouse. *Carcinogenesis.* 1996; 17:1757-1760.

[156] Barnes CJ, Lee M. Chemoprevention of spontaneous intestinal adenomas in the adenomatous polyposis coli Min mouse model with aspirin. *Gastroenterology.* 1998; 114:873-877.

[157] Torrance CJ, Jackson PE, Montgomery E, et al. Combinatorial chemoprevention of intestinal neoplasia. *Nat Med.* 2000; 6:1024-1028.

[158] Smalley WE, DuBois RN. Colorectal cancer and nonsteroidal anti-inflammatory drugs. *Adv. Pharmacol.* 1997; 39:1-20.

[159] Kawamori T, Rao CV, Seibert K, Reddy BS. Chemopreventive activity of celecoxib, a specific cyclooxygenase-2 inhibitor, against colon carcinogenesis. *Cancer Res.* 1998; 58:409-412.

[160] Steinbach G, Lynch PM, Phillips RK, et al. The effect of celecoxib, a cyclooxygenase-2 inhibitor, in familial adenomatous polyposis. N Engl J Med. 2000; 342:1946-1952.

[161] Smigel K. Arthritis drug approved for polyp prevention blazes trail for other prevention trials. *J Natl Cancer Inst.* 2000; 92:297-299.

[162] Pirollo KF, Bouker KB, Chang EH. Does p53 status influence tumor response to anticancer therapies? *Anticancer Drugs.* 2000; 11:419-432.

[163] Jernvall P, Makinen MJ, Karttunen TJ, Makela J, Vihko P. Loss of heterozygosity at 18q21 is indicative of recurrence and therefore poor prognosis in a subset of colorectal cancers. *Br J Cancer.* 1999; 79:903-908.

[164] Shibata D, Reale MA, Lavin P, *et al.* The DCC protein and prognosis in colorectal cancer. *N Engl J Med.* 1996; 335:1727-1732.

[165] Saito M, Yamaguchi A, Goi T, *et al.* Expression of DCC protein in colorectal tumors and its relationship to tumor progression and metastasis. *Oncology.* 1999; 56:134-141.

[166] Mehlen P, Rabizadeh S, Snipas SJ, Assa-Munt N, Salvesen GS, Bredesen DE. The DCC gene product induces apoptosis by a mechanism requiring receptor proteolysis. Nature. 1998; 395:801-804.

[167] Mcleod HL, Murray GI. Tumour markers of prognosis in colorectal cancer. *Br J Cancer.* 1999; 79:191-203.

[168] Pirollo KF, Bouker KB, Chang EH. Does p53 status influence tumor response to anticancer therapies? Anticancer Drugs. 2000; 11:419-432.

[169] Soussi T. The p53 tumor suppressor gene: from molecular biology to clinical investigation. *Ann N Y Acad Sci.* 2000; 910:121-137.

[170] Ahnen DJ, Feigl P, Quan G, *et al.* Ki-ras mutation and p53 overexpression predict the clinical behavior of colorectal cancer: a Southwest Oncology Group study. *Cancer Res.* 1998; 58:1149-1158.

[171] Grady WM. Genetic testing for high-risk colon cancer patients. *Gastroenterology.* 2003; 124:1574-1594.

[172] Laken SJ, Petersen GM, Gruber SB, *et al.* Familial colorectal cancer in Ashkenazim due to a hypermutable tract in APC. *Nat Genet.* 1997; 17:79-83.

[173] Lothe RA, Hektoen M, Johnsen H, *et al.* The APC gene I1307K variant is rare in Norwegian patients with familial and sporadic colorectal or breast cancer. *Cancer Res.*1998; 58:2923-2924.

[174] Boland CR, Thibodeau SN, Hamilton SR, *et al.* A National Cancer Institute Workshop on Microsatellite Instability for cancer detection and familial predisposition: development of international criteria for the determination of microsatellite instability in colorectal cancer. *Cancer Res.* 1998; 58:5248-5257.

[175] Lawes DA, SenGupta S, Boulos PB. The clinical importance and prognostic implications of microsatellite instability in sporadic cancer. *Eur J Surg Oncol.* 2003; 29:201-212.

[176] Kornmann M, Link KH, Lenz HJ, *et al.* Thymidylate synthase is a predictor for response and resistance in hepatic artery infusion chemotherapy. *Cancer Lett.* 1997; 118:29-35.

[177] Spears SP, Gustavsson BG, Mitchell MS, *et al.* Thymidylate synthase inhibition in malignant tumors and normal liver of patients given intravenous 5-fluorouracil. *Cancer Res.* 1984; 44:4144-4150.

[178] Peters GJ, Van der Wilt CL, Van Groeningen CJ, Smid K, Meijer S, Pinedo HM: Thymidylate synthase inhibition after administration of fluorouracil with or without leucovorin in colon cancer patients: implication for treatment with fluorouracil. *J Clin Oncol.* 1994; 12:2035-2042.

[179] Peters GJ, Van der Wilt CL, Van Groeningen CJ, *et al.* Effect of different leucovorin formulations on 5-fluorouracil induced thymidylate synthase inhibition in colon tumors and normal tissues from patients in relation to response to 5-flourouracil. In: Pfleiderer W, Rokos H, eds. *Chemistry and Biology of Pteridines and Folates, Proc 11th International Symposium.* Berling: Blackwell Science; 1997:145-150.

[180] Leichman L, Lenz H-J, Leichman CG, *et al.* Quantitation of intratumoral thymidylate synthase expression predicts for resistance to protracted infusion of 5-fluorouracil and weekly leucovorin in disseminated colorectal cancers: preliminary report from an ongoing trial. *Eur J Cancer.* 1995; 31:1306-1310.

[181] Leichman CG, Danenberg PV, Tan M, *et al.* Quantitation of intratumoral thymidylate synthase expression predicts for disseminate colorectal cancer response and resistance to protracted-infusion fluorouracil and weekly leucovorin. *J Clin Oncol.* 1997; 15:3223-3229.

[182] Edler D, Hallstrom M, Johnston PG, Magnusson I, Ragnhammar P, Blomgren H. Thymidylate synthase expression: an independent prognostic factor for local recurrence, distant metastasis, disease-free and overall survival in rectal cancer. *Clin Cancer Res.* 2000; 6:1378-1384.

[183] Yamachika T, Nakanishi H, Inada K-I, *et al.* A new prognostic factor for colorectal carcinoma, thymidylate synthase, and its therapeutic significance. *Cancer*. 1998; 82:70-77.

[184] Farrugia DC, Ford HE, Cunningham D, Danenberg KD, Danenberg PV, Brabender J, McVicar AD, Aherne GW, Hardcastle A, McCarthy K, Jackman AL. Thymidylate synthase expression in advanced colorectal cancer predicts for response to raltitrexed. *Clin Cancer Res*. 2003; 9:792-801.

[185] Johnston PG, Drake JC, Trepel J, Allegra CJ: Immunological quantitation of thymidylate synthase using the monoclonal antibody TS-106 in 5-fluorouracil-sensitive and -resistant human cancer cell lines. *Cancer Res*. 1992; 52:4306-4312.

[186] Takenoue T, Nagawa H, Matsuda K, *et al.* Relation between thymidylate synthase expression and survival in colon carcinoma, and determination of appropriate application of 5-Fluorouracil by immunohistochemical method. *Ann Surg Oncol*. 2000; 7:193-198.

[187] Edler D, Glimelius B, Hallstrom M, *et al.* Thymidylate synthase expression in colorectal cancer: a prognostic and predictive marker of benefit from adjuvant fluorouracil-based chemotherapy. *J Clin Oncol*. 2002; 20:1721-1728.

[188] Lane DP. p53, guardian of the genome. *Nature*. 1992; 358:15-16.

[189] Kastan MB, Canman CE, Leonard CJ. p53, cell cycle control and apoptosis: implications for cancer. *Cancer Metas Rev*. 1995; 14:3-15.

[190] Hollstein M, Sidransky D, Vogelstein B, Harris CC. p53 mutations in human cancers. *Science*. 1991; 253:49-53.

[191] Lenz HJ, Danenberg KD, Leichman CG, *et al.* p53 and thymidylate synthase (TS) expression in untreated stage II colon cancer: association with recurrence, survival and tumor site. *Clin Cancer Res*. 1998; 4:1227-1234.

[192] Lenz HJ, Hayashi K, Salonga D, *et al.* p53 point mutations and thymidylate synthase messenger RNA levels in disseminated colorectal cancer: an analysis of response and survival. *Clin Cancer Res*. 1998; 4:1243-1250.

[193] Longley DB, Latif T, Boyer J, Allen WL, Maxwell PJ, Johnston PG. The interaction of thymidylate synthase expression with p53-regulated signaling pathways in tumor cells. *Semin Oncol*. 2003; 30(3 Suppl 6):3-9.

[194] Ward SA, Joel SP, Papamichael D, Slevin ML, Glynne-Jones R: Thymidylate (TS) and P53 protein expression in patients with rectal cancer treated with pre-operative 5-fluorouracil (5-FU) based chemo-radiotherapy (CRT). *Proc Am Assoc Clin Oncol*. 1998;17:#1040.

[195] Longley DB, Boyer J, Allen WL, *et al.* The role of thymidylate synthase induction in modulating p53-regulated gene expression in response to 5-fluorouracil and antifolates. *Cancer Res*. 2002; 62:2644-2649.

[196] Cascinu S, Catalano V, Aschele C, *et al.* Immunohistochemical determination of p53 protein does not predict clinical response in advanced colorectal cancer with low thymidylate synthase expression receiving a bolus 5-fluorouracil-leucovorin combination. *Ann Oncol*. 2000; 11:1053-1056.

[197] Kawakami K, Salonga D, Park JM, *et al.* Different lengths of a polymorphic repeat sequence in the thymidylate synthase gene affect translational efficiency but not its gene expression. *Clin Cancer Res.* 2001; 7:4096-4101.

[198] Peters GJ, Backus HH, Freemantle S, *et al.* Induction of thymidylate synthase as a 5-fluorouracil resistance mechanism. *Biochim Biophys Acta.* 2002; 1587:194-205.

[199] Zinzindohoue F, Ferraz JM, Laurent-Puig P. Thymidylate synthase promoter polymorphism. *J Clin Oncol.* 2001; 19:1779-1786.

[200] Kawakami K, Omura K, Kanehira E, Watanabe Y. Polymorphic tandem repeats in the thymidylate synthase gene is associated with its protein expression in human gastrointestinal cancers. *Anticancer Res.* 1999; 19:3249-3252.

[201] Luo HR, Lu XM, Yao YG, *et al.* Length polymorphism of thymidylate synthase regulatory region in Chinese populations and evolution of the novel alleles. *Biochem Genet.* 2002; 40:41-51.

[202] Marsh S, McKay JA, Cassidy J, Mcleod HL. Polymorphism in the thymidylate synthase promoter enhanced region in colorectal cancer. *Int J Oncol.* 2001; 19:383-386.

[203] Ulrich CM, Robien K, Sparks R. Pharmacogenetics and folate metabolism -- a promising direction. *Pharmacogenomics.* 2002; 23:299-313.

[204] Skibola CF, Smith MT, Hubbard A, *et al.* Polymorphisms in the thymidylate synthase and serine hydroxymethyltransferase genes and risk of adult acute lymphocytic leukemia. *Blood.* 2002; 99:3786-3791.

[205] Park DJ, Stoehlmacher J, Zhang W, Tsao-Wei D, Groshen S, Lenz HJ. Thymidylate synthase gene polymorphism predicts response to capecitabine in advanced colorectal cancer. *Int J Colorectal Dis.* 2002; 17:46-49.

[206] Krajinovic M, Costea I, Chiasson S. Polymorphism of the thymidylate synthase gene and outcome of acute lymphoblastic leukaemia. *Lancet.* 2002; 359:1033-1034.

[207] Steiner M, Schuff-Werner P, Freund M, Kohne CH. Combined Chemotherapy Trials Require Combined Pharmacogenetic Approaches. *J Clin Oncol.* 2002; 20:1425-1430.

[208] Innocenti F, Ratain MJ. Update on pharmacogenetics in cancer chemotherapy. *Eur J Cancer.* 2002; 38:639-644.

[209] Sekine I, Saijo N. Polymorphisms of metabolizing enzymes and transporter proteins involved in the clearance of anticancer agents. *Ann Oncol.* 2001; 12:1515-1525.

[210] Milano G, Mcleod HL. Can dihydropyrimidine dehydrogenase impact 5-fluorouracil-based treatment? *Eur J Cancer.* 2000; 36:37-42.

[211] Haring JS, Pewe LL, Perlman S. Bystander CD8 T cell-mediated demyelination after viral infection of the central nervous system. *J Immunol.* 2002; 169:1550-1555.

[212] Ezzeldin H, Okamoto Y, Johnson MR, Diasio RB. A high-throughput denaturing high-performance liquid chromatography method for the identification of variant alleles associated with dihydropyrimidine dehydrogenase deficiency. *Anal Biochem.* 2002; 306:63-73.

[213] Mattison LK, Johnson MR, Diasio RB. A comparative analysis of translated dihydropyrimidine dehydrogenase cDNA; conservation of functional domains and relevance to genetic polymorphisms. *Pharmacogenetics.* 2002; 12:133-144.

[214] Johnson MR, Wang K, Diasio RB. Profound dihydropyrimidine dehydrogenase deficiency resulting from a novel compound heterozygote genotype. *Clin Cancer Res.* 2002; 8:768-774.

[215] Kornmann M, Schwabe W, Sander S, Kron M, Strater J, Polat S, Kettner E, Weiser HF, Baumann W, Schramm H, Hausler P, Ott K, Behnke D, Staib L, Beger HG, Link KH. Thymidylate synthase and dihydropyrimidine dehydrogenase mRNA expression levels: predictors for survival in colorectal cancer patients receiving adjuvant 5-fluorouracil. *Clin Cancer Res*. 2003; 9:4116-4124.

In: Focus on Colorectal Cancer Research
Editor: Julia D. Martinez, pp. 209-240
ISBN #1-59454-101-9

Chapter IX

Laparoscopic Surgery for Colon and Rectal Cancer

Oded Zmora **and Danny Rosin**
Department of Surgery and Transplantation,
Sheba Medical Center, Tel Hashomer, Israel
Sakler School of Medicine, Tel Aviv University, Tel Aviv, Israel

Abstract

The application of laparoscopic techniques for curative resection of colorectal cancer is controversial, mainly owing to reports of cancer recurrence at the port site wounds. Despite research efforts of clinical studies and animal models, neither the actual rate nor the mechanisms causing port site metastasis are known. In this review, we gathered data from clinical series of laparoscopic surgery for colorectal cancer, having more then 50 patients each. The port site recurrence in 3901 patients participated in these series was approximately 0.67%. Although the methods and patient selection in these studies varies, this numbers may be comparable to the incidence reported for other malignancies, and in laparotomies for colorectal cancer.

This chapter reviews the technical aspects relative to laparoscopic resection of colorectal cancer, and summarizes the research regarding the potential causes for port site metastasis, and suggested protective measures.

This review suggests that wound recurrence may possibly be a result of an unfortunate learning curve, rather then an inherited concern. The final results of the large randomized studies will hopefully solve this question in the near future.

The introduction of laparoscopic techniques, at the end of the 1980's, was one of the most significant events in the evolution of general surgery in the 20th century. In just a few years, advanced laparoscopic techniques have been developed for the treatment of most intra-

* Corresponding author: Oded Zmora, MD, Department of Surgery and Transplantation, Sheba Medical Center, Tel-Hashomer 52621, Israel. Tel: (972-3) 530 2247; Fax: (972-3) 534 1097; E-mail: ozmora@post.tau.ac.il

abdominal pathologies. Advanced laparoscopic procedures require specific skills and expertise, which are only partially translatable from the respective "open" procedure.

With the rapid application of advanced laparoscopy at the beginning of the 1990's, laparoscopic colon and rectal procedures were also developed [1, 2, 3]. Advances in technology ensured a high quality image, and the development of consistently reliable laparoscopic staplers and energy sources have permitted a secure intracorporeal division of major vessels. Laparoscopic surgical techniques have been developed to dissect the colon and rectum and safely anastomose the ends in the manner used in laparotomy. Technical advances and increased experience have considerably reduced iatrogenic complications and the need to convert to laparotomy. With experience, a significant reduction in the operative time has been reported, and although the operative cost of laparoscopic surgery is higher, this may be offset by a shorter length of hospital stay and earlier return to work [4, 5, 6].

The use of laparoscopic colon and rectal surgery for benign diseases has been widely accepted as a safe and effective approach, with the potential advantages of improved cosmetics, reduced postoperative pain, shorter length of hospital stay, and earlier return to normal activity [7, 8, 9]. Older patients may specifically gain advantage from this technique, as reduced surgical trauma may be of increased importance in these patients [10, 11]. The utilization of this technique for colon and rectal cancer however, remained controversial long after its acceptance for benign conditions. Surgery for non-metastatic colorectal cancer is aimed at cure, and cure rates following laparotomy are generally favorable. When evaluating the laparoscopic approach for the treatment of cancer, it is crucial to show that oncologic principles are not compromised, and that overall rates of local and distal recurrence and survival are comparable or better than those rates after laparotomy. Few concerns regarding laparoscopy for colon and rectal cancer have been voiced. The extent of resection, proximal, distal and radial margins, and lymph node clearance need to be comparable to or better than those achieved by laparotomy. In treating rectal cancer, the ability to perform an adequate laparoscopic total mesorectal excision with coloanal anastomosis may be technically challenging, mainly in applying the distal staple line at the level of the pelvic floor. Difficulty localizing small lesions laparoscopically has been solved by the use of preoperative ink-marking (tattooing). However, still a matter of concern is the port site recurrence, a poorly understood phenomenon, which may adversely affect survival rates following laparoscopic resection for attempted cure of cancer. The potential benefits of laparoscopic surgery, such as less pain, a shorter hospital stay, and earlier return to full activity become irrelevant if either survival or cure are compromised.

Laparoscopic Colon Resection - Can Adequate Resection Be Achieved?

One of the controversies related to resections for cancer is whether adequate proximal and distal margins, and clearance of the lymph node basin of the tumor can be laparoscopically achieved. It is generally believed, that adherence to these oncologic principles is directly related to improved cure rates. Thus, if laparoscopic surgery is considered for the attempted curative treatment of cancer, adherence to these principals needs to be definitely proven.

In fact, adequate proximal and distal margins can usually be achieved by either laparoscopy or laparotomy, as long as the tumor is correctly localized. Intraoperative localization of colonic lesions in laparotomy relies largely on palpation of the tumor and its relations to adjacent organs. In laparoscopic surgery, tactile sensation is reduced, and palpation of the colon is blunted. Thus, intraoperative assessment of the colon relies mainly on the visual appearance of the colon during laparoscopy. Colonic pathology however, may often be confined to the mucosa and submucosa, and therefore may not be adequately assessed by visualizing the serosal surface. Difficulties in correct localization of the diseased segment during laparoscopy led to early reports of resection of the wrong segment of the colon [12]. In an early survey of the members of the American Society of Colon and Rectal Surgeons, 6.5% of the responders had experienced at least one case of mistakenly resecting the wrong segment, requiring conversion to a standard laparotomy to perform the correct operation [13]. Thus, when laparoscopic surgery is planned for early colon cancer, preoperative colonoscopic marking should be considered. This goal may be achieved by injection of India ink, or other dye substances, at 4 quadrants of the colonic wall [14]. Since it is impossible during colonoscopy to know which wall is mesenteric and which is antimesenteric, the ink should be injected in a circumferential pattern at four 90 degrees intervals adjacent to the lesion. If preoperative marking was not performed, or if laparoscopic exploration does not identify the lesion, intraoperative colonoscopy may be performed for tumor localization. Care should be taken to gently occlude the distal small bowel to prevent its insufflation. The laparoscopic light source may need to be reduced in intensity to permit the colonoscopist to navigate the lumen and subsequently to transilluminate the appropriate segment. The area can then be marked with clips, sutures, or cautery marks by the laparoscopic team. The colon should be fully desufflated as the colonoscope is withdrawn. Predicting which patient will require intraoperative colonoscopy is difficult, although small and flat tumors or polyps are more likely to be difficult to locate. Intraoperative colonoscopy should be immediately available for such cases.

Indeed, series which have examined the margins achieved during laparoscopic resection for colon cancer, reported that if the lesion was correctly localized, adequate margins were achieved in all cases [15-19].

Adequate lymph node clearance depends on an appropriate mesenteric resection. In order to achieve adequate cancer resection, mesenteric resection to the base of the mesentery should be performed. Several series of laparoscopic colon resection for cancer have evaluated the adequacy of lymph node clearance, most of them were compared to historical laparotomy results (Table 1). Lord et al [20], in a single institution experience, compared the number of lymph nodes laparoscopically harvested in 55 patients with cancer, to patients in whom the procedure was converted to laparotomy. The average number of lymph nodes was 9 when the procedure was completed laparoscopically, compared to 7.1 when conversion was performed. Gellman et al [21] in another single institution experience, found a mean of 9.3 lymph nodes in 58 patients who had laparoscopic colectomy for cancer, compared to a mean of 9.5 lymph nodes in 705 patients in whom the resection was performed by laparotomy. Kockerling et al [16], in a prospective multicenter study in German speaking countries in Europe, found a mean of 13 lymph nodes laparoscopically harvested. However, There was a significant difference among hospitals in the number of lymph nodes harvested, which slightly increased with experience. Franklin et al [17], in a multicenter study, allowed patients to select having their colon resection for cancer done either by laparoscopy or by laparotomy. The mean number of lymph nodes was 18 in the laparoscopic group, compared to 15 in the laparotomy group.

In cases of laparoscopically assisted right colectomy, most surgeons prefer an itracorporeal division of the ileocolic vessel, as the excision at the base of the mesentery may be technically difficult through the small incision. However, even with early colonic mobilization, followed by an open mesenteric division through a small incision, adequate oncologic resection is often possible. Moore et al [33] compared the specimens resected in laparoscopic assisted right colectomy, as compared to the same procedure via laparotomy, and found no difference in the number of lymph nodes harvested.

In conclusion, it appears that when principals of oncologic resection are respected, colon resection can be adequately performed laparoscopically.

Laparoscopic Rectal Resection - Can Adequate Total Mesorectal Excision be Performed?

The concept of total mesorectal excision for cancer of the mid and lower rectum was first introduced by Heald in 1982 [34]. Using this technique, he reported local recurrence rate of less than 5% with 5-year survival rate of nearly 80% [35]. These results reflect a great improvement over the results of the prior traditional techniques. In light of these results, total mesorectal excision has been widely adopted as the standard technique for curative rectal resection. Data from few subsequent series revealed that applying total mesorectal excision resulted in a significant reduction in the local recurrence rates [36-38]. In McCall's [39] review of the literature, the median local recurrence rate was 18.5% in 10,465 patients; however, in 1033 patients who underwent total mesorectal excision the local recurrence rate was only 7.1%.

The technical feasibility of performing a laparoscopic total mesorectal excision has been repeatedly established [23, 24, 18, 20, 40]. The tissue planes for TME are avascular, and with the appropriate retraction, laparoscopy provides excellent visualization of the pelvis, facilitating the pelvic dissection. Although the operative time is significantly longer when laparoscopy is used [24, 29], the morbidity rate is comparable to those following laparotomy. Table 2 summarizes the reported complication rate following laparoscopic total mesorectal excision.

Table 1: Lymph Nodes Harvesting

Author	Procedure	Laparoscopy (n)	Laparotomy (n)	Nodes retrieved (mean (range))	
				Laparoscopy	Laparotomy
Croce et al [15]	Colectomy	134		12.8(1-41)	
Kockerling et al [16]	Various	231		13 (5-28)	
Franklin et al [17]	Various	84	110	15.8(13-18)	14.7(13-16)
Croce et al [18]	Various	129		12.8(1-41)	
Lord et al [20]	Various	55	14 (conversion)	9(1-34)	7.1(0-34)
Gellman et al [21]	Various	58	705	9.3(NS)	9.5(NS)
Huscher et al [22]	Various	196		12.1(1-32)	
Seow-Choen et al [23]	APR	16	11	10 (6-16)	10 (6-32)
Iroatulam et al [24]	APR	7	7	9 (3-18)	9.5 (3-16)
Ramos et al [25]	APR	18	18	11.1(3-23)	7.8(1-27)
Larach et al [26]	APR	4		4.8(1-8)	
Wu et al [27]	APR	17		13(4-37)	
Darzi et al [28]	APR	12	16	9.5(6-19)	6 (4-14)
Fleshman et al [29]	APR	33	152	9.7(0-37)	7.9(0-43)
Schwander et al [30]	Anterior resection	19	19	12.7(±3.6)	13.7(±5.2)
	APR	13	13	13.2(±6.9)	12.2(±2.8)
Bokey et al [31]	Anterior resection	2			
	APR	8		10.5(±5.2)	
Lujan et al [32]	Various	102		6.6 (0-22)	

APR= Abdominoperineal resection

Table 2. Complications Following Laparoscopic and Conventional Total Mesorectal Excision

	Laparoscopy				Laparotomy			
Author	**Number of Patients**	**Mortality (%)**	**Major complications (%)**	**Overall morbidity (%)**	**Number of patients**	**Mortality (%)**	**Major complications (%)**	**Overall morbidity (%)**
Schwander et al [30]	32	0	3 (9)	10 (31.3)	32	1 (3)	4 (12)	10 (31.3)
Seow-Choen et al [23]	16	0	1 (6)	3 (18)	11	0	1 (9)	6 (55)
Iroatulam et al [24]	7	0	1 (14)	2 (25)	7	0	0	3 (43)
Ramos et al [25]	18	0	4 (22)	8 (44)	18	1 (5.5)	3 (16)	12 (66)
Darzi et al [28]	12	1 (8)	1 (8)	4 (33)	16	1 (6)	3 (18)	
Hartley et al [41]	21	0	4 (19)	6 (28)	22	0	1 (5)	4 (18)
Chung et al [40]	5	0	0	2 (40)				

Technique of Laparoscopic Rectal Resection

When total mesorectal excision is combined with abdominoperineal resection, it is amenable to laparoscopy, as the specimen can be retrieved through the perineal incision, thus obviating the need for any abdominal incision or pelvic anastomosis. In brief, mobilization of the sigmoid colon and upper rectum may be performed prior to mesenteric division (lateral to medial approach), or after the base of the mesentery is divided (medial to lateral approach). The right side of the peritoneum is incised near the inferior mesenteric vessels. After dissecting the inferior mesenteric artery close to its origin from the aorta, the vessel is divided using large clips, an endoscopic linear cutting vascular stapler or the Ligasure™ device. In the same fashion, the inferior mesenteric vein is divided near the inferior border of the pancreas. Care should be taken to identify and protect the left ureter, before the division of the mesenteric vessels. The dissection is continued along the base of the mesentery into the retrorectal space using either electrocautery or the ultrasonic scalpel. The peritoneum is incised on both sides of the rectum and the mesorectum is mobilized from the sacrum, taking care to identify and preserve the autonomic nerves at the sacral promontory and along the pelvic sidewalls. The peritoneum of the rectovaginal or rectovesical pouch is incised, as is the fascia of Denonvillier's. The rectum is completely freed from the seminal vesicles and prostate or vagina. Again, care is taken to protect the parasympathetic nerves at this distal lateral location. When using the medial to lateral approach, full mobilization of the sigmoid colon is than completed.

In females, the uterus and fallopian tubes can be temporarily secured to the anterior abdominal wall to facilitate exposure. Insertion of a blunt obturator into the uterine cavity has been described in order to assist retraction of the uterus [37], but is infrequently used. In abdominoperineal resection the perineal part of the procedure is undertaken in the traditional fashion, and the specimen is removed through the perineal incision.

When a low anterior resection with coloanal anastomosis is performed, a few technical difficulties are encountered. In addition to the pelvic dissection, sphincter saving total mesorectal excision requires creation of a safe anastomosis. This procedure in conventional laparotomy at present usually uses the double-stapling technique. Ideally, the rectum is transected perpendicular to its axis, at the level of the anorectal junction, often caudal to the levator ani muscles. With the laparoscopic staples, low division of the rectum is difficult, and usually results in a resection line which is not perpendicular to the axis of the rectum, but rather at an acute angle to its axis. Thus, a potentially poorly vascularised antimesenteric corner may result.

Several techniques have been developed in an attempt to overcome this technical difficulty. Inserting a "regular" 55mm stapler through a small pfannensteil incision allows transection of the distal rectum in an open fashion [42]. The specimen is retrieved from the suprapubic incision and the rectosigmoid junction is transected at the location chosen for the proximal side of the anastomosis. An anvil of a circular stapler is inserted into the sigmoid colon and secured with a purse-string. This limb is now returned to the abdominal cavity, the pfannensteil incision is closed, pneumoperitoneum reestablished, and a double stapled anastomosis constructed. Recently introduced modern laparoscopic equipment may enable the surgeon to achieve the same goal laparoscopically. Reticulating staplers are now available, as well as 90 degrees linear cutting staplers, design specifically for this purpose.

The triple stapled anastomosis, originally described by Steichen in 1988 [43] was adopted by several authors for laparoscopic sphincter saving total mesorectal excision [43, 44]. This technique allows complete intracorporeal anastomosis, transanally removing the specimen. When performing total mesorectal excision for cancer, however, removing the specimen transanally may violate oncologic principles.

Adequacy of the Rectal Excision

When correctly performed, laparoscopic TME provides lymph node clearance comparable to that reported after laparotomy (Table 1). Some concerns regarding the adequacy of the distal margins have certainly been highlighted by a variety of studies. Tate et al [46] compared 11 patients whose tumors were at a mean height of 20 cm from the anal verge as compared to 14 patients whose tumors were at a mean height of 15cm. Even though the location of these tumors was in the upper rectum or even lower sigmoid, the distal margin in the laparoscopic group was as small as 5mm. Lord et al [20] compared 19 patients who underwent laparoscopic anterior resection to 30 patients who underwent anterior resection by laparotomy. The margins in the former group were 4.9cm as compared to 2.5cm in a latter. However, neither the height of the tumor nor of the anastomosis was stated. Thus, one could assume that the larger margin in the laparoscopic group was the result of selection of patients with lesions in the upper portion of the rectum for the laparoscopic procedures. Conversely, patients with tumors in the lower rectum may have been directed towards laparotomy thereby resulting in shorter margins. The study by Goh et al [47] suffers from the same problem in that, although the distal margins were 4.0 (range, 2-8) cm in the laparoscopic group and 4.5 (range, 3-7.5) cm in the laparotomy group, neither the height of the tumor nor the level of the anastomosis was stated. In addition to some problems with distal margins, Darzi et al [28] noted an approximately 50% reduction in the tumor-free lateral margin in a group of 12 patients who underwent laparoscopic abdominoperineal resection when compared to 16 patients who underwent abdominoperineal resection by laparotomy. Seow-Choen [23] assessed 16 patients who underwent laparoscopic abdominoperineal resection in comparison to 11 patients who underwent abdominoperineal resection by laparotomy. Although they did not measure the lateral margin in millimeters, none of the lateral margins were involved by tumor in any of the 27 patients in the study. Thus, although it is possible to obtain adequate tumor-free distal and lateral margins, some compromise may occur perhaps as the result of technical limitations imposed by the instruments. The use of a 30-degree camera, the magnification afforded by laparoscopy, and the ultrasonic dissector which allows a meticulous hemostatic field ensure an adequate total mesorectal excision with wide lateral clearance. Nonetheless, one must be cognizant of the potential to "cone down" and have resultant inadequate margins.

If the mesorectum is not violated, and the specimen is removed through the perineum, or when the rectal transaction is performed at the level of the pelvic floor, at the distal end of the mesorectum, oncologic principles are not compromised using laparoscopy. Thus, although laparoscopic low anterior resection is technically difficult, laparoscopy can permit, at least technically, an oncologic excision comparable to laparotomy.

Comparative Studies

The acceptance of laparoscopic colorectal surgery as a safe and effective modality for the surgical treatment colon and rectal cancer will ultimately depend on the availability of established scientific data. Although much of the published data available today is still based on non-randomized series, several large randomized prospective trials are underway, and the evidences provided by smaller prospective trials are accumulating [48, 49, 50].

The Barcelona trial [51], published in 2002, included 219 patients, of which 119 were operated laparoscopically. Earlier recovery and lower morbidity were noted in the laparoscopic group. Interestingly, reduced risk of tumor relapse and increased survival were noted in the laparoscopic group, mainly due to differences in recurrence in patients with stage III disease.

The CLASICC trial (Conventional vs. Laparoscopic Assisted Surgery for Colorectal Cancer) is a muti-center UK based study, of which short-term results were recently announced. Morbidity, mortality and oncologic parameters of resection were similar in the laparoscopic and the open groups. Long term oncologic outcome however is still pending.

The COLOR trial (Colon cancer Laparoscopic or Open Resection) is a European multi-center trial [52] in which enrolment was closed on March 2003, after recruiting 1108 patients. 550 patients were included in the laparoscopic resection group. Preliminary report showed that the laparoscopic procedure, despite being longer, is safe and associated with earlier recovery.

In the United States, the COST study (Clinical Outcome of Surgical Therapy) recently published assessment of quality of life, and found only minimal short-term benefits with the laparoscopic resection compared with standard open resection [53]. Improvements in quality of life were more apparent in the laparoscopic group when a successful procedure was accomplished, but the presence of post-operative complications negated this advantage in the overall analysis.

The NCI trial (National Cancer Institute) was supposed to include 1200 patients [54], but enrolment was closed in September 2001 after 890 patients were accrued. No long term follow-up data is available yet.

Port Site Metastasis - A Myth or a Real Concern?

In 1993, two years after the introduction of laparoscopic colon resection, the first sporadic cases of port site metastasis were reported. Alexander et al [55] were the first to report, in a letter to the Lancet, on a 67-year male who presented with port site metastasis following laparoscopic assisted right colectomy for Dukes' C adenocarcinoma. This report was followed by one from O'Rourke et al [56], who described an 82-year old female with two port site metastasis, following resection for a Dukes' B adenocarcinoma. Cirocco et al [57] suggested that there was an "alarming rate" of wound recurrences in laparoscopic colectomy for cancer, compared to laparotomy. In the next two years at least 35 cases of port site recurrence were reported in the literature [58], raising the possibility that laparoscopic surgery with curative intent for colorectal cancer may actually have compromise cure.

Incidence of Port Site Metastasis in Laparoscopic Colon and Rectal Cancer Resection

Wound implantation is not unique to either laparoscopic or to colorectal surgery. However, the rapid accumulation of reports of port site metastasis in the first years, compared to the total number of laparoscopic colon resections performed during the early 1990's, suggested that there was an extraordinary high rate of wound recurrence in colorectal surgery. This fear turned the enthusiasm from the laparoscopic advantages into a more prudent and careful attitude. Many surgeons have limited their laparoscopic practice only to benign conditions, or to patients with metastatic disease on presentation. The trepidation was elucidated in a statement published by the American Society of Colon and Rectal Surgeons, that laparoscopic colorectal surgery should be undertaken only in a setting of an approved study with prospective retrieval of the data [59].

The information regarding port site metastasis in colorectal surgery was based on early case reports, while the actual incidence or prevalence of wound seeding remained unknown. Since 1996, there has been a marked reduction in the number of sporadic case reports; whether this phenomenon presents a real decline in the occurrence of port site metastasis is unclear. Since many surgeons do not perform laparoscopic colorectal surgery for cancer, it is difficult to compare the estimated rate of port site metastasis in the first years, with the actual rate published in the more recent literature.

The first published series of laparoscopic colon resection, included a relatively limited number of patients. For instance, although Berends et al [50] reported a 21% port site metastasis, the denominator was only 14 laparoscopic procedures. This small series probably reflects the preliminary experience of this group, and may be adversely influenced by the learning curve of this technically demanding procedure. As more experience was gained, larger series were recently published. Table 3 summarizes several series published in the English language literature, each with more then 50 patients who underwent laparoscopic colectomy for attempted cure of cancer. Smaller series were eliminated, as they may have reflected the learning curve of the authors. The rate of port site metastasis in these series was between zero and 1.7%. A summary of the data presented in Table 3 shows that a total number of 3901 patients who had laparoscopic resection of colorectal cancer in these series, 19 of whom had developed port site metastasis. Although the methods and patient selection is very varied, the overall wound recurrence rate in these series is approximately 0.7%.

Although such a rate of port site metastasis is not negligible, it may be comparable to the incidences reported for other malignancies, and to the 0.6-0.8% reported by Hughes [80] and by Reilly [81] for laparotomy for colorectal cancer. Several prospective randomized trials comparing laparoscopic versus laparotomy resections for cancer are currently underway. These studies are designed to determine whether laparoscopic colectomy is an adequate oncologic surgery, and to clarify any benefits and advantages of this procedure in terms of life quality and cost.

Table 3. Port Site Metastasis Laparoscopic Colorectal Resections for Carcinoma (series with >50 patients)

Authors	Year	*n* Patients	Number PSM*	% of PSM*
Guillou et al [61]	1993	59	1	1.7
Franklin et al [62]	1996	191	0	0
Gellman et al [21]	1996	58	1	1.7
Kwok et al [63]	1996	83	1	1.2
Vokasin et al [64]	1996	451	5	1.1
Fleshman et al [65]	1996	372	4	1.1
Lacy et al [66]	1997	106	0	0
Fielding et al [67]	1997	149	2	1.3
Larach et al [12]	1997	108	0	0
Croce et al [15]	1997	134	1	0.9
Khalili et al [68]	1998	80	0	0
Bouvet et al [69]	1998	91	0	0
Kawamura et al [70]	1999	67 (gasless)	0	0
Leung et al [71]	1999	217	1	0.65
Poulin et al [72]	1999	172	0	0
Schiedeck et al [73]	2000	399	1	0.25
Balli et al [74]	2000	320	0	0
Lezoche et al [75]	2000	112	2	1.8
Hong et al [76]	2001	98	0	0
Hahnloser [19]	2002	103	3	3
Lechaux [77]	2002	206	1	0.5
Lumley [78]	2002	154	2	1.1
Patankar [78]	2003	172	1	0.6
Total		3901	26	0.67

*PSM= Port site metastasis

The United States trial includes intended randomization of 1200 patients with potentially curable carcinomas of the right, left, or sigmoid colon, to colectomy by either laparoscopy or laparotomy, with a follow up of up to 8 years. Hopefully, this and other randomized studies will provide some valid information to determine the role of laparoscopic surgery for colorectal cancer.

Wound Recurrence in Open Surgery

The fact that most experienced surgeons have never seen a case of wound site recurrence after laparotomy for curative resection of colorectal cancer intimates its rarity. In fact, there are only two large retrospective series that have analyzed the incidence of wound recurrence after laparotomy. Hughes et al [80] reviewed 1603 patients, and found only 11 cases with abdominal scar recurrence, and another 5 cases with stoma or drain site recurrence. The total rate of wound recurrence in their series was 0.8%, and most of these patients had diffuse carcinomatosis at the time of recurrence. This report was the only large series specifically dealing with the issue of wound recurrence, until laparoscopic surgery drew attention to this problem. During the laparoscopic era and perhaps in defense of laparoscopy, Reilly et al [81] reviewed 1711 cases of patients participating in other clinical trials, and found 11 patients (0.6%) with wound recurrence. Only four of these patients were clinically diagnosed, as the remaining were incidentally diagnosed during laparotomy.

Care should be taken however, when comparing these retrospective series, to the recently published series of laparoscopic colon resections, where all wound recurrences were clinically significant. Conversely, the retrospective series of laparotomies included all patients who underwent colon resections, whereas the laparoscopic series included only selected patients who were judged to be good candidates for laparoscopic resection. Hence, selection bias may influence the comparative results.

Port Site Recurrence in Other Malignancies

Port site recurrence after laparoscopic procedures for malignant diseases is not unique to colon and rectal cancer. Although more then 60 cases of port site metastasis following colon resections were reported, they have also been noted following laparoscopic procedure for other malignancies.

Gynecologic surgeons have reported on sporadic cases of port site recurrence since the mid 1980's [82, 83]. In a recent study, four out of 25 patients who had laparoscopic surgery for malignant gynecologic diseases had port site metastasis [84]. In general surgery, there are numerous reports of port site metastasis of occult gallbladder carcinoma, after cholecystectomy for presumed cholelithiasis. Three recent large series found that once this rare tumor is diagnosed following laparoscopic cholecystectomy, the chance of port site metastasis is 14-32% [85, 86, 87].

Interestingly, port site metastases have also been reported following laparoscopic procedures without any manipulation of the tumor itself. Such reports have included recurrence after laparoscopic ultrasound for staging of pancreatic cancer [88], and of occult colon or pancreatic carcinoma after laparoscopic cholecystectomy [89, 90]. Mintz et al [91] reported on a case of port site metastasis of adenocarcinoma of an unknown primary focus, where despite thorough investigation, including exploratory laparotomy, no source was ever identified.

Port site metastases were also reported following video assisted thoracoscopic procedures for cancer. Downey et al [92] surveyed members of the Video-Assisted Thoracic Surgery Study Group, and found 17 wound recurrences. Unlike the abdominal wall, the thorax is rigid, and when the lung is collapsed, the pleural space is kept opened without need for a high pressure or gas rapid insufflation. Some proposed mechanisms for port site metastasis, which are based on gas pressure and insufflation, could not explain tumor recurrence in thoracoscopic wounds.

Proposed Mechanism for Port Site Metastasis

The pathophysiology leading to port site metastasis in laparoscopic surgery for cancer is poorly understood. Much basic research was done in the past decade, mainly on animal models, trying to identify mechanisms that may be responsible for this phenomenon. Animal models for laparoscopy have used both large animals, such as pigs or dogs, and small animals like rabbits, hamsters and mice. When large animal models are used, laparoscopic instruments and ports can be used in a similar fashion as used in human beings. Because of the expense, the number of animals used in most series is small. Although operations on small animals may be technically more difficult, they provide a more economical model that can be easily repeated on a larger number of animals. In vitro models, using chambers with carbon dioxide insufflation, have also been used to study cell movement during pneumoperitoneum. These animal and in vitro models have several drawbacks however, which may limit the application of their results to the understanding of the mechanism of port site metastasis in humans. Ideally, the model should use a cell type which resembles human colon cancer, maintain cultures in the host animal, and form a solid intraluminal colonic growth which resembles human colon cancer. The laparoscopic procedure should mimic laparoscopic colon resection. Different animal models have been applied, most of which have only partially fulfilled these criteria. In most of these models, the cells were introduced as a suspension or inoculum into the peritoneal cavity. These models may have limited relevance to colorectal cancer biology. Allardyce et al [93] used a porcine model of colon resection, and found that the incidence of port site metastasis was higher when cells suspension was intraperitoneally introduced, compared to transanal or to intramural injection. In other models, cells suspensions were injected trans rectally to the colon. Cells were also directly injected into the bowel wall, to simulate solid colon cancer [93], or to other solid organs as the spleen [94] or pancreas [95]. The latter models may also have a limited teleologic relevance.

Because of the technical difficulty of laparoscopic colon resection in animal models, especially in a small animals model, most experimental laparoscopic surgical procedures were limited to creation of pneumoperitoneum, or laparoscopic manipulation of a solid tumor, or organ containing a tumor.

Since port site metastasis is an infrequent event, investigational models have been undertaken in artificial conditions, where the rate of port site metastasis was intentionally much higher. Although this higher incidence was necessary in order to demonstrate any significant decrease in the treatment group, it may limit practical conclusions in humans.

The proposed mechanisms which were investigated may be divided into two main groups: mechanisms which are related to the pneumoperitoneum, and mechanisms related to tissue handling.

Mechanisms Related to Pneumoperitoneum

Free tumor cells, exfoliated from a colorectal tumor, have been found in the peritoneal cavity of patients undergoing cancer resection [96]. Since laparoscopic surgery is associated with constant flow of gas, it was postulated that these cells may be aerosolized, and implanted in port sites in the event of sudden loss of pneumoperitoneum, causing a sudden rush of gas through the trocar site. The return of intra-abdominal gas may also cause a plume with shedding of cells into the port site. Hewett et al [97] developed an in vivo model using radiolabeled tumor cells, introduced to the peritoneal cavity of pigs. The cells movement was detected in real time using a gamma camera. Tumor cells moved throughout the peritoneal cavity in a faster rate with pneumoperitoneum. Cavina et al [98] have clearly demonstrated intraperitoneal flow of cells, and Jones et al [99] have suggested that pneumoperitoneum predispose to port site metastasis. Knolmayer et al [100] analyzed the expelled gas from the peritoneal cavity during laparoscopy, by allowing the escaping gas to bubble in saline, and found a significant number of cells in the saline samples. However, Hewett et al [101] used filters to analyze the expelled gas, and found that only one of 30 filters was positive for tumor cells. Wittich et al [102] used a tubing system to connect the abdominal cavities of pairs of rats, one was injected with tumor cells and insufflated with gas. Tumor cells were found in the recipient rat only with a very high innoculum of cells to the donor animal. Whelan et al [103] used an in vitro chamber, as well as in vivo model, and did not find aerosolization of cells. Thus, contingent upon both methodology and model, the findings relative to aerosolization have been quite variable.

Although the theory of aerosolization was unproven, it is possible that pneumoperitoneum induce port site metastasis through other pathways. Many different studies have examined the poorly understood effect of pneumoperitoneum on port site metastasis, but the results of these studies are contradictory. A few studies found that pneumoperitoneum increases the rate of port site metastasis following intraperitoneal installation of cell suspension [104-106], and with injection of tumor cells to the kidneys [107], spleen [108], cecal mesentery [109], or subcutaneous tissue [110]. Other investigators found that pneumoperitoneum had no effect on the rate of port site metastasis [111, 112], and few studies even suggested that pneumoperitoneum may have a "protective effect", reducing the rate of port site metastasis compared to an open surgery [111-115]. Both laparoscopy by CO_2 pneumoperitoneum and laparotomy result in portal and venous distant dissemination of neoplastic cells, without any significant difference between the two methods [116].

CO_2 pneumoperitoneum was shown in a few modems to induce conditions which may stimulate tumor cells growth and invasiveness. Ridgway [117] showed in vitro that exposure of colon cancer cells to CO2 resulted in increased invasiveness through Matrigel coated filters.

Leister [118] used in animal model in which colon carcinoma sets were implanted in the upper abdomen. Tumor growth, as well as expression of propane is known to be associated with tumor growth and progression where significantly increased when pneumoperitoneum was used, compared to laparotomy. On the other hand, Tomita [119] injected colon cancer cell to the cecum of rats, and could not demonstrate increased in the original tumor size or liver metastases rate after laparoscopy and pneumoperitoneum in comparison to laparotomy.

Likewise, Lecuru [120] used an abdominal of ovarian cancer cells carcinomatosis model in rats, and found no difference in omental weight and abdominal wall spread between animals who had laparoscopic and those with laparotomy.

Pneumoperitoneum may be associated with changes in abdominal wall and systemic blood flow, which may influence on tumor spread in port site metastasis. Brundell [121] injected tumor cells into the jugular vein of rats at the time of laparoscopy or laparotomy. Abdominal wounds were harvested 15 days later. No tumor spread to the abdominal wall was found in the laparotomy group, whereas port site metastasis were found in the laparoscopy one. In another study by the same author [122], abdominal wall blood flow was evaluated using a radiolabeled albumin. Abdominal wall blood flow was significantly increased with pneumoperitoneum creation with CO2.

CO_2 induces local conditions such as change in the intraperitoneal pH and vasodilatation. Wildbrett [123] measured pH and partial oxygen tension in the abdominal wall laparoscopic wounds in rats undergoing laparoscopic with different gas mixtures, as well as the pH of colon carcinoma cell suspension installed into the peritoneal cavity. CO2 pneumoperitoneum resulted in a significant decrease in partial oxygen tension and pH, and an increase in intracellular Calcium levels, as well as a significant decrease in the carcinoma cell suspension pH.

Because the problem may be CO_2 specific, which may promote port site metastasis, some authors have suggested that other types of gases, such as Helium [124], may reduce the rate of wound recurrence.

Gas temperature and humidity may also affect tumor growth. Nduka [125] used cold or warmed CO2 and found increased tumor growth with the use of cold gas. Both cold and the warm gases used for laparoscopy were associated with significantly increased tumor growth in comparison to animals that did not have laparoscopy.

Intra-abdominal pressure by itself may have an effect on inducing of port site metastasis, and few authors suggested that increased pressure may be associated with increased risk of port site metastasis [100, 109]. Others suggested that the increase in port site metastasis rate is related to gas flow. Zayyan [126] found significant increase in port site implants in rats who had rapid flow insufflation of CO2, compared to those who had slow insufflation or gasless laparoscopy. Brundell [121] found that increased volumes of gas insufflation caused increased abdominal movement of tumor cells in rats, although this did not translate to higher rate of port site involvement. Surprisingly, decreased insufflation pressures resulted in this study in increased contamination of port sites.

Recently, Yamaguchi et al [127] found that pneumoperitoneum increased the levels of Hyaluronic acid in the peritoneal cavity, and injection of Hyaluronic acid into the abdomen increase the rate of port site metastasis in a murine model. However, the cause and effect and clinical implications of these findings are not clear yet.

Mechanisms Related to Tissue Handling

One of the first mechanisms which was blamed for port site metastasis was specimen handling. After using potentially traumatic instruments to grasp the bowel, the specimen is removed through a limited skin incision. Contact of the specimen with the abdominal wall is obvious, and frequently accompanied by manipulation of the specimen to assist "squeezing" the tumor through the wound. These mechanisms became potential suspects in facing the initial reports of port site metastasis.

Although the dissection in laparoscopic colon surgery is similar to that in laparotomy, the tissue handling and manipulation may be different. Palpation of the specimen is blunted with the long laparoscopic instruments, and perception is distorted with the two dimensional optics. Lee et al [94] studied the impact of laparoscopic tissue manipulation on colon adenocarcinoma cells injected into the spleen in a murine model, and found that manipulation of the tumor before splenectomy increased the incidence of abdominal wound tumor implantation, independent of the presence or absence of pneumoperitoneum. Mathew et al [128] manipulated abdominal wall tumors, and found that wound metastasis was 5 times more likely in rats who had laparoscopic manipulation. Conversely, Mutter et al [95] injected cancer cells into rats pancreas, and found that tumor manipulation via laparoscopy did not increase tumor implantation, whereas laparotomy did cause an increase.

Others have investigated the role of the laparoscopic surgical tools, and found that the instruments were contaminated with tumor cells, more so for the operating surgeon then the assisting surgeon [99, 129]. Wilkinson [130] in the kidneys solid tumor model found that ports used for laparoscopic surgical instruments were associated with much higher rate of port site metastasis in comparison to ports used for the camera. Recently, Brundell [131] found that metal laparoscopic ports are associated with higher number of tumor cells adhered to the port, in comparison to plastic ports, but this did not translate to statistically significant difference in port site metastasis rate and laparoscopic wounds. Nduka et al [132] hypothesized that the ultrasonic scalpel waves may release viable airborne cancer cells, but found no difference in the cell count in aspirated smoke flume with harmonic scalpel compared to cautery. Subsequently, the Harmonic scalpel has been shown as a superior dissecting tool which products less trauma then do diathermy. Thus, tumor cell implantation should theoretically be less likely after ultrasonic dissection [133].

Local abdominal trauma due to the trocar itself causing ischemia has also been suggested as a possible cause of port site metastasis. Tseng et al [134] induced local tissue trauma by crushing half of the port sites. In this rat model a significant increase in the incidence and size of the port site recurrences was noted in the induced ischemia group. A subsequent study by Farrel et al [135] confirmed that traumatized tissue surfaces may have been more predisposed to tumor cell implantation. Indeed, in their study implantation was much more common in the pneumoperitoneum than in the control group. Recently, Hirabayashi [136] examined port sites under light and electron microscope in fixed time intervals after laparoscopy and injection of gastric cancer cells. On the day of surgery, the abdominal peritoneum was found to be peeled of and the muscular layer was damaged in all port sites, and several tumor cells were attached to the injured tissue. Three days postoperatively, the injured tissue contained granulation tissue, and several cancer cells were observed. On post operative date 8, a small nodule was macroscopically visible at the port sites, which microscopically was proved to be port site metastasis covered by mesothelial cells.

Results of the basic science data regarding possible mechanisms of port site recurrence are summarized in Table 4.

Table 4. Proposed Mechanisms of Port Site Metastasis

Mechanism	Supporting evidence	Non supporting evidence
Creation of pneumoperitoneum	Jones et al [99]	Pauels et al [138]
	Wu et al [137]	Paik et al [139]
	Bouvy et al [107, 114]	Hubens et al [140]
	Mathew et al [104, 141]	Allardyce et al [93, 111]
	Dorrance et al [105]	Gutt et al [113]
	Chen et al [108]	Southall et al [112]
	Jacobi et al [106, 109]	Moriera et al [142]
	Cavina et al [98]	
Aerosolization of tumor cells	Hewett et al [97, 101]	Whelan et al [103]
	Knolmayer et al [100]	
	Wittich et al [143]	
Tissue manipulation	Mathew et al [128]	Mutter et al [95]
Trocar site trauma	Tsang et al [134]	
Tumor manipulation	Lee et al [94]	
Instrument contamination	Hewett et al [101]	Nduka et al [132]
	Allardyce et al [111, 129]	

PREVENTIVE MEASUREMENTS

Although the cause of post site metastasis is not understood, a few preventive measures have been suggested, base on the presumed aforementioned mechanisms.

- *Wound Protectors.* The assumption that the withdrawal of a large specimen through a small wound may lead to port site metastasis, led to the use of plastic wound protectors and specimen bags. The fact that wound recurrences have been found in protected sites and in sites which have had no direct contact with the specimen however, questions the benefit of these measurements [115]. Since the protectors are simple to use, inexpensive, and without known morbidity, they are probably the most common preventives currently in use.
- *Gasless Laparoscopy.* In the light of some of the investigational evidence that the creation of pneumoperitoneum may be responsible for wound recurrences, a few authors have suggested the use of gasless laparoscopy. However, the experimental results with this technique are controversial. Some authors have found a significantly decrease in the occurrence of port site metastasis with gasless laparoscopy in an animal model [107, 114], but others could not repeat these results [113, 144]. A group from the University of Tokyo in Japan reported on a series of 67 patient who underwent colon resection with the gasless laparoscopy technique [70]. In a mean follow up of two years, none of them developed port site metastasis. It should be mentioned however, that unlike rats' abdominal walls, in human patients lifting systems are causing local pressure and tissue trauma at the abdominal wall, and technical problems make laparoscopic resections difficult. Thus, improved lifting

systems must be developed before the widespread of this technique can be applied to patients with colorectal cancer.

- *Type of Gas:* the hypothesis that CO_2 may lead to an environmental change which contributes to wound recurrence, led Neuhaus et al [124] to compare different gas types for pneumoperitoneum in an animal model. Only helium was found to reduce the rate of wound metastasis significantly. These findings were supported by Jacobi et al [106], who found that CO_2 promotes growth and attenuates the immunologic response, compared to helium or air. More recently, Gupta [143] compared tumor spread after laparoscopy with four different gases after intraperitoneal installation of tumor cells in a rat model. Laparoscopy with helium resulted in the lower rate of port site metastasis, whereas argon and nitrogen pneumoperitoneum were associated with the highest rate, and the effect CO2 insufflation was intermediate. However, Dorrance et al [105], found that laparoscopy promotes tumor growth, independent of the gas type used, and more recently Hopkins [144] found no difference in port site recurrence rate in a rat model after pneumoperitoneum with either CO_2, helium, or nitrous oxide. Currently, in the absence of complete concordance among studies and the unknown effect of helium pneumoperitoneum in humans, CO_2 remains the most commonly used gas.
- *Wound Excision.* Assuming that cancer cells are implanted in the wound during surgery, it seems logical that excision of the wound will eliminate, or at least reduce the rate of wound recurrence. Wu et al [148], in an animal model, found that wound excision reduced the rate of port site metastasis from 89% to 78%, but did not completely eliminate wound recurrence. On the other hand, Watson [149] surprisingly found that wound excision significantly increased port site metastasis in a rat model. Thus, to date, data are contradicting, and this protected measure cannot yet be recommended.
- *Peritoneal and Port Site Irrigation:* Some authors have suggested that irrigation of the peritoneal cavity or the trocar wounds with various solutions, may reduce the occurrence of wound metastasis. Animal studies have shown that peritoneal irrigation with Povidone-Iodine [150, 151], Heparin [152], Methotrexate [151], and Cyclophosphamid [146], all reduced the rate of port site metastasis. Eshraghi et al [153] irrigated the port sites with various agents, and found that 5-FU reduced the rate of wound recurrence. These agents however are potentially hazardous, and the application of these results to humans does not seem to be currently acceptable.

Recently, several authors suggested peritoneal irrigation with taurolidine, a derivate of the amino acid taurine, which is thought to inhibit tumor growth by the inhibition of interleukin production by peritoneal macrophages. Wenger [154] use a chemically induced pancreatic cancer model in rats who underwent diagnostic laparoscopy and biopsies. The use of taurolidine significantly decreased pancreatic tumor size, as well as liver and Port site metastasis. Opitz [155] used laparoscopic cecal resection in rats, where tumor cells were injected into the peritoneal cavity at time of surgery, and found that peritoneal installation of taurolidine in combination with heparin significantly decreased peritoneal tumor spread. Volz [156] found that peritoneal injection of taurolidine mixed with heparin significantly increased survival time in rats after peritoneal installation of tumor cells. Further study with these agents however is required to determine its usefulness and potential risks, before human studies can be performed.

Hamzaoglu [157] have recently challenged an interesting and unique concept of application of honey on wounds in order to prevent wound tumoral growth. Sixty rats underwent standard posterior neck incisions and cancer cells were applied to the wounds. In half of the animals, the wounds were coated with honey before and after tumor inoculation, whereas the second group served as control. Tumor implants were evident macroscopically and microscopically in all control groups' rats, whereas macroscopic implants were not detected in any of the treatment group animals, and microscopic deposits were found only in 26% of the treatment group.

The results of these experimental studies in port site implantation reduction are summarized in Table 5.

Table 5. Port Site Metastasis Preventative Measures

	Supporting data	Non supporting data
Wound protectors	Montorsi [115]	
Gasless laparoscopy	Bouvy et al [107, 114]	Gutt et al [113]
	Watson et al [147]	Iwanaka et al [146]
	Kawamura et al [70]	
Different gas	Neuhaus et al [124]	Dorrance et al [105]
	Jacobi et al [106]	Farrell et al [158]
	Gupta [143]	Hopkins [144]
Wound excision	Wu et al [148]	Watson [149]
Peritoneal irrigation		
Iodine	Lee et al [150]	
	Neuhaus et al [151]	
Heparin	Neuhaus et al [152]	
Cytotoxic agents	Neuhaus et al [151]	
	Iwanaka et al [146]	
	Jacobi et al [159]	
Taurolidine	Wenger [154]	
	Opitz [155]	
	Volz [156]	
Wound irrigation	Eshraghi et al [153]	
	Hamzaoglu [157]	

Because of the potential multifactorial etiology of port site implantation, it is important to employ as many "protective measures" as possible. The decrease from the early port site implantation incidence of over 3% (range, 0% - 21%) to the more recent mean of 0.7% (range 0% - 1.7%) is probably due to both technique and technical improvements. The importance of these protective measures was highlighted by Schneider et al [160]. In this study, 18 pigs underwent laparoscopic sigmoid resection by a "senior" laparoscopic surgeons. In the control group, "standard" dissection was undertaken where no great protective efforts were made. In the "protective measures" group, the trocars were deliberately fixed in place, gas leaks were prevented, all instruments, ports and trocars were rinsed with povidine-iodine and a mini-laparotomy with deliberate wound edge protection was undertaken. The tumor recurrence rate in the control group was 63% which was significantly higher than the 13.8% in the group in which protective measures was undertaken. Thus, the routine use of protective measures in patients undergoing laparoscopic resection for attempted cure of colorectal cancer should be considered. These measures include gentle handling of the tissue, deliberate avoidance of handling the tumor itself, making the specimen extraction incision large enough to avoid tearing or forcing the lesion through the delivery site, protecting the wounded site with some type of wound protectors, and irrigating the wound at the conclusion of the procedure.

Immune System Response to Laparoscopic Surgery

A variety of studies have demonstrated less depression in the immune system in laparoscopic colorectal surgery, compared to laparotomy. This may be beneficial for patients with malignant disease, minimizing intraoperative tumor spread and implantation. Allendorf et al [161, 162], in an animal model, found that skin reaction to an antigen was significantly reduced when open cecal resection was performed, compared to laparoscopic resection, or to a control group having only anesthesia. Schwenk et al [163] noted less depression of the interleukin 1, interleukin 6 and C-reactive protein levels in laparoscopy, as compared to laparotomy. Similarly, Da Costa et al [164] found significantly greater tumor growth after laparotomy than after laparoscopy. There was a greater decrease in lymphokine activated killer and natural killer cells activity after laparotomy as compared to laparoscopy and controls. More recently, Ordemann [165] randomized 40 patients with colon cancer to either laparoscopic surgery or laparotomy. Post operative cell immunity, assessed by measuring the white blood cell (WBC) count, the CD4+ and CD8+ lymphocytes, the CD4+/CD8+/ratio, the HLA-DR expression of CD14+ monocytes, and the production of interleukin-6 (IL-6) and TNF-a, was better preserved after laparoscopic surgery as compared to laparotomy. However, not all studies have been as enthusiastically optimistic about laparoscopy. Fukushima et al [166] reported no differences between patients who underwent sigmoid colectomy using gasless laparoscopy or laparotomy, relative to either interleukin 6, glucagon, or C-reactive protein levels. However, there was a correlation between the length of surgery and the depression in these immune parameters. Since laparoscopy usually requires longer operative time, laparotomy would seem to be favored in this regard. More recently, Wu [167] measured proinflammatory cytokines in peritoneal drains and blood of 28 patients were randomized 40 either laparoscopic surgery or laparotomy for colon cancer. The immediate levels of proinflammatory cytokines in the serum were significantly lower in the laparoscopic group, but the same cytokines locally produced in the peritoneal cavity showed no differences, which suggests that the two intra-abdominal approaches are equally traumatic. No differences in cellular response were observed between the groups.

Although the issue of immune response to laparoscopic surgery is not yet clear, laparoscopy may, at least theoretically, offer some benefits to patients undergoing attempted curative resection of colorectal cancer. Indeed, in a recent study by Lacy [51], 219 patients with colon cancer were prospectively randomized to laparoscopic resection or laparotomy. Probability of cancer related survival was higher in the laparoscopic group, with reduced rate of tumor recurrence. The authors of the study postulated that the attenuated immune response associated with the laparoscopic surgery may be responsible for these results. However, large multicenter studies, with the appropriate power to detect differences in survival, are still underway. Hopefully, the results of these studies will allow firm conclusion in this issue.

Conclusions

Laparoscopic colon and rectal surgery has potential advantages of improved cosmesis, reduced postoperative pain, earlier recovery, and less immune compromise. However, when applying this technique for attempted cure colorectal cancer, it is crucial to show that all oncologic surgery principals are strictly maintained, and survival and recurrence rates are not compromised. Series of patients who had laparoscopic surgery for cancer show that oncologic resections, with adequate proximal, distal and circumferential margins can be technically achieved. An exception of this rule may be the laparoscopic low anterior resection, where distal laparoscopic application of the stapler may be technically difficult.

Despite extensive research efforts, neither the incidence of port site metastasis after laparoscopic surgery for cancer, nor its causes are known. The data grouped in this review suggest that the recent rate of port site metastasis is much lower than the initial reported rate, probably due to technical and technique improvement. Thus, port site metastasis may not be inherited detriment of laparoscopic colectomy, but rather an unfortunate sequelae of the learning curve of the application of laparoscopy for colorectal cancer. Indeed, Lee et al [168] have recently showed that the rate of port site metastasis in an animal model decreases with increase of experience. Numerous consecutive recent reports failed to confirm the unacceptably high incidence of port site recurrence initially reported, further supporting the hypothesis that learning curve, surgical experience, good judgment and technique, and appropriate use of this new technology are important factors in this regard. The final results of the large randomized prospective studies which are currently underway, and information drawn from the continuous basic science efforts, will hopefully solve this question in the near future. The safest approach in the interim is to only offer laparoscopic colorectal resections for attempted cure of carcinoma within prospectively randomized externally monitored peer reviewed trials. When patients are randomized to the laparoscopic procedures, precautions such as wound protection and irrigation should be employed.

References

[1] Schlinkert RT. Laparoscopic-assisted hemicolectomy. *Dis Colon Rectum* 1991, 34(11):1030-1031.

[2] Corbitt JD. Preliminary experience with laparoscopic-guided colectomy. *Surg Laparosc Endosc.* 1992, 2(1):79-81.

[3] Jacobs M, Verdeja JC, Goldstein HS. Minimally invasive colon resection (laparoscopic colectomy). *Surg Laparosc Endosc.* 1991, 1(3):144-150.

[4] Bouvet M, Mansfield PF, Skibber JM, Curley SA, Ellis LM, Giacco GG, Madary AR, Ota DM, Feig BW. Clinical, pathologic, and economic parameters of laparoscopic colon resection for cancer. *Am J Surg.* 1998, 176(6):554-558.

[5] Lumley JW, Fielding GA, Rhodes M, Nathanson LK, Siu S, Stitz RW. Laparoscopic-assisted colorectal surgery. Lessons learned from 240 consecutive patients. *Dis Colon Rectum.* 1996, 39(2):155-159.

[6] Delaney CP, Kiran RP, Senagore AJ, Brady K, Fazio VW. Case-matched comparison of clinical and financial outcome after laparoscopic or open colorectal surgery. *Ann Surg.* 2003 Jul;238(1):67-72.

[7] Chen HH, Wexner SD, Weiss EG, Nogueras JJ, Alabaz O, Iroatulam AJ, Nessim A, Joo JS. Laparoscopic colectomy for benign colorectal disease is associated with a significant reduction in disability as compared with laparotomy. *Surg Endosc.* 1998, 12(12):1397-1400.

[8] Lawrence DM, Pasquale MD, Wasser TE. Laparoscopic versus open sigmoid colectomy for diverticulitis. *Am Surg.* 2003 Jun;69(6):499-503.

[9] Bemelman WA, Dunker MS, Slors JF, Gouma DJ. Laparoscopic surgery for inflammatory bowel disease: current concepts. *Scand J Gastroenterol Suppl.* 2002;(236):54-9.

[10] Senagore AJ, Madbouly KM, Fazio VW, Duepree HJ, Brady KM, Delaney CP. Advantages of laparoscopic colectomy in older patients. *Arch Surg.* 2003 Mar;138(3):252-6.

[11] Law WL, Chu KW, Tung PH. Laparoscopic colorectal resection: a safe option for elderly patients. *J Am Coll Surg.* 2002 Dec;195(6):768-73.

[12] Larach SW, Patankar SK, Ferrara A, Williamson PR, Perozo SE, Lord AS. Complications of laparoscopic colorectal surgery. Analysis and comparison of early vs. latter experience. *Dis Colon Rectum.* 1997, 40(5):592-596.

[13] Wexner SD, Cohen SM, Ulrich A, Reissman P. Laparoscopic colorectal surgery--are we being honest with our patients? *Dis Colon Rectum.* 1995, 38(7):723-727.

[14] Botoman VA, Pietro M, Thirlby RC. Localization of colonic lesions with endoscopic tattoo. *Dis Colon Rectum.* 1994 Aug;37(8):775-776.

[15] Croce E, Azzola M, Russo R, Golia M, Olmi S. Laparoscopic colectomy: the absolute need for a standard operative technique. *J Soc Laparoendosc Surg.* 1997, 1(3):217-224.

[16] Kockerling F, Reymond MA, Schneider C, Wittekind C, Scheidbach H, Konradt J, Kohler L, Barlehner E, Kuthe A, Bruch HP, Hohenberger W. Prospective multicenter study of the quality of oncologic resections in patients undergoing laparoscopic colorectal surgery for cancer. The Laparoscopic Colorectal Surgery Study Group. *Dis Colon Rectum.* 1998, 41(8):963-70.

[17] Franklin ME, Rosenthal D, Norem RF. Prospective evaluation of laparoscopic colon resection versus open colon resection for adenocarcinoma. A multicenter study. *Surg Endosc.* 1995, 9(7):811-816.

[18] Croce E, Olmi S, Azzola M, Russo R, Di Bonifacio M . Laparoscopic colectomy: indications, standardized technique and results after 6 years experience. *Hepatogastroenterology* 2000, 47(33):683-691.

[19] Hahnloser D, Chanson Ch, Nassiopoulos K, Wahl P, Petropoulos P. Laparoscopic surgery of colorectal cancer. Apropos of 103 interventions *Swiss Surg.* 2002;8(5):203-8.

[20] Lord SA, Larach SW, Ferrara A, Williamson PR, Lago CP, Lube MW. Laparoscopic resections for colorectal carcinoma. A three-year experience. *Dis Colon Rectum.* 1996, 39(2):148-154.

[21] Gellman L, Salky B, Edye M: Laparoscopic assisted colectomy. *Surg Endosc* 1996, 10(11):1041-1044.

[22] Huscher C, Silecchia G, Croce E, Farello GA, Lezoche E, Morino M, Azzola M, Feliciotti F, Rosato P, Tarantini M, Basso N. Laparoscopic colorectal resection. A multicenter Italian study. *Surg Endosc.* 1996, 10(9):875-879.

[23] Seow-Choen F, Eu KW, Ho YH, Leong AFPK. A preliminary comparison of a consecutive series of open versus laparosocpic abdomino-perineal resection for rectal adenocarcinoma. *Int J Colorect Dis* 1997;12:88-90.

[24] Iroatulam AJN, Agachan F, Alabaz O, Weiss EG, Nogueras JJ, Wexner SD. Laparosocpic abdominoperineal resection for anorectal cancer. *Am Surg* 1998, 64:12-18.

[25] Ramos JR, Petrosemolo RH, Valory EA, Polania FC, Pecanha R. Abdominoperineal resection: laparoscopic versus conventional. *Surg Laparosc Endosc* 1997, 7:148-152.

[26] Larach SW, Salomon MC, Williamson PR, Goldstein E. Lapaorscopic assisted abdominoperineal resection. *Surg Laparosc Endosc* 1993, 3:115-118.

[27] Wu JS, Birnbaum EH, Fleshman JW. Early experience with laparoscopic abdominoperineal resection. *Surg Endosc* 1997, 11:449-455.

[28] Darzi A, Lewis C, Menzies-Gow N, Guillou PJ, Monson JRT. Laparosocpic abdominoperineal excision of the rectum. *Surg Endosc* 1995, 9:414-417.

[29] Fleshman JW, Wexner SD, Anvari M, LaTulippe JF, Birnbaum EH, Kodner IJ, Read TE, Nogueras JJ, Weiss EG. Laparoscopic vs. open abdominoperineal resection for cancer. *Dis Colon Rectum* 1999, 42:930-939.

[30] Schwander O, Schiedeck THK, Killaitis C, Bruch HP. A case-control study comparing laparoscopic versus open surgery for rectosigmoid and rectal cancer. *Int J Colorect Dis* 1999, 14:158-163.

[31] Bokey EL, Moore JWE, Keating JP, Zelas P, Chapuis PH, Newland RC. Laparoscopic resection of the colon and rectum for cancer. *Br J Surg* 1997, 84:822-825.

[32] Lujan HJ, Plasencia G, Jacobs M, Viamonte M 3rd, Hartmann RF. Long-term survival after laparoscopic colon resection for cancer: complete five-year follow-up. *Dis Colon Rectum.* 2002 Apr;45(4):491-501.

[33] Moore JW, Bokey EL, Newland RC, Chapuis PH. Lymphovascular learance in laparoscopically assisted right hemicolectomy is similar to open surgery. *Aust N Z J Surg.* 1996 Sep, 66(9):605-7.

[34] Heald RJ, Husband EM, Ryall RD. The mesorectum in rectal cancer surgery--the clue to pelvic recurrence? *Br J Surg.* 1982, 69(10):613-616.

[35] MacFarlane JK, Ryall RDH, Heald RJ. Mesorectal excision for rectal cancer. *Lancet* 1993, 341:457-460.

[36] Dahlberg M, Glimelius B, Pahlman L. Changing strategy for rectalcancer is associated with improved outcome. *Br J Surg* 1999, 86:379-384.

[37] Arbman G, Nilsson E, Halbook O, Sjodahl R. Local recurrence following total mesorectal excision for rectal cancer. *Br J Surg* 1995, 18:375-379.

[38] Enker WE, Thaler HT, Cranor ML, Polyak T. Total mesorectal excision in the operative treatment of carcinoma of the rectum. *J Am Coll Surg* 1995, 18:335-346.

[39] McCall JL, Cox MR, Wattchow DA. Analysis of local recurrence rates after surgery for rectal cancer. *Int J Colorect Dise* 1995, 10:126-132.

[40] Chung CC, Ha JP, Tsang WW, Li MK. Laparoscopic-assisted total mesorectal excision and colonic J pouch reconstruction in the treatment of rectal cancer. *Surg Endosc*. 2001 Oct;15(10):1098-101.

[41] Hartley JE, Mehigan BJ, Qureshi AE, Duthie GS, Lee PW, Monson JR. Total mesorectal excision: assessment of the laparoscopic approach. *Dis Colon Rectum*. 2001, 44:315-321.

[42] Lezoche E, Paganini AM, Feliciotti F. A new technique to facilitate laparosocpic resection of low rectal tumors. *Surg Laparosc Endos* 997, 7:9-12.

[43] Steichen FM. Changing concepts in surgical techniques. In: Ravitch MM, Steichen FM, Wlter R (eds). *Current Practice of Surgical stapling. Proceedings of the second international symposium and first European congress on stapling in surgery*. Luxembourg, 1988. Lea & Febiger, Philadephia, 1990, 23-27.

[44] Fleshman JW, Brunt LM, Fry RD. Laparoscopic anterior resection of the rectum using a triple stapled intracorporeal anastomosis in the pig. *Surg Laparosc Endosc* 1993, 3:119-126.

[45] Vasilescu C, Tomulescu V, Calin I, Nuraltay E. Anterior resection of the rectum via laparoscopy. *Chirurgia (Bucur)* 1998, 93:43-48.

[46] Tate JJ, Kwok S, Dawson JW, Lau WY, Li AK. Prospective comparison of laparoscopic and conventional anterior resection. *Br J Surg*. 1993, 80:1396-1398.

[47] Goh YC, Eu KW, Seow-Choen F. Early postoperative results of a prospective series of laparoscopic vs. Open anterior resections for rectosigmoid cancers. *Dis Colon Rectum*. 1997, 40:776-780.

[48] Feliciotti F, Paganini AM, Guerrieri M, Sanctis A, Campagnacci R, Lezoche E. Results of laparoscopic vs open resections for colon cancer in patients with a minimum follow-up of 3 years. *Surg Endosc*. 2002 Aug;16(8):1158-61.

[49] Lezoche E, Feliciotti F, Paganini AM, Guerrieri M, De Sanctis A, Minervini S, Campagnacci R. Laparoscopic vs open hemicolectomy for colon cancer. *Surg Endosc*. 2002 Apr;16(4):596-602.

[50] Champault GG, Barrat C, Raselli R, Elizalde A, Catheline JM. Laparoscopic versus open surgery for colorectal carcinoma: a prospective clinical trial involving 157 cases with a mean follow-up of 5 years. *Surg Laparosc Endosc Percutan Tech*. 2002 Apr;12(2):88-95.

[51] Lacy AM, Garcia-Valdecasas JC, Delgado S, Castells A, Taura P, Pique JM, Visa J. Laparoscopy-assisted colectomy versus open colectomy for treatment of non-metastatic colon cancer: a randomised trial. *Lancet*. 2002 Jun 29;359(9325):2224-9.

[52] Hazebroek EJ; Color Study Group. COLOR: a randomized clinical trial comparing laparoscopic and open resection for colon cancer. *Surg Endosc.* 2002 Jun;16(6):949-953.

[53] Weeks JC, Nelson H, Gelber S, Sargent D, Schroeder G; Clinical Outcomes of Surgical Therapy (COST) Study Group. Short-term quality-of-life outcomes following laparoscopic-assisted colectomy vs open colectomy for colon cancer: a randomized trial. *JAMA*. 2002 Jan 16;287(3):321-8.

[54] Nelson H. Laparoscopic colectomy for colon cancer--a trial update. *Swiss Surg.* 2001;7(6):248-51.

[55] Alexander RJ, Jaques BC, Mitchell KG. Laparoscopically assisted colectomy and wound recurrence. *Lancet* 1993, 341(8839), 249-250 (letter).

[56] O'Rourke N, Price PM, Kelly S, Sikora K. Tumor inoculation during laparoscopy. *Lancet* 1993, 342(8867), 368 (letter).

[57] Cirocco WC, Schwartzman A, Golub RW. Abdominal wall recurrence after laparoscopic colectomy for colon cancer. *Surgery* 1994, 116(5):842-846.

[58] Cohen SM, Wexner SD. laparoscopic colorectal resection for cancer: The Cleveland Clinic Florida experience. *Surg Oncol* 1993, 2(suppl):35s-42s.

[59] American Society of Colorectal Surgeons: Policy statement. *Dis Colon rectum* 1992, 35:5A.

[60] Berends FJ, Kazemier G, Bonjer HJ, Lange JF. Subcutaneous metastases after laparoscopic colectomy. *Lancet* 1994, 334(8914):58 (letter).

[61] Guillou PJ, Darzi A, Monson JR. Experience with laparoscopic colorectal surgery for malignant disease. *Surg Oncol* 1993, 2 (suppl):43S-49S.

[62] Franklin ME, Rosenthal D, Abrego-Medina D, Dorman JP, Glass JL, Norem R, Diaz A. Prospective comparison of open Vs. laparoscopic colon surgery for carcinoma. Five-year results. *Dis Colon Rectum* 1996, 39(10suppl):35S-46S.

[63] Kwok SP, Lau WY, Carey PD, Kelly SB, Leung KL, Li AK. Prospective evaluation of laparoscopic-assisted large bowel excision of cancer. *Ann Surg* 1996, 223(2):170-176.

[64] Vukasin P, Ortega AE, Greene FL, Steele GD, Simons AJ, Anthone GJ, Weston LA, Beart RW. Wound recurrence following laparoscopic colon cancer resection. *Dis Colon Rectum* 1996, 39(10 suppl):21S-23S.

[65] Fleshman JW, Nelson H, Peters WR, Kim HC, Larach S, Boorse RR, Ambroze W, Leggett P, Bleday R, Stryker S, Christenson B, Wexner S, Senagore A, Rattner D, Sutton J, Fine AP. Early results of laparoscopic surgery for colorectal cancer. Retrospective analysis of 372 patients treated by Clinical Outcomes of Surgical Therapy (COST) study group. *Dis Colon Rectum* 1996, 39(10suppl):53S-58S.

[66] Lacy AM, Garcia-Valdecasas JC, Delgado S, Grande L, Fuster J, Tabet J, Ramos C, Pique JM, Cifuentes A, Visa J. Postoperative complications of laparoscopic-assisted colectomy. *Surg Endosc* 1997, 11(2):119-122.

[67] Fielding GA, Lumley J, Nathanson L, Hewitt P, Rhodes M, Stitz R. Laparoscopic colectomy. *Surg Endosc* 1997,11(7):745-749.

[68] Khalili TM, Fleshner PR, Hiatt JR, Sokol TP, Manookian C, Tsushima G, Phillips EH. Colorectal cancer: comparison of laparoscopic with open approaches. *Dis Colon Rectum* 1998, 41(7):832-838.

[69] Bouvet M, Mansfield PF, Skibber JM, Curley SA, Ellis LM, Giacco GG, Madary AR, Ota DM, Feig BW. Clinical, pathologic, and economic parameters of laparoscopic colon resection. *Am J Surg* 1998, 176(6)554-558.

[70] Kawamura YJ, Sawada T, Sunami E, Saito Y, Watanabe T, Masaki T, Muto T. Gasless laparoscopic assisted colonic surgery. *Am J Surg* 1999, 177(6): 515-517.

[71] Leung KL, Yiu RY, Lai PB, Lee JF, Thung KH, Lau WY. Laparoscopic-assisted resection of colorectal carcinoma: five year audit. *Dis Colon Rectum* 1999, 42(3):327-332.

[72] Poulin EC, Mamazza J, Schlachta CM, Gregoire R, Roy N. Laparoscopic resection does not adversely affect early survival curves in patients undergoing surgery for adenocarcinoma. *Ann Surg* 1999, 229(4):487-492.

[73] Schiedeck THK, Schwandner O, Baca I, Baehrlehner E, Konradt J, Kockerling F, Kuthe A, Buerk C, Herold A, Bruch HP. Laparoscopic surgery for the cure of colorectal cancer. Results of a german five center study. *Dis Colon Rectum* 2000, 43(1):1-8.

[74] Balli JE, Franklin ME, Almeida JA, Glass JL, Diaz JA, Reymond M. How to prevent port-site metastases in laparoscopic colorectal surgery. *Surg Endosc.* 2000, 14(11):1034-1036.

[75] Lezoche E, Feliciotti F, Paganini AM, Guerrieri M, Campagnacci R, De Sanctis A. Laparoscopic colonic resections versus open surgery: a prospective non-randomized study on 310 unselected cases. *Hepatogastroenterology*. 2000, 47(33):697-708.

[76] Hong D, Tabet J, Anvari M. Laparoscopiv vs. open resection for colorectal adenocarcinoma. *Dis Colon Rectum* 2001, 44(1):10-18.

[77] Lechaux D, Trebuchet G, Le Calve JL. Five-year results of 206 laparoscopic left colectomies for cancer. *Surg Endosc*. 2002 Oct;16(10):1409-12.

[78] Lumley J, Stitz R, Stevenson A, Fielding G, Luck A. Laparoscopic colorectal surgery for cancer: intermediate to long-term outcomes. *Dis Colon Rectum.* 2002 Jul;45(7):867-72.

[79] Patankar SK, Larach SW, Ferrara A, Williamson PR, Gallagher JT, DeJesus S, Narayanan S. Prospective comparison of laparoscopic vs. open resections for colorectal adenocarcinoma over a ten-year period. *Dis Colon Rectum.* 2003 May;46(5):601-11.

[80] Hughes ES, McDermott FT, Poliglase AL, Johnson WR. Tumor recurrence in the abdominal wall scare tissue after large bowel cancer surgery. *Dis Colon Rectum* 1983, 26(9):571-572.

[81] Reilly WT, Nelson H, Schroeder G, Wieand HS, Bolton J, O'Connell MJ. Wound recurrence following conventional treatment of colorectal cancer. A rare but perhaps underestimated problem. *Dis Colon Rectum* 1996, 39(2):200-207.

[82] Stockdale AD, Pocock TJ: Abdominal wall metastases following laparoscopy: a case report. *Eur J Surg Oncol* 1985, 11(4):373-375.

[83] Hsiu J, Given FT, Kemp GM: Tumor implantation after diagnostic laparoscopic biopsy of serous ovarian tumors of low malignant potential. *Obstet Gynecol* 1986, 68(3 suppl): 90S-93S.

[84] Kadar N: Port-site recurrence following laparoscopic operations for gynecological malignancies. *Br J Obstet Gynecol* 1997, 104(11):1308-1313.

[85] Z'graggen K, Birrer S, Maurer CA, et al: Incidence of port site recurrence after laparoscopic cholecystectomy for preoperatively unsuspected gallbladder carcinoma. *Surgery* 1998, 124(5):831-838.

[86] Lundberg O, Kristoffersson A: Port site metastasis from gallbladder cancer after laparoscopic cholecystectomy. Results of a Swedish survey and review of published reports. *Eur J Surg* 1999, 165(3):215-222.

[87] Winston CB, Chen JW, Fong Y, et al: Recurrent gallbladder carcinoma along laparoscopic cholecystectomy port tracks: CT demonstration. *Radiology* 1999, 212(2):439-444.

[88] Jorgensen JO, McCall JL, Morris DL: Port site seeding after laparoscopic ultrasonographic staging of pancreatic carcinoma. *Surgery* 1995, 117(1):118-119 (letter).

[89] Ugarte F: Laparoscopic cholecystectomy port seeding from a colon carcinoma. *Am Surg* 1995, 61(9):820-821.

[90] Lane TM, Cook AJ: Port site metastasis after laparoscopic cholecystectomy for benign disease. *J Laparoendosc Adv Surg Tech A* 1999, 9(3):283-284.

[91] Mintz Y, Lotan C, Goitein D, et al: Laparoscopic port site metastasis of an undetected primary tumor. *Surg Laparosc Endosc* 1999, 9(1):68-69.

[92] Downey RJ, McCormack P, LoCicero J: Dissemination of malignant tumors after video-assisted thoracic surgery: a report of twenty-one cases. The Video-Assisted Thoracic Surgery Study Group. *J Thorac Cardiovasc Surg* 1996, 111(5):954-960.

[93] Allardyce RA, Morreau PN, Frizelle FA, Bagshaw PF. Tumor cell wound distribution after colectomy in a porcine model. *Aust N Z J Surg.* 1998 May;68(5):363-366.

[94] Lee SW, Southall J, Allendorf J, Bessler M, Whelan RL. Traumatic handling of the tumor independent of pneumoperitoneum increases port site implantation rate of colon cancer in a murine model. *Surg Endosc* 1998, 12(6):828-834.

[95] Mutter D, Hajri A, Tassetti V, Solis-Caxaj C, Aprahamian M, Marescaux J. Increased tumor growth and spread after laparoscopy vs laparotomy: influence of tumor manipulation in a rat model. *Surg Endosc.* 1999, 13(4):365-370.

[96] Solomon MJ, Egan M, Roberts RA, Philips J, Russell P. Incidence of free colorectal cancer cells on the peritoneal surface. *Dis Colon Rectum.* 1997 Nov;40(11):1294-1298.

[97] Hewett PJ, Texler ML, Anderson D, King G, Chatterton BE. In vivo real-time analysis of intraperitoneal radiolabeled tumor cell movement during laparoscopy. *Dis Colon Rectum* 1999, 42(7):868-875.

[98] Cavina E, Goletti O, Molea N, Buccianti P, Chiarugi M, Boni G, Lazzeri E, Bianchi R. Trocar site tumor recurrences. May pneumoperitoneum be responsible? *Surg Endosc.* 1998, 12:1294-1296.

[99] Jones DB, Gue LW, Rienhard MK Soper NJ, Philpott GW, Connett J, Fleshman JW. Impact of pneumoperitoneum on trocar site implantation on colon cancer in hamster model. *Dis Colon Rectum* 1995, 38(11):1182-1188.

[100] Knolmayer TJ, Asbun HJ, Shibata G, Bowyer MW. An experimental model of cellular aerosolization during laparoscopic surgery. *Surg Laparosc Endosc.* 1997, 7(5):399-402.

[101] Hewett PJ, Thomas WM, King G Eaton M. Intraperitoneal cell movement during abdominal carbon dioxide insufflation and laparoscopy. *Dis Colon Rectum* 1996, 39(10suppl):62s-66s.

[102] Wittich P, Marquet RL, Kazemier G, Bonjer HJ. Port-site metastases after CO_2 laparoscopy. Is aerosolization of tumor cells a pivotal factor? *Surg Endosc.* 2000, 14(2):189-192.

[103] Whelan RL, Sellers GJ, Allendorf JD, Gleason NR, Donahue J, Laird D, Bessler MD, Treat MR. Trocar site recurrence is unlikely to result from aerosolization of tumor cells, *Dis Colon Rectum* 1996, 39(10 suppl): 7S-13S.

[104] Mathew G, Watson DI, Ellis TS, Jamieson GG, Rofe AM. The role of peritoneal immunity and the tumour-bearing state on the development of wound and peritoneal metastases after laparoscopy. *Aust N Z J Surg.* 1999, 69(1):14-18.

[105] Dorrance HR, Oien K, O'Dwyer PJ. Effects of laparoscopy on intraperitoneal tumor growth and distant metastases in an animal model. *Surgery.* 1999, 126(1):35-40.

[106] Jacobi CA, Sabat R, Bohm B, Zieren HU, Volk HD, Muller JM. Pneumoperitoneum with carbon dioxide stimulates growth of malignant colonic cells. *Surgery.* 1997, 121(1):72-78.

[107] Bouvy ND, Giuffrida MC, Tseng LN, Steyerberg EW, Marquet RL, Jeekel H, Bonjer HJ Effects of carbon dioxide pneumoperitoneum, air pneumoperitoneum, and gasless laparoscopy on body weight and tumor growth. *Arch Surg* 1998, 133(6):652-656.

[108] Chen WS, Lin W, Kou YR, Kuo HS, Hsu H, Yang WK. Possible effect of pneumoperitoneum on the spreading of colon cancer tumor cells. *Dis Colon Rectum* 1997, 40(7):791-797.

[109] Jacobi CA, Wenger FA, Ordemann J, Gutt C, Sabat R, Muller JM. Experimental study of the effect of intra-abdominal pressure during laparoscopy on tumour growth and port site metastasis. *Br J Surg.* 1998, (10):1419-1422.

[110] Paik PS, Misawg T, Chiang M, Towson J, Im S, Ortega A, Beart RW. Abdominal incision tumor implantation following pneumoperitoneum. Laparoscopic procedure versus standard open incision in asyngenetic rate model. *Dis Colon Rectum* 1998;41(4):419-422.

[111] Allardyce R, Morreau P, Bagshaw P. Tumor sell distribution following laparoscopic colectomy in a porcine model. *Dis Colon Rectum* 1996;39(10s):S47-S52.

[112] Southall JC, Lee SW, Allendorf JD, Bessler M, Whelan RL. Colon adenocarcinoma and B-16 melanoma grow larger following laparotomy vs. pneumoperitoneum in a murine model. *Dis Colon Rectum.* 1998, 41(5):564-569.

[113] Gutt CN, Riemar V, Kim ZG, Jacobi CA, Paolucci V, Lorenz M. Impact of laparoscopic colonic resection on tumor growth and spread in an experimental model. *Br J Surg* 1999, 86(9):1180-1184.

[114] Bouvy ND, Marquet RL, Jeekel H, Bonjer HJ. Impact of gas(less) laparoscopy and laparotomy on peritoneal tumor growth and abdominal wall metastasis. *Ann Surg* 1996, 224(6):964-700.

[115] Montorsi M, Fumagalli U, Rosati R, Bona S, Chella B, Huscher C. Early parietal recurrence of adenocarcinoma of the colon after laparoscopic colectomy. *Br J Surg* 1995, 82(8):1036-1037.

[116] Bessa X, Castells A, Lacy A, Elizadle JI, Delgado S, Boix L, Pinol V, Pellise M, Garcia-Valdecasas JC, Pique J. Laparoscopic-assisted Vs. open colectomy for colorectal cancer: influence on neoplastic cell mobilization. *J Gastrointest Surg* 2001, 5:66-73.

[117] Ridgway PF, Smith A, Ziprin P, Jones TL, Paraskeva PA, Peck DH, Darzi AW. Pneumoperitoneum augmented tumor invasiveness is abolished by matrix metalloproteinase blockade. *Surg Endosc.* 2002 Mar;16(3):533-6.

[118] Leister I, Manegold S, Schuler P, Alves F, Becker H, Fuzesi L, Markus PM. Effect of laparotomy and CO(2) pneumoperitoneum on tumor growth of human colon carcinoma and expression pattern of tumor-associated proteins in the SCID mouse. *Int J Colorectal Dis.* 2003

[119] Tomita H, Marcello PW, Milsom JW, Gramlich TL, Fazio VW. CO2 pneumoperitoneum does not enhance tumor growth and metastasis: study of a rat cecal wall inoculation model. *Dis Colon Rectum.* 2001 Sep;44(9):1297-301.

[120] Lecuru F, Agostini A, Camatte S, Robin F, Aggerbeck M, Jais JP, Vilde F, Taurelle R. Impact of pneumoperitoneum on tumor growth. *Surg Endosc.* 2002 Aug;16(8):1170-4.

[121] Brundell S, Ellis T, Dodd T, Watson DI, Hewett PJ. Hematogenous spread as a mechanism for the generation of abdominal wound metastases following laparoscopy. *Surg Endosc.* 2002 Feb;16(2):292-5.

[122] Brundell SM, Tsopelas C, Chatterton B, Touloumtzoglou J, Hewett PJ. Experimental study of peritoneal blood flow and insufflation pressure during laparoscopy. *Br J Surg.* 2002 May;89(5):617-22.

[123] Wildbrett P, Oh A, Naundorf D, Volk T, Jacobi CA. Impact of laparoscopic gases on peritoneal microenvironment and essential parameters of cell function. *Surg Endosc.* 2003 Jan;17(1):78-82.

[124] Neuhaus SJ, Ellis T, Rofe AM, Pike GK, Jamieson GG, Watson DI. Tumor implantation following laparoscopy using different insufflation gases. *Surg Endosc* 1998, 12(11):1300-1302.

[125] Nduka CC, Puttick M, Coates P, Yong L, Peck D, Darzi A. Intraperitoneal hypothermia during surgery enhances postoperative tumor growth. *Surg Endosc.* 2002 Apr;16(4):611-5.

[126] Zayyan KS, Christie-Brown JS, Van Noorden S, Yiu CY, Sellu DP, Mathie RT. Rapid flow carbon dioxide laparoscopy disperses cancer cells into the peritoneal cavity but not the port sites in a new rat model. *Surg Endosc.* 2003 Feb;17(2):273-7.

[127] Yamaguchi K, Hirabayashi Y, Suematsu T, Shiraishi N, Adachi Y, Kitano S. Hyaluronic acid secretion during carbon dioxide pneumoperitoneum and its association with port-site metastasis in a murine model. *Surg Endosc.* 2001 Jan;15(1):59-62.

[128] Mathew G, Watson DI, Rofe AM, Rowland R, Rofe AM, Pike GK, Mathew G, Jamieson GG. Wound metastasis following laparoscopic and open surgery for abdominal cancer in a rat model. *Br J Surg* 1996;83(8):1087-1090

[129] Allardyce RA, Morreau P, Bagshaw PF. Operative factors affecting tumor cell distribution following laparoscopic colectomy in procine model. *Dis Colon Rectum* 1997, 40(8):939-945.

[130] Wilkinson NW, Shapiro AJ, Harvey SB, Stack RS, Cornum RL. Port-site recurrence reproduced in the VX-2 rabbit carcinoma model: an in vivo model comparing laparoscopic port sites and open incisions. *JSLS*. 2001 Jul-Sep;5(3):221-6.

[131] Brundell S, Tucker K, Chatterton B, Hewett PJ. Experimental study of the material composition of laparoscopic ports on tumour cell adherence. *Br J Surg*. 2002 Jul;89(7):928-32.

[132] Nduka CC, Poland N, Kennedy M, Dye J, Darzi A. Does the ultrasonically activated scalpel release viable airborne cancer cells? *Surg Endosc* 1998, 12(8):1031-1034.

[133] Bergamaschi R, Marvik R. Laparoscopic intracorporeal bowel resection with ultrasound versus electrosurgical dissection. *JSLS*. 2001,5:17-20.

[134] Tseng LN; Berends FJ; Wittich P, Bouvy ND, Marquet RL, Kazemier G, Bonjer HJ. Port-site metastases. Impact of local tissue trauma and gas leakage. *Surg Endosc* 1998;12 (12):1377-80.

[135] Farrel TM, Johnson AB, Metreveli RE, Smith CD, Hunter JG: Facial closure limits incision metastasis after pneumoperitoneum. *Surg Endosc* 1999, 13:S33.

[136] Hirabayashi Y, Yamaguchi K, Shiraishi N, Adachi Y, Kitamura H, Kitano S. Development of port-site metastasis after pneumoperitoneum. *Surg Endosc*. 2002 May;16(5):864-8.

[137] Wu JS, Bransfield EB, Guo LW, Ruiz M, Connett JM, Philpott GW, Jones DB, Fleshman JW. Implantation of colon cancer at trocar sites is increased by low pressure pneumoperitoneum. *Surgery* 1997, 122(1): 1-7.

[138] Pauwels M, Lauwers P, Hendriks J, et al: The effect of CO2 pneumoperitoneum on the growth of a solid colon carcinoma in rats. *Surg Endosc*. 1999 Oct;13(10):998-1000.

[139] Paik PS, Misawg T, Chiang M, Towson J, Im S, Ortega A, Beart RW. Abdominal incision tumor implantation following pneumoperitoneum. Laparoscopic procedure versus standard open incision in asyngenetic rate model. *Dis Colon Rectum* 1998;41(4):419-422.

[140] Hubens G, Panwels M, Hubens A, Vermeulen P, Van Marck E, Eyskens E. The influence of a pneumoperitoneum on the peritoneal implantation of free intraperitoneal colon cancer cells. *Surg Endosc* 1996;10(8):809-812.

[141] Mathew G, Watson DI, Ellis T, De Young N, Rofe AM, Jamieson GG. The effect of laparoscopy on the movement of tumor cells and metastases to surgical wounds. *Surg Endosc* 1997;11(12):1163-1166.

[142] Moreira H Jr, Yamaguchi T, Wexner S, Singer L, Zhao R, Baig MK, Mack JA, Xiong H, Abramson S. Effect of pneumoperitoneal pressure on tumor dissemination and tumor recurrence at port-site and midline incisions. *Am Surg*. 2001, 67:369-673.

[143] Gupta A, Watson DI, Ellis T, Jamieson GG. Tumour implantation following laparoscopy using different insufflation gases. *ANZ J Surg*. 2002 Apr;72(4):254-7.

[144] Hopkins MP, von Gruenigen V, Haller NA, Holda S. The effect of various insufflation gases on tumor implantation in an animal model. *Am J Obstet Gynecol*. 2002 Oct;187(4):994-6.

[145] Wittich P, Marquet RL, Kazemier G, Bonjer HJ. Port-site metastases after CO_2 laparoscopy. Is aerosolization of tumor cells a pivotal factor? *Surg Endosc*. 2000, 14(2):189-192.

[146] Iwanaka T, Arya G, Ziegler MM. Mechanism and prevention of port-site tumor recurrence after laparoscopy in a murine model. *J Pediatr Surg* 1998, 33(3):457-461.

[147] Watson DI, Mathew G, Ellis T, et al: Gasless laparoscopy may reduce the risk of port site metastases following laparoscopic tumor surgery. *Arch Surg* 1997, 132(2):166-168.

[148] Wu JS, Guo LW, Ruiz MB, Pfister SM, Connett JM, Fleshman JW. Excision of trocar sites reduces tumor implantation in an animal model. *Dis Colon Rectum* 1998, 41(9):1107-1111.

[149] Watson DI, Ellis T, Leeder PC, Neuhaus SJ, Dodd T, Jamieson GG. Excision of laparoscopic port sites increases the likelihood of wound metastases in an experimental model. *Surg Endosc.* 2003 Jan;17(1):83-5.

[150] Lee SW, Gleason NR, Bessler M, Whelan RL. Peritoneal irrigation with povidone-iodine solution after laparoscopic-assisted splenectomy significantly decrease port-tumor recurrence in a murine model. *Dis Colon Rectum* 1999, 42(3):319-326.

[151] Neuhaus SJ, Watson DI, Ellis T, Rofe AM, Jamieson GG. Influence of cytotoxic agents on intraperitoneal tumor implantation after laparoscopy. *Dis Colon Rectum* 1999, 42(1):10-15.

[152] Neuhause SJ, Ellis T, Jamieson GG, Watson DI. Experimental study of the effect of intraperitoneal heparin on tumor implantation following laparoscopy. *Br J Surg* 1999, 86(3):400-404.

[153] Eshraghi N, Swanstrom LL, Bax T, Jobe B, Horvath K, Sheppard B, Deveney C. Topical treatment of laparoscopic port site can decrease the incidence of incisional metastasis. *Surg Endosc* 1999, 13(11):1121-1124.

[154] Wenger FA, Kilian M, Braumann C, Neumann A, Ridders J, Peter FJ, Guski H, Jacobi CA. Effects of taurolidine and octreotide on port site and liver metastasis after laparoscopy in an animal model of pancreatic cancer. *Clin Exp Metastasis.* 2002;19(2):169-73.

[155] Opitz I, Veen HC, Braumann C, Ablassmaier B, Fuhrer K, Jacobi CA. The influence of adhesion prophylactic substances and taurolidine/heparin on local recurrence and intraperitoneal tumor growth after laparoscopic-assisted bowel resection of colon carcinoma in a rat model. *Surg Endosc.* 2003 Apr 28 [Epub ahead of print]

[156] Volz J, Volz-Koster S, Kanis S, Klee D, Ahlert C, Melchert F. Modulation of tumor-induced lethality after pneumoperitoneum in a mouse model. *Cancer.* 2000 Jul 15;89(2):262-6.

[157] Hamzaoglu I, Saribeyoglu K, Durak H, Karahasanoglu T, Bayrak I, Altug T, Sirin F, Sariyar M. Protective covering of surgical wounds with honey impedes tumor implantation. *Arch Surg.* 2000 Dec;135(12):1414-7.

[158] Farrell TM, Metreveli RE, Johnson AB, Smith CD, Hunter JG. Choice of insufflating gas influences on wound metastasis. *Surg Endosc.* 2000, 14(11):1047-1049.

[159] Jacobi CA, Peter FJ, Wenger FA, Ordemann J, Muller JM. New therapeutic strategies to avoid intra- and extraperitoneal metastases during laparoscopy: results of a tumor model in the rat. *Dig Surg.* 1999, 16(5):393-399.

[160] Schneider C, Reymond MA, Tannapfel A, Franklin ME, Morel Ph, Kockerling F. The surgeon is a major factor in the incidence of port site recurrence. *Surg Endosc* 1999, 13:S5.

[161] Allendorf JD, Bessler M, Whelan RL, Trokel M, Laird DA, Terry MB, Treat MR. Postoperative immune function varies inversely with the degree of surgical trauma in a murine model. *Surg Endosc.* 1997, 11:427-430.

[162] Allendorf JD, Bessler M, Whelan RL, Trokel M, Laird DA, Terry MB, Treat MR. Better preservation of immune function after laparoscopic-assisted vs. open bowel resection in a murine model. *Dis Colon Rectum.* 1996, 39(Suppl):S67-72.

[163] Schwenk W, Jacobi C, Mansmann U, Bohm B, Muller JM. Inflammatory response after laparoscopic and conventional colorectal resections - results of a prospective randomized trial. *Langenbecks Arch Surg.* 2000, 385:2-9.

[164] Da Costa ML, Redmond HP, Finnegan N, Flynn M, Bouchier-Hayes D. Laparotomy and laparoscopy differentially accelerate experimental flank tumour growth. *Br J Surg.* 1998, 85:1439-1442.

[165] Ordemann J, Jacobi CA, Schwenk W, Stosslein R, Muller JM. Cellular and humoral inflammatory response after laparoscopic and conventional colorectal resections. *Surg Endosc.* 2001 Jun;15(6):600-8. Epub 2001 Apr 03.

[166] Fukushima R, Kawamura YJ, Saito H, Saito Y, Hashiguchi Y, Sawada T, Muto T. Interleukin-6 and stress hormone responses after uncomplicated gasless laparoscopic-assisted and open sigmoid colectomy. *Dis Colon Rectum.* 1996, 39:S29-34.

[167] Wu FP, Sietses C, von Blomberg BM, van Leeuwen PA, Meijer S, Cuesta MA. Systemic and peritoneal inflammatory response after laparoscopic or conventional colon resection in cancer patients: a prospective, randomized trial. *Dis Colon Rectum.* 2003 Feb;46(2):147-55.

[168] Lee SW, Gleason NR, Bessler M, Whelan RL. Port site tumor recurrence rates in a murine model of laparoscopic splenectomy decreased with increased experience. *Surg Endosc.* 2000 Sep;14(9):805-11.

In: Focus on Colorectal Cancer Research
Editor: Julia D. Martinez, pp. 241-285
ISBN #1-59454-101-9

Chapter X

DEVELOPMENT AND APPLICATION OF A NEW TRIAL DESIGN FOR THE ANALYSIS OF AN IMMUNE MODULATOR – G-CSF (GRANULOCYTE-COLONY STIMULATING FACTOR) FOR IMPROVEMENT OF POSTOPERATIVE OUTCOME IN HIGH RISK COLORECTAL CANCER PATIENTS PROTOCOL FOR A RANDOMIZED CONTROLLED CLINICAL TRIAL DEVELOPED BY CONSENSUS OF AN INTERNATIONAL STUDY GROUP

A. Bauhofer[1,*], W. Lorenz[1], B. Stinner[2], A. Torossian[3], U. Plaul[4], M. Koller[1], H. Sitter[1], I. Celik[1] and Lucerne Group for Consensus-assisted Development of the Study Protocol on Prevention of Abdominal Sepsis: Example G-CSF[5]

[1] Institute of Theoretical Surgery, Philipps-University of Marburg, Germany
[2] Clinic of Visceral-, Thorax- and Vascular Surgery, Elbe Clinic Stade, Germany
[3] Clinic of Anesthesia and Intensive Care Medicine, Philipps-University Marburg
[4] Clinic of Visceral-, Thorax- and Vascular Surgery, Philipps-University Marburg
[5] Bartscherer (Marburg), Bauer (Altötting), Black (Bristol), Dietz (Delmenhorst), Duda (Mainz), Encke (Frankfurt), Fagniez (Paris), Feifel, Menger (Homburg Saar), Fingerhut (Poissy), van Goor, Goris (Nijmegen), Greger (Lichtenfels), Hanisch (Dortmund), Hartel (München), Hay (Colombes), Hesterberg (Kassel), Hönemann (Stade), Horeyseck

---

[*] Corresponding author: Dr. Artur Bauhofer, Institute of Theoretical Surgery, University of Marburg, Baldingerstrasse, 35033 Marburg, Germany, Tel.: +49 6421 28 6251, FAX: +49 6421 28 68926, e-mail: bauhofer@mailer.uni-marburg.de

(Siegburg), Izbicki, Schneider, (Hamburg), Klose (Marburg), Lacaine (Paris), Lorijn (Luzern), Margolis, Pliskin (Beer Sheva), Middeke (Marburg), Neugebauer, Lefering (Cologne), Nyström (Linköping), Platzer (Basle), Reemst (Nijmegen), Rothmund, Schäfer, Voigt (Marburg), Schein (New York), Solomkin (Cincinatti), Troidl (Kolone), Volk (Berlin), Wittmann (Milwaukee), Wyatt (London), Wendel, Hartung (Konstanz), Werdan (Halle), Willatts (Bristol).

Abstract

A new trial design for a surgical outcome trial with an immune modulator was developed by consensus of an international study group. Granulocyte-colony stimulating factor (G-CSF, filgrastim) was tested in a randomized, controlled trial for prevention of postoperative infectious complications and a sub-optimum recovery from operation in patients with colorectal cancer and increased perioperative risk (ASA 3 and 4). The rationale for the trial and the design of the randomized, placebo controlled, double-blinded trial (n = 40 patients for each group) is described in this chapter.
This prototype trial includes the following elements:

- The study population was restricted to patients with high risk (ASA 3 and 4) and left sided surgical resection of colorectal cancer.
- Clinic modeling randomized trials (CMRTs) in rodents were used to help to define trial conditions.
- Patients were allocated by random to the control or treatment group (n = 40/group). Two antibiotics (A = cefuroxime/metronidazole and B = ofloxacin/metronidazole) were balanced, randomized in a 2 x 2 design (G-CSF/placebo x antibiotic A/B) in the trial. The double blinding strategy of the trial was assessed by psychometric indices.
- A new endpoint construct (integrated outcome concept) was evaluated with quality of life (EORTC-QLQ-C30 and QLQ-C38 cancer module) and a recovery index (Mc Peek index) were used as primary endpoints. Qualitative analysis of clinical relevance was performed by both patients and doctors.
- A confirmatory statistical model with quality of life as the first primary endpoint in the hierarchic test procedure is used. Statistical analysis uses an area under the curve (AUC) model for improvement of quality of life at discharge from hospital, two and six months after operation. The second primary endpoint is the McPeek index.
- The management of postoperative complications was directed by an evidence based guideline.

A new trial design for preoperative prophylaxis and postoperative recovery was developed and used to avoid previous methodological failures. The trial was performed in three centers within two years plus an additional half year for follow up. At present it can be concluded that the trial protocol is feasible and can therefore be used to test other immune-modulators in complex clinical scenarios. Data analysis will demonstrate the effect of G-CSF on the different endpoints.

1. Introduction

In order to investigate the effectiveness of recombinant human granulocyte-colony stimulating factor (rhG-CSF, filgrastim) in the prevention of postoperative infectious complications and of sub-optimum recovery from operation we formed the Lucerne Group for Consensus-Assisted Development of a Study Protocol on Prevention of Abdominal Sepsis with G-CSF. This group consists of clinicians, theoretical surgeons [1], basic scientists, statisticians and social psychologists, as well as experts in formal organization of a protocol for FDA approval and the corresponding EU administration. Their names are listed on the front page of this article. Five years were needed for development and publication of the study protocol in three parts before conducting the study in a time period of two years [2-4]. This procedure was accompanied by many discussions and controversies in sepsis trials [5-16] but much appreciated by Balk and Bone [17]: "The concept of developing an experimental protocol and then submitting it to full a priori review by the knowledgeable and interested medical community was a novel approach and was likely to pay dividends in study quality." This concept had justified the long lasting work of the Lucerne Study Group and was proposed for the outline of surgical trials [18] and by the CONSORT statement [19,20].

At first the "rationale and hypothesis" on perioperative prophylaxis with G-CSF (granulocyte-colony stimulating factor) to prevent postoperative infectious complications and sub-optimum recovery after colorectal operation was presented. Then the design of the trial including novel features like control of the blinding procedure, the use of a quality of life endpoint construct and the Mc Peek recovery index, qualitative analysis of clinical relevance of the endpoints by both patients and doctors, and the management of postoperative complications directed by an evidence based guideline are demonstrated.

Now the trial is finished and in the analytic process. With the knowledge of the trial conditions and the actual literature the protocol is updated. Only little changes have to be introduced between the published protocol and clinical reality.

2. Rationale for the Selection of G-CSF as Immune Modulator

Many biological response modifiers were used in pre-clinical and clinical investigations. In most trials the aim of these drugs was a reduction in the frequency and extension of SIRS, sepsis, septic shock, multiorgan failure and, finally death [21,22]. G-CSF was injected primarily not to block endotoxin or a proinflammatory cytokine like TNF-α or IL-1 which are essential for the induction of the SIRS reaction [10]. However, it was demonstrated that G-CSF down-regulates the expression and release of TNFα and other proinflammatory cytokines in response to endotoxin and bacterial products [23-25]. Even more important was the induction of the primary and non-specific host-defense reaction by increasing chemotaxis, bacterial binding and cytotoxicity against microbes with oxygen and nitrogen radicals [26-28]. These effects can be obtained directly by stimulation of these defense functions of PMNs (polymorphonuclear neutrophils) or indirectly by increasing the number of PMNs in peripheral blood and tissues. The increase in number is achieved by stimulating the proliferation of PMN precursors in the bone-marrow and reducing apoptosis of these cells [29,30].

2.1 G-CSF in Clinic Modeling Randomized Trials (CMRTs)

In order to predict more successfully the clinical effectiveness of a study drug the concept of clinic modeling randomized trials (CMRTs) in animals [31-33] (Table 1) was developed. In contrast to traditional, reductionistic animal experiments, in CMRTs complex clinical interactions (anesthesia, antibiotic-, heparin-, antihistamine- prophylaxis, operation, infection and surgical management) with the study drug were analyzed. These interactions are even more important than species differences in the assessment of new drugs. The usefulness of CMRTs had already been demonstrated for perioperative prophylaxis with antihistamines against cardiorespiratory instability: CMRTs in dogs were followed by the development of a consensus-assisted trial protocol [34] and a definitive randomized clinical trial [35], which demonstrated the benefits of a H_1/H_2 antagonist prophylaxis in the post-induction period of general anesthesia [35].

The biological response modifier recombinant human granulocyte-colony stimulating factor (G-CSF, filgrastim) was tested in more than 30 clinic modeling randomized trials in rats. These CMRTs carefully analyzed the response to G-CSF for appropriate dosing [24,31], combination with various antibiotics, and operative procedures. In addition these trials suggested clinical conditions in which G-CSF might be effective and other circumstances in which it might not help. For example, in combination with ceftriaxone or ceftriaxone/metronidazole G-CSF prophylaxis resulted in a trend to a decreased survival [31]. The most active combination with G-CSF was cefuroxime/metronidazole. In these CMRTs G-CSF prophylaxis down regulated proinflammatory cytokines like TNF-α and IL-6 systemically and at the site of infection – the peritoneum [24,33] and stimulated innate immunity for clearance of bacteria [36].

Additionally, in CMRTs endpoints beside of mortality rate, cellular functions and cytokine expression were analyzed. Sickness behavior, the animal equivalent to quality of life [37] in humans, was assessed. We analyzed core body temperature, heart rate, blood pressure, food and water intake, locomotor activity and circadian rhythm of these parameters in freely moving rats with the technique of radiotelemetry. Most of these functions were restored to normal values in septic rats earlier by the addition of a G-CSF prophylaxis [37,38].

These trials gave rationales for the clinical trial with regard to dosing, timing, combination with antibiotics, other prophylactic principles (e.g. heparin- and H_1/H_2-antagonist prophylaxis) and they were promising positive results with regard to a postoperative improvement of quality of life. Based on this knowledge we tested whether G-CSF may work in patients under prophylactic clinical conditions modeled by a team of clinical experts from the previously established Lucerne study group. We hope that the results of this clinical trial demonstrate once again the benefit of this strategy.

Table 1. Clinic modeling randomized trials (CMRTs) in rats with peritoneal contamination and infection for the analysis of clinical conditions before the start of the clinical trial

Assessed clinical condition	n	Survival rate [%] control	inter-vention	intervention + G-CSF	p <
Risk factors simulating ASA 3 and 4					
Blood loss with co-amoxiclav					
– pre-operative blood loss	18	33*	17	50	0.1
– intra-operative blood loss	18	56*	17	66	0.01
Diabetes mellitus	6	100	33	-	0.05
Interaction of prophylaxes					
Antibiotics: positive results					
– cefuroxime/metronidazole	12	16	50	92	0.01
– co-amoxiclav	18	-	44	83	0.05
– amikacin/metronidazole	18	-	44	83	0.05
– ofloxacin/metronidazole	18	-	50	83	0.05
– levofloxacin/metronidazole	40	-	38	59	0.05
– cefotaxime/metronidazole	18	-	35	66	0.07
– imipenem	12	-	75	100	0.07
Antibiotics negative results					
– ofloxacin	12	-	33	50	0.4
– cefotaxime	12	-	50	75	0.2
– ceftriaxone	12	-	42	33	0.7
– ceftriaxone/metronidazole	11	16	55	45	0.2
Heparin					
– with levofloxacin/metronidazole	18	39*	56	83	0.05
H_1/H_2 antihistamines					
– with co-amoxiclav	30	40*	67	-	0.05
– with levofloxacin/metronidazole	30	30*	17	52	0.05

The result of each study were used for designing the features of the clinical trial. For further explanation of CMRTs see reference (28). n = number/group. Since all numbers per group have to be multiplied by 3 according to the design, a total of 820 rats with individual operations were involved in the project listed here, much like a large multicenter trial. In trials in which only two groups are shown, the third group consisted of G-CSF as a single dose, whereas all results shown here refer to three G-CSF applications, with each dose administered at 24 hour intervals. The number of animals/group in each trial was calculated by the formula of Friedman (78):

$$n = \frac{p_1\ (1-p_1)\ +\ p_2\ (1-p_2)}{(p_2-p_1)^2} f(\alpha,\beta),$$ where p_1 = success rate in the control group, p_2 = success rate in the test group, $p_2 - p_1 = \delta$ (estimated effect of the test intervention), $f(\alpha, \beta)$ = function of α, β ($2\alpha = 0.05$, $\beta = 0.2$). δ as the difference between the control and test group was obtained from pilot studies before the definitive CMRT. Statistical test: chi^2-test with k-samples in all of the CMRTs; * control group in these studies also received antibiotics. (Reproduced with permission form Ref. 3).

2.2 G-CSF in Clinical Trials

G-CSF showed significant benefits in curing diabetic foot infections in the trial of Gough [39] and reduced the rate of amputations in another trial [40], but showed no effect in the trial of Yonem [41]. G-CSF attenuates the inflammatory response in Crohn's disease [42], the rate of opportunistic infections in HIV patients [43-45] and as co-treatment in surgical infections [46,47]. Hartung et al, showed that a G-CSF prophylaxis in surgical patients was beneficial with regard to cellular functions and the inflammatory cytokine response [48]. The most promising data of G-CSF were demonstrated by Stephans [49] who showed a reduction of the mortality rate in patients with septic shock from 73 % to 31 % due to *Burholderia pseudomalei* infections. In patients admitted to the clinic with community-acquired pneumonia G-CSF reduced the subsequent occurrence of acute respiratory distress syndrome and disseminated intravascular coagulation [50]. In a further study with 480 patients with community-acquired multilobular pneumonia no improvement in survival or reduced organ dysfunction was found by the G-CSF treatment [51].

For more than 10 years now G-CSF (filgrastim) had been used without marked side effect [52] as a crucial cytokine in the prevention and treatment of neutropenia and febrile neutropenia in patients undergoing cancer therapy. A recent systematic Cochrane review [53] shows that in patients with malignant lymphoma and conventional chemotherapy G-CSF prophylaxis reduces not only the relative risk of neutropenia and febrile neutropenia but also for infections. As expected, there was no effect on the remission rate and on the survival rate [53].

3. Key Elements for a Prototype Study

Protocols of well-known multicenter trials on the treatment of sepsis with biological response modifiers were analyzed, including anti-endotoxin antibody [22] and IL-1ß receptor antagonist [21] in advance to identify study design problems. Five major components seemed deficient and were listed here as key elements for the current study and future trials in perioperative risk and sepsis:

3.1. Selection of a Study Population Close to the Clinical Scenario

Previous trials tried to satisfy the methodologists with epidemiological, biochemical or molecular biological entry criteria, but the capability for generalization (external validity) and applicability were inversely neglected, a particularly danger in surgical trials [54]. We therefore chose the opposite strategy, a defined, frequent operation – left-sided colorectal cancer surgery.

3.2 Selection of Trial Conditions in Accordance with Clinic Modeling Randomized Trials (CMRTs) in Animals

The planed clinical trial was pre-tested [31,33,55] in complex experimental scenarios (CMRTs) in an animal model. Their results were used for designing the clinical trial.

3.3 Assessment of Patients and Surgeons Expectations

Blinding procedures in clinical trials [56] were essential to minimize bias. However, blinding had not always worked well when its effectiveness was measured empirically [35], particularly in trials with biological response modifiers when patients had well-known reactions such as hyperglycaemia or leukocytosis. In addition, recent work in social psychology had shown that patients' and surgeons' expectations regarding treatment effects may go beyond the classical placebo theories [57]. Therefore, in addition to blinding procedures to reduce bias, expectations of patients and surgeons were assessed [58].

3.4 Outcome Assessment with Mechanistic Variables, Quality of Life and the True Endpoint Concept

Following extensive theoretical work [15,58-60] it was proposed that outcome analysis in surgery should be based on three obligatory elements:

- a quality of life index, self-reported and assessed by the patient, free from foreign observer interference [15,61].
- the surgeon's assessment of recovery and health status by an index (clinical, mechanistic variables determined with the McPeek index) [62,63].
- analysis of clinical relevance of the endpoints in both groups of variables by patients and doctors with methods of qualitative research (true endpoint concept) [64].

The development of this concept was strongly promoted by the two consensus conferences and further interactions of the Lucerne Study Group and was published recently [15].

3.5 Assessment of Adherence to Clinical Practice Guidelines

The main reasons why sepsis trials failed in the past were heterogeneity of management and treatment of patients. The Lucerne Study Group dedicated most effort in two Consensus meetings to analyses heterogeneity of patient management in colorectal cancer and postoperative anastomotic leakage. Clinical algorithms were developed from individual cases [65,66], and the heterogeneity of clinical management among centers was analyzed in a Nominal Group Process (NGP) [65]. A final consensus for one guideline for all centers was however not achieved [66]. It was agreed that adherence to one guideline for the three in the trial participating centers was necessary to show similarities in both treatment arms.

These five key elements in the design of this study protocol had justified its publication [2-4] as a prototype protocol rather then yet another proposal for trials in surgical infection and sepsis. Experience gained from the planned study should be reliable - probably even more than any significant or non-significant result in favor of or against a new biological response modifier for preoperative prophylaxis.

4. Design of the G-CSF Prophylaxis Trial

4.1 Description of the Study Type

The study was planned with several prospective features, including classical ones such as randomization and risk factor analysis by a logistic regression model [35], other relatively modern features include systematic adherence to the special type of preclinical trials, CMRTs in rats [31] (Table 1), interpretation of the positive/negative effects of the drug by covariance analysis with doctor's and patient's expectations and the negative affect of the patients are going beyond the placebo effect [58], assessment and comparison of the clinical practice guideline adherence and analysis of the outcome model by sensitivity analysis. Exploratory analysis played a considerable role, not only for generating new hypotheses, but also for interpreting and understanding the analyzed results using inferential statistics.

Such a trial, with several new features, naturally bears an increased risk for failure. Hence feasibility had been tested in a randomized pilot study made up of six patients who had been enrolled according to the protocol after approval by the ethical committee. To avoid the hazards of small studies [67], a sample size of between 50 and 100 patients was planned for the full-scale study and for restriction of treatment heterogeneity the study was restricted to no more than three study centers and for feasability to a time-span of no more than two years.

4.2 Definition of the Study Population

Selection of patients for randomized trials with biological response modifiers is the most critical issue [9] when negative (not significant) results had been obtained in studies on postoperative infections and sepsis [9-11,68-72]. Principles for eligibility of the patients had therefore been developed with a certain hierarchy based on the rationale of the study including several CMRTs (Table 1).

4.2.1. Colorectal Carcinoma including Left Side Resection

The surgical conditions for eligibility included elective interventions, but were not otherwise restricted (Table 2). Re-operations, palliative operations, patients with hereditary non-polyposis colorectal cancer (HNPCC) and with familial adenomatous polyposis (FAP) were included. For the latter positive results with G-CSF had been reported [73]. Operative conditions included low anterior resection (total mesorectal excision, TME) and all types of operation used electively for left-sided colorectal cancer: segmental colonic resection, left hemicolectomy, sigmoid resection, Hartmann's procedure, low anterior resection (LAR), abdominoperineal resection (APR), proctocolectomy and subtotal colectomy. Staging criteria were important only for one category: UICC 0 was excluded because the gut is not dissected. Beside of several types and techniques of operation, patients with and without adjuvant chemo- or radiotherapy were included. The study was not restricted to only a few surgeons, but included all surgeons routinely involved in the department for such an operation - to reflect clinical reality.

Table 2.Criteria for patient inclusion: the study population

Main items	Specification
Primary disease	Colorectal cancer UICC I-IV including FAP and HNPCC
Concomitant diseases	ASA 3 and 4: increased risk for non-optimum recovery, absence of acute infections or ileus
General conditions	All ages ≥ 18 years Mentally fit - Both sexes
Surgical conditions	-Undergoing elective surgery (1) dissecting the gut (2) left-sided or including left side (3) any type of operation indicated (4) first operation in study period (5) first intervention or reintervention (6) curative or palliative (7) including subsequent adjuvant chemotherapy or radiotherapy
Anaesthetic conditions	General anaesthesia Pain management with or without epidural catheter

(Reproduced with permission form Ref. 3).

No emergency patients were included for reasons of feasibility since the first G-CSF administration occurred 12 h before operation. Patients with acute infections, preoperative ileus or SIRS were likewise excluded, but patients with chronic obstructive lung disease (COLD) were included. Data from recent studies did not support the assumption of a risk with G-CSF in those patients [74].

4.2.2 Co-morbidity and Immune Alteration

Selection of ASA 3 and 4 patients was a priority and more important for sub-optimum outcome than either type or extent of operation, extent of blood loss or surgical skills (Figure 1). Internal consistency was tested and found excellent by comparing ASA classes with mortality rates and complications in 3000 patients for two years [75]. The ASA classification is in regular use in the clinics of the study for continued medical education, audit and feedback (e.g. mortality and morbidity conferences), and reminders (e.g. part of the patient record file).

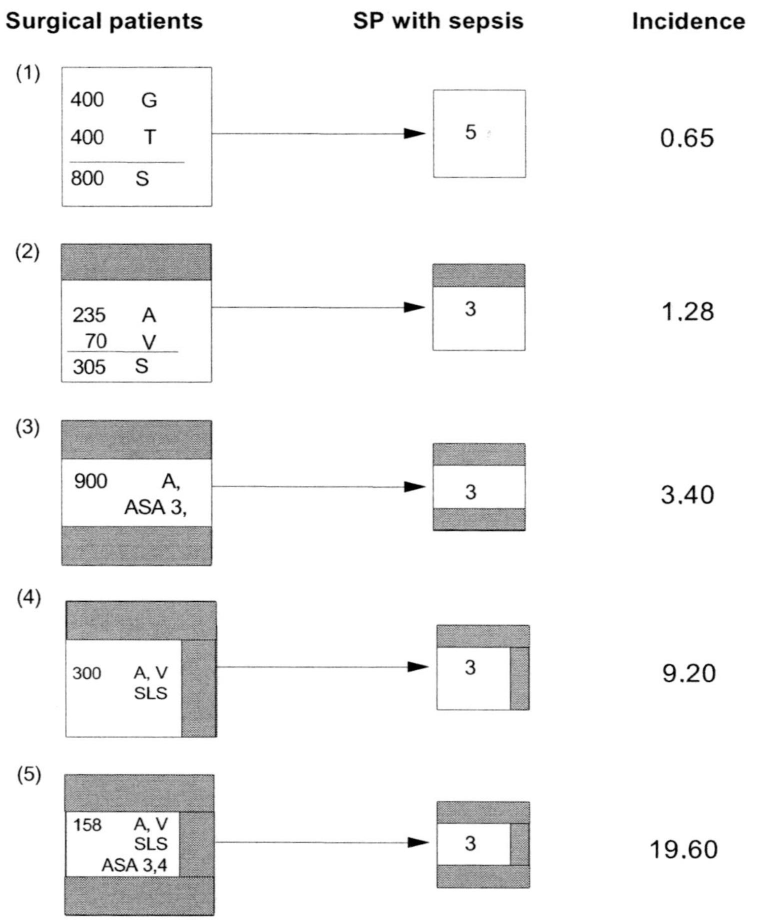

Figure 1. Analysis of the surgical ICU population from University Marburg of one year. Decision support for the study population selection. The white area is the set of available patients, the dark area represents the reduction of patients from this set, if an additional selection criterion is introduced. 1-5 = steps of selection. Abbreviations: G = general surgery, T = trauma surgery, ASA = American Society of Anaesthesiology score, A = abdominal surgery, V = vascular surgery, SLS = situations having led to sepsis: left-sided colorectal surgery and surgery for aortic aneurysms. Only colorectal surgery was selected for the present study. (Reproduced with permission form Ref. 3).

Since the ASA classification is an important selection step ASA classification must follow the rules developed for surgical trials [76]. In the trial the ASA classification was performed independently by three persons: first by the duty anesthetist who is often biased towards higher ASA classes [35], second by a trained trial observer and third by a trained study anesthetist who had the final decision about the ASA class of the individual patient.

Biochemical indicators for an adversely effected immunological state, such as *ex vivo* cellular ability to produce cytokines and surface antigens, were not used for eligibility, but only for base-line comparison and secondary endpoints.

Adherence to these two main principles lead to a study population characterized in Table 2. The key issues were ASA 3 and 4, left-sided colorectal cancer and elective surgery with a type of operation for dissecting the gut and usually resulting in an anastomosis. This classification was easily rememberable, clinically applicable and close to an everyday clinical scenario.

4.2.3 Categories of Excluded Patients: Escapes and Withdrawals

Patients with colorectal cancer who were not recruited were escapes and hamper generalization, but were less of a problem than withdrawals (standard less than 10% [77]).

The first goal of the strategy for defining escape clauses was to **avoid withdrawals**. A relevant problem in this study relates to the early enrolment (first application of G-CSF 12-16 hours before operation).

The second goal was **feasibility** of such a complex study as explained in the rationale, so that only one patient/day was enrolled and was pre-tested for possible co-operation on quality of life issues. Experience with 119 patients with rectal cancer in a systematic tumor – follow-up [78] supported by the German Ministry of Health (FB 2-43332-70/6) had demonstrated that, in contrast to breast cancer patients, those with rectal cancer more often do not answer quality of life questionnaires within the first month after operation. Feasibility included a well-designed organizational structure for the afternoon before operation as well as weekend and holiday strategies. For this reason observer clinicians were established. This strategy had worked well in three other situations [35,79,80] also including up to 16 escape clauses.

Time for enrolment of the single patient was about 2.00 pm to 8.00 pm on the preoperative day, but only one patient was included per day. These primary aims, avoiding withdrawals and warranty feasibility, defined and explained the items listed in Table 3 for escape clauses. Patients with AIDS and hepatitis were not excluded, since they do not have an increased risk for postoperative infections [81,82]. The present experience had been that they do well with G-CSF [83]. There was no escape for women and minority group members (NIH criteria, McKneally in [1]), except for those who were pregnant or lactating and children below the age of 18 because the risks in this trial outweigh the benefits.

There were considerable risks of withdrawals due to short-term effects (in the perioperative period) and relatively long-term effects (six months after operation for quality of life). In addition, doctor-related health status and patient self-reported quality of life consisted of a wide spectrum of variables, so that missing values or missing actions should not automatically lead to withdrawals. The recommendations of Friedman et al. were followed for missing data [84]: "act vigorously and keep the missing values to a minimum, especially the preoperative values in order to make analysis of covariance credible and, in particular, the preoperative values of quality of life".

There were three main causes for withdrawals: operation cancelled, refusal of consent and technical reasons as explained in Table 4.

Table 3. List of escape clauses and coding (Reproduced with permission form Ref. 3)

Category of clauses	Specification	Coding
None	• Patient included	00
General	• Holidays on weekdays	01
	• Failure of application and assessment capabilities (e.g. health status, sample taking, first G- CSF)	02
	• Errors in applying exclusion rules	03
	• Not the first patient elected/day	04
	• Not the first operation for treatment of colorectal cancer in study period	05
	• Age less than 18 years	06
	• Pregnancy or lactation period	07
Disease-related	• ASA 1, 2 and 5, but left-sided colorectal cancer	08
	• Diagnosis of colorectal cancer uncertain	09
	• Left-side not included preoperatively	10
	• Local resections	11
	• Staging UICC 0	12
	• Squamous cell cancer of the anus	13
	• Not elective (ileus, bleeding emergency)	14
	• Concomitant acute infection	15
	• Known adverse reaction to G-CSF	16
Patient-doctor relationship	• Absence of written consent by patient	17
	• Patient's incapability or unwillingness to fill out quality of life questionnaire	18
	• Patient enrolled in another trial, especially with another biological response modifier	19
	• Patient excluded by surgeon (e.g. private patient)	20
	• Ethical dilemma with G-CSF (e.g. with gene technology)	21
	• Patient rejects consent	22
Others	• Unforeseen, to avoid any harm to an individual patient.	23
	• Decision only by group of principle investigators	
	• Other reasons not listed	24

Enrolment of patients followed a clinical algorithm. A strong organizational structure for enrolment was necessary, made up of several study clinicians with considerable experience. The operation schedule for the next day was completed at about 2 pm. Selection of patients for the trial must guarantee consideration of all patients submitted to hospital and the greatest possible avoidance of bias.

Table 4. Categories of exclusion

Withdrawal	No withdrawal
Operation cancelled after inclusion in study: e.g. an elective case becomes an emergency case	Death of the patient. In this case quality of life value will be 0 on all dimensions at each time point of measurement after death had occurred
Refusal of consent	Exclusion due to apparent side-effects of study drugs
Technical reasons: observer and/or equipment are not available after inclusion, especially during hospitalisation. (Consensus decision of the principal investigators is necessary in this case)	Non adherence to guidelines including new medications (new trials) within six months after operation
	Operation delayed beyond the day following the first dose of G-CSF
	Violation of conditions defined for quality of life measurement (handled as missing values)

- **First step:** A member of the trial staff identified all patients for elective colorectal cancer surgery on the schedule and ranked them by labeling with numbers, starting with patient one in any theatre in the first row of the time schedule, then working through the theatres, following with the next row of time schedule using the same procedure and so on. No more than three patients fulfilled the criteria for the first step at a single day.
- **Second step:** An observer clinician established first willingness of each patient identified to participate and their mental fitness for quality of life assessment. The patient record file (PRF) was then checked for risk assessment and ASA 3 and 4. Enrolment was then decided at this stage and the observer explained the decision in a written, short comment.
- **Third step:** The observer informed the patient - in detail - about the benefits of quality of life (QL) assessment. After introducing the method of QL assessment the patient completed the QL questionnaire by him/herself without any interaction with the doctor. Major difficulties in understanding and completing the questionnaire constitutes an escape case, because initial difficulty indicated poor subsequent compliance.
- **Fourth step:** When the result was positive, the observer left the patient for some time and asked for written informed consent not earlier than at 8.00 pm 12-16 hours before the start of operation. With the informed consent, the first injection of G-CSF or placebo was performed.

All patients with colorectal cancer not enrolled (escapes) were followed up to capture the data on survival, hospital stay and postoperative complications. From patients enrolled but who were withdrawn as much data as possible were collected especially survival, complications and hospital stay. In the trial only one patient was withdrawn, due to cancellation of the operation after assignment to the trial. Missing data due to problems with general practitioners, were minimized by visits of a study clinician. In advance the feasibility of the entire procedure was confirmed in a pilot trial with six patients lasting for eight months before the main trial was started.

4.3 G-CSF- and Control Group

The G-CSF Prophylaxis Group

G-CSF was administered in a dose of 5 μg/kg s.c. (with no preference for the adipose tissue of abdomen, upper arm, or thigh) three times as a prophylaxis. This occurred the first time 12-16 hours before the start of operation and as a treatment 12 hours and 36 hours after operation (Figure 2). Patients received one hour before skin incision by random cefuroxime/metronidazole or ofloxacin/metronidazole (2 x 2 design, 20 patients with one and 20 with the other antibiotic). Further prophylaxis for all patients were low-dose un- or fractionated heparin, crystalloid volume substitution and antihistamine H_1- + H_2-prophylaxis with 0.1 mg/kg dimetindene and 5 mg/kg cimetidine i.v. at least 15 min before induction of anesthesia [34,35].

The decision with regard to dosing of G-CSF, route, administration frequency and possible combination with antibiotics, heparin, volume substitution and antihistamines used in the trial were based on three components: systematically performed clinic modeling randomized trials (CMRTs) in rats [31], other clinical G-CSF trials and concepts developed at two consensus meetings of the Lucerne group (January 1995 and 1997).

The dose of G-CSF is derived from the CMRTs (Table 1), using roughly 1/5 of the rat dose for human subjects, and from clinical trials with other indications [47,85-93]. The subcutaneous route is more convenient than the intravenous infusion [47], especially on a normal ward and the clearance of G-CSF is not as fast as after infusion [48]. The first injection at -12 hours had been derived from CMRTs [31], (Figure 2) and the 24 hour intervals of further injections were in line with the optimum time course of stimulation of the bone marrow by G-CSF and with the activity of granulocytes following G-CSF application [94-96]. This regime was very successful in the CMRTs [31], (Table 1). The selection of the antibiotics and other types of prophylaxes were derived directly from the large number of CMRTs shown in Table 1, indicating best effectivity with cefuroxime/metronidazole and to a lesser extent for ofloxacin/metronidazole in combination with G-CSF. In addition G-CSF had been demonstrated to increase the uptake of fluoro-quinolones into granulocytes [97].

Although G-CSF had been proven to be safe in patients with different underlying diseases, its possible side-effects include pulmonary inflammation [98], thrombocytopenia [99] and bone pain [100]. Careful monitoring of possible side effects of the study drugs was part of this trial.

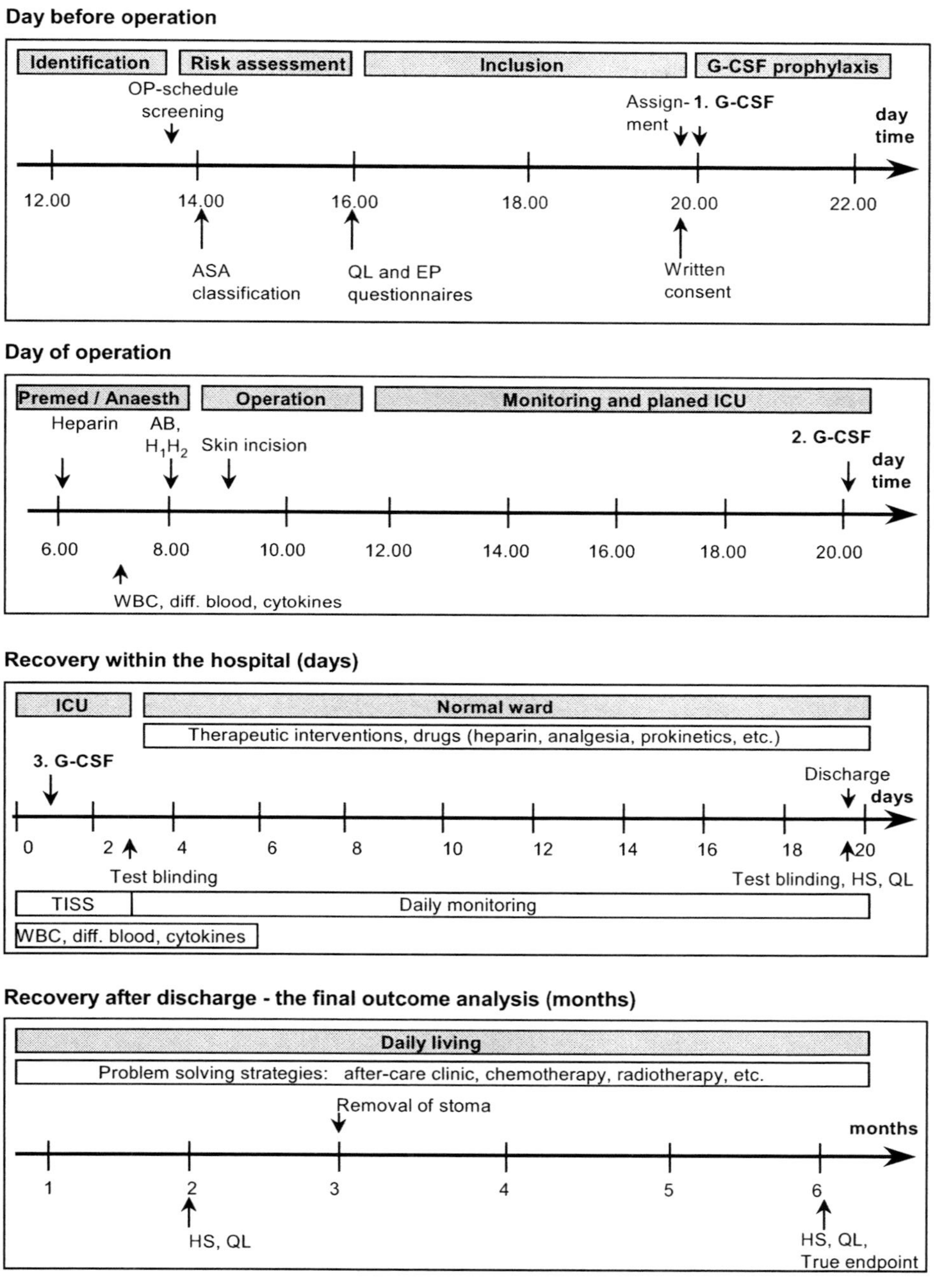

Figure 2. Protocol of the individual patient (Reproduced with permission form Ref. 4). Anaesth = anaesthesia; AB = i.v. antibiotic prophylaxis (cefuroxime/metronidazole or ofloxacin/ metronidazole); ASA = American society of Anaesthesiologists score; assignment = random allocation to control or test group; cytokines = blood sampled in the morning for cytokine determination; diff. blood = differential blood count; EP = expectancy from patient and surgeon; G-CSF = filgrastim or placebo; HS = health status; H_1H_2 = anti histamines for H1 and H2 receptors; ICU = intensive care unit; premed = prae-midication; QL = estimation of quality of life with the EORTC-QLQ-CR30/CR38, true endpoint = true endpoint concept measured by structured interview; TISS = Therapeutic Intervention Scoring System with 28 items; WBC = white blood count; written consent = written informed consent about the trial.

The Placebo Group

Intervention in the control group was replacement of G-CSF by saline and also included three placebo injections and the same antibiotic combinations in the 2 x 2 design with balanced, randomized allocation of cefuroxime/metronidazole and ofloxacin/metronidazole. Low-dose heparin was administered in the morning before operation, as well as colloidal and crystalloid volume substitution according to clinical rules and on-demand, a strategy to minimize blood transfusion. Antihistamine H_1- + H_2-prophylaxis was injected at least 15 minutes before induction of anesthesia [34,35]. Anesthesia und pain management were also standardized by balanced anesthesia (sevoflurane, fentanyl) and an epidural catheter when appropriate.

The use of a control group involves analyzing the opinion of whether the drug G-CSF was indeed received. On day three and at discharge from hospital, questions to the responsible surgeon, observer clinician and patient in the PRF were asked, what they feel the patient had received - placebo or active drug. This procedure had been successfully performed in a former trial [35] and is necessary in this trial to control influences on quality of life assessment [101] and other endpoints.

Randomisation: Strategy and Procedure

This complex trial had many baseline and process variables and - for reasons of feasibility - a restricted sample size. Thus, it needed an allocation mechanism which distributed prognostic factors equally to the two arms of the study. There were randomization procedures available which avoid major inequalities in prognostic factors such as the biased coin method [102]. Furthermore, stratification for sex [103,104] and localization of the tumor (rectum vs. more proximal localization in the intestinal tract) [105] were discussed to avoid inequalities in these risk factors for an adverse outcome. Finally, an unbalanced randomization (G-CSF: placebo = 2:1) was considered to overcome some disadvantages of the small sample size. However, following the rationale and major goals of this study, a simple randomization procedure was chosen to increase clinical confidence in this design.

For a total of 80 patients, a balanced randomization in two random permuted blocks of 40 subjects was performed, similar to a previous study on perioperative risk [34]. Randomisation was performed with a PC using the SAS software [106]. Each arm of the trial was subdivided by balanced block randomization (2 x 2 design) in 20 subjects with cefuroxime/ metronidazole and 20 with ofloxacin/metronidazole prophylaxis. To minimize doubt about the credibility of trial results when prognostic factors were imbalanced, prospective risk factors for a sub-optimum postoperative recovery were defined. Besides epidemiological factors like age, sex, tumor size and comorbidity, for the first time other factors such as patient expectance, negative affect and surgeon's adherence to guidelines were included into the risk profiles. Logistic regression will be performed with step-wise forward (entry of covariates into the model) coding of nominal data as 2/1 for present/absent and $\alpha = 0.2$, as in the previous trial [35].

4.4 Reducing Variance and Bias from Expectations: Partial Blinding and Application of a Psychometric Index for Analysis of Covariance

A remarkable contradiction is observed in some clinical trials on sepsis when the principle of (observed versus expected) is applied to characterization and selection of patients using APACHE scoring [107], but is not applied to the analysis of treatment effectiveness. The reason why - observed versus expected - was introduced as an outcome measure was the marked heterogeneity of patients in ICUs [108]. However, not only diagnostic variables but also treatment options show heterogeneity in their magnitude and intensity on the outcomes. They had such a considerable influence on mortality that they were used as a criterion of quality for ICUs [109]. More importantly, they depend considerably on expectations of patients and surgeons in outcome which were not uniform and unidirectional, and can influence outcome both positively [110] and negatively [111]. This nuisance variable [112] can exceed the placebo effect in importance [113]. Expectation and its influence on outcome (health status and quality of life) can be measured quantitatively by psychometric indices and can be analyzed for variations. This technique was therefore used in this trial for analysis of covariance. As long as it fulfils certain criteria, such as that of similarity of variance in both groups [112], covariance analysis will be used to calculate adjusted means for both major outcome variables quality of life and the recovery index. Since there is no experience with the magnitude of variance by the study patients with colorectal cancer, the analysis of variance is performed additionally and not included in the confirmatory statistical model.

In addition to randomization, a series of measures were proposed to reduce variance, bias and influences from the placebo effect and from expectations in this trial:

Double-Blinding Concept and Technique

Although double-blinding may not be entirely successful because G-CSF induces leukocytosis, it may be partially effective if properly conducted. The responsible pharmacist and statistician were the only persons who knew the randomization list. The pharmacist prepared 20 sets of consecutively numbered study drugs containing: 3 vials with G-CSF or NaCl, the antibiotics, H_1 antagonist dimetindene and H_2 antagonist cimetidine. Each time when two sets were left, he prepared the next 20 sets. This was done with regard to the expiration date of the drugs. Each vial containing the placebo or active drug was covered in a sealed envelope with the random number on it and on the vial (e.g 3.1 = patient 3, first application). At the time of application, the envelope was handed out to a nurse on the ward of the patient. In the absence of the study observer, the seal of the envelope was broken. A 1 ml syringe was prepared by the nurse containing the study drug or placebo. The empty vials were left in the empty envelope which was then sealed again and stored in the study center. The application of the drug was then performed by the study observer.

In advance the syringes with active drug and placebo had been tested 50-times to be indistinguishable even after shaking. An addition of human albumin had been tested to be not necessary.

The information about the placebo and active drug distribution was not given to the investigators before primary data analysis had been completed [35]. Also additional assessors of the data were blinded at this time. This corresponds to a triple blinding design.

On day 3 after operation (Figure 2) when the patient had received G-CSF 36 h after operation for the last time, the operating surgeon, the study observer and the surgeon responsible for the patient had to rate and write down in the PRF whether they feel the patient had received the placebo or active drug. The size of any selection bias, statistically tested with a Phi-coefficient [35,114] will demonstrate the success of the blinding technique.

Measurement of Expectations by Patients and Surgeons and Covariance Analysis

According to a recent concept of outcome analysis [1,15,59,115], surgeons must objectively assess the health status of their patients after operation and patients must deliver independent self-reports about their postoperative quality of life. Both groups, however, had different expectations about the effectiveness of cancer treatment regimes, as shown in a study on cancer radiotherapy [101]. Most patients expected a complete recovery from the life-threatening disease, whereas surgeons were more cautious and most expected only pain relief and a reduction in the tumor size. If expectations significantly influence outcome, then it is necessary to measure them quantitatively and to analyze their influence on outcome by an analysis of covariance [112]. The expectation scale developed in another study [101] was used in the present trial (Table 5) on the day before operation, almost immediately before administration of the first dose of G-CSF.

Table 5. Expectations scale for patients with colorectal cancer therapy

	yes	no
1. stop tumor growth	☐	☐
2. reduce tumor size	☐	☐
3. healing	☐	☐
4. prevent metastases	☐	☐
5. prevent tumor relapse	☐	☐
6. prevent increase of pain	☐	☐
7. pain relief	☐	☐
8. free of pain without medication	☐	☐
9. relief of tumor-related symptoms	☐	☐
10. psychological stabilisation	☐	☐

The scale was developed not for pure statistical means, but for the individual patient. It can be used by the affected patient himself and by his/her responsible doctor. This psychometric scale was subjected to extensive reliability and structural validity testing (Cronbach's Alpha and other multivariate tests (95)). Patients and doctors are asked:

- *Patient:* Which of the following describes your personal expectations toward your cancer therapy? You may check one or several of the following items.
- *Doctor:* Which of the following describes your personal expectations toward the cancer therapy of the present patient. You may check one or several of the following items.

(Reproduced with permission form Ref. 3).

Neither all responses on the expectation scale, nor all of the outcome variables following cancer treatment, can be used for an analysis of covariance. In patients, the expectation of a full recovery is the most prominent variable (Figure 3) and was chosen and will be analyzed in covariance analysis against self-reported quality of life. By analogy, the surgeons' expectations of reduction in tumor size will be used in covariance analysis against the health status assessment using the McPeek index [62]. Analysis of covariance, including a comparison of the variation of the covariables in the G-CSF and placebo group, will be performed using both the method of Hays [112] and SPSS statistical software [116]. The covariance analysis is planned and will be performed in addition to the confirmatory statistical analysis, but will not be used to reject the null-hypotheses.

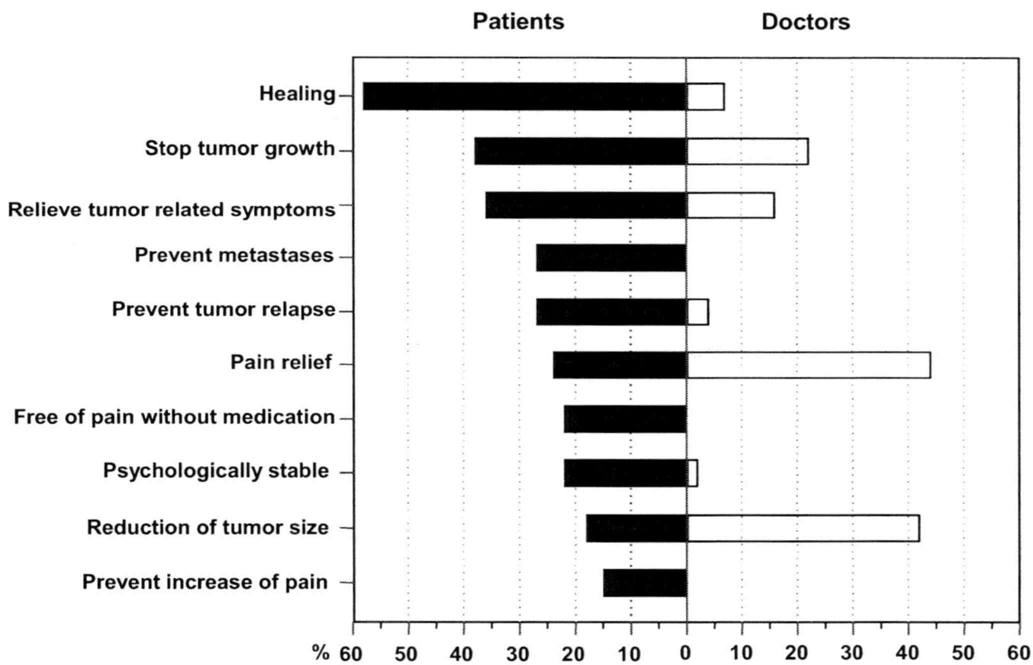

Figure 3. Analysis of the tumor therapy-related expectations of patients and doctors. Expectations was assessed in 55 patients. Checking of multiple expectations was possible. The results represent percentages of yes-responses to the expectation scale which in this study will be administered immediately before the beginning of G-CSF prophylaxis at the afternoon before operation. Patients = affected patients themselves, doctors = physicians or surgeons mainly responsible for the patients. Adopted from Koller et al. [137]. (Reproduced with permission form Ref. 3).

4.5 Definition of Endpoint Constructs and of Base-Line Characteristics

Endpoint Constructs

Since the outcome of surgical interventions is such a fundamental problem in medicine, it is not surprising that there are numerous endpoints for postoperative sub-optimum and optimum recovery. In general, mortality and morbidity after operation had been well defined by Nyström et al. [6] or by Rangel-Fausto et al. [117], leading to a clear sequence of sepsis, severe sepsis, septic shock, end-organ dysfunction and death. To reduce outcome variation Zimmerman et al. [118] measured the standardized mortality ratio based on APACHE scoring. An additional dimension of perioperative mortality was, however, introduced by classifying each death as "expected" or "unexpected" surgical mortality [119], thus encompassing the whole clinical system. This endpoint was further investigated by Rosenberg et al. [120] who studied circadian rhythm. Many studies had been dedicated to perioperative mortality and morbidity, such as cardiac morbidity [121-126]. However, such morbidity can not unambiguously be differentiated from the consequences of SIRS, including infectious and non-infectious activation of the neuro-endocrine immune systems, leading to various postoperative complications. Pulmonary complications after general surgery pose particularly severe postoperative outcomes [127].

Additionally, organ-specific definitions of sub-optimum recovery, such as after colorectal operations as in this study, were carefully investigated by Mc Lauchlan et al. [104] and Dawes et al. [128]. On a more pathobiochemical basis, immunological dissonance as an undesirable outcome had been stressed by Bone [129] and Jiminez et al. [130], and was closely related to the proposal in this trial.

Finally, several other principles of outcome classification in postoperative recovery and severe infections included cultural influences [131], patient preferences for outcomes [132], a complex model of outcome using a specific index [133] and quality of life [134].

In this study, however, a new model of outcome – the integrated outcome model - was used the first time in a randomized, controlled trial [59,60]. Based on conceptual work, outcome analysis depends on three obligatory elements [15,59,60]:

1. A quality of life index self-reported by the patient and assessed by him or her independently from observation by others (family members, doctors)
2. A doctor's assessment of recovery and health status through a corresponding index (McPeek Index)
3. Analysis of clinical relevance of the endpoints in both groups is performed with the method of qualitative research (true endpoint concept).

After these three necessary steps - bridging theory to practical establishment - the set of primary endpoints is listed and their assessment and measurement explained.

Primary Endpoint No. 1: Patient's Assessment of Recovery Using a Self-Reported Quality of Life Index (EORTC-QLQ-C30) with an Organ-Specific Module for Colorectal Cancer (EORTC-QLQ-CR38)

This well-known index of quality of life [135] was based on a modular approach, whereby a 30-item score questionnaire was supplemented by a 38-item colorectal cancer module [136]. This renders the index very suitable for a specific assessment of health-related quality of life, fulfilling many of the conceptual demands [15,64,115] for outcome analysis and the practical demands for constructing a clinically readable quality of life profile [137,138] (Figure 4).

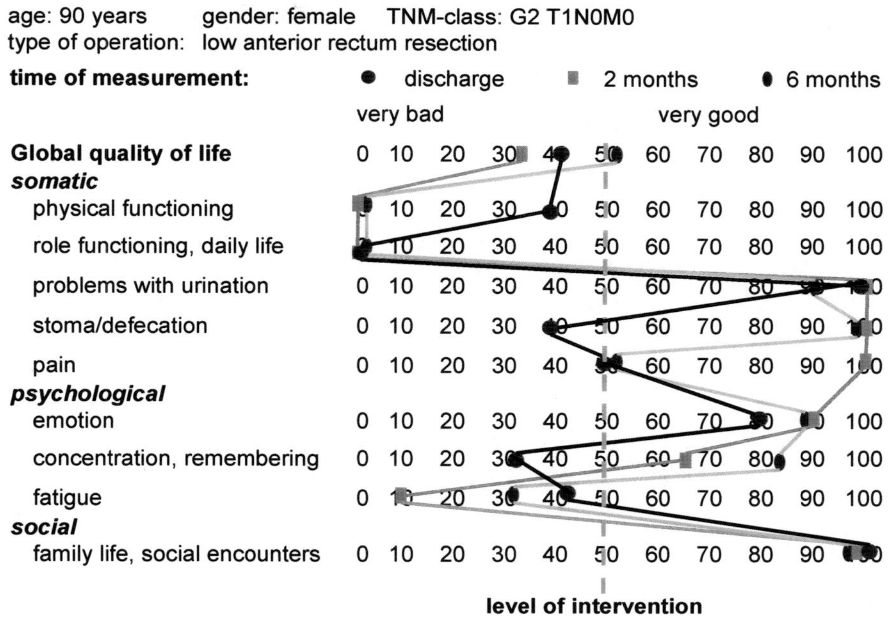

Patient A

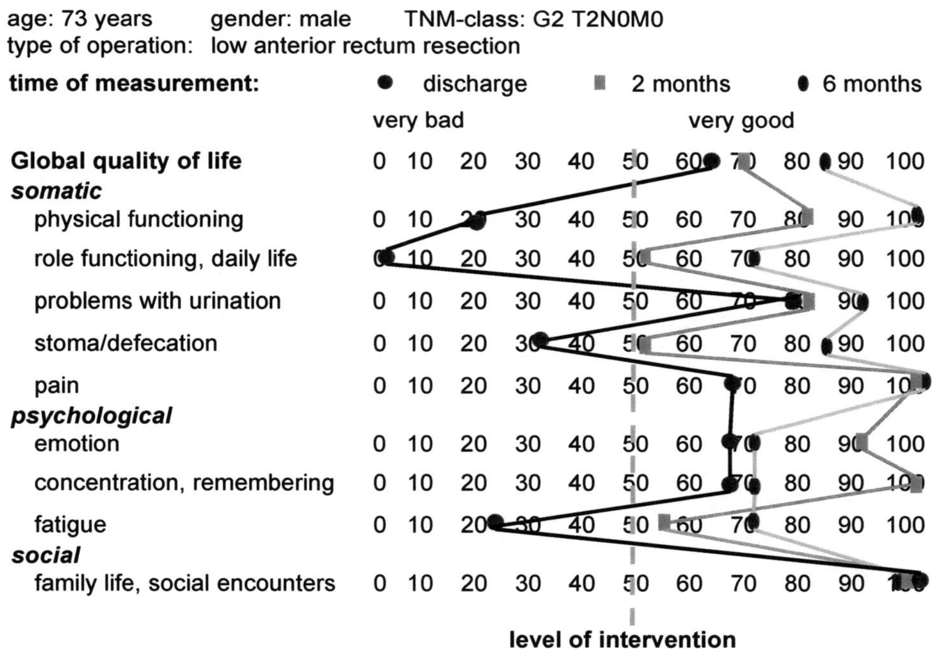

Patient B

Figure 4. Quality of life profiles from two patients of this trial. Qualtity of life profiles were obtained by transformation of the Likert-scaled items of the EORTC-QLQ-30 index into continuous scales. Cero indicates a very poor quality of life (QL) and 100 an excellent QL. At 50 points is the level of intervention to improve Ql of the patient at the different domains. Patient A did not improve in the different domains during the 6 moth follow up but patient B. The later is one who recovered as expected in the hypothesis for QL measurement (see figure 5).

Quality of life as a clinically relevant [139], conceptually and analytically valid endpoint can and must be assessed by the patient himself, without interference by health professionals (surgeons, physicians) or socially related subjects (relatives, friends) [140]. Furthermore, it can and must be assessed with consideration of influences which were not related to health as a theoretical concept [141,142], but which belong to other domains of the human psyche - in particular to negative affect, social desirability and expectations [101,137,143].

In this randomized trial, global quality of life was used as the primary endpoint. Means calculated from two items which were measured in seven-interval Likert scales and then combined and transformed into a scale between 0 and 100 points according to Koller et al. [144] will be compared between the two treatment groups and between the four groups with the different antibiotics in the 2 x 2 design. Quality of life was assessed at discharge from the surgical clinic (when the patient either goes home or to an oncology clinic), at two months and at six months after operation. Global quality of life as a primary endpoint was measured as a summary measure over six months according to Fairclough [145]. When death occurred during the study period of six months quality of life was defined as zero.

The information obtained from the quality of life profiles in the somatic, pain, psychological and social domains will be analyzed as secondary endpoints and help us to understand the primary endpoint variable, global quality of life. From the background of social psychology, in particular studies about coping [146], it cannot be expected that even excellent quality of life scores 100 points. A profile which always scores 100 points corresponds to a psychological state of repression or simply to an artifact or a process of denying or lying by an individual patient. Scores of ≥ 80 points after recovery were considered normal and values < 50 points indicated the need of support in the effected quality of life domains. The number of patients in each study arm with more than 50 points in global quality of life will be calculated.

Primary Endpoint No. 2: Doctor's Assessment of Recovery Using the McPeek Recovery Index

The McPeek recovery index (Table 6) combines several attributes for the concept of outcome: variables which stand for themselves and were - in one way or an other - also proxy variables for very undesirable states or processes. The extent of undesirability is weighted by a scoring system which is simple and understandable from a clinical point of view. The original index was created by an experienced anesthesiologist and statistician who built up a clinical measurement team over many years [62]. Its validity was assessed against major external standards: age, sex, race, body build, perioperative physical status (ASA), hospital status, cardiovascular and respiratory complications, starting time of operation (day and month of the year), principal anesthetic drug combination and the experience of the anesthetist. The McPeek index was recently evaluated in three independent prospective trials with a total of 669 patients [63]. The McPeek score demonstrated to be a reliable, valid, sensitive and practicable instrument for outcome analysis of operations including mortality and ICU treatment. The score includes further a criterion of value judgment, which is a necessary part in the integrated outcome concept.

Table 6. Doctor's assessment of postoperative recovery: the modified McPeek index (59)

Patient characteristics	Score
Patient who died	
• in the operating room	0
• in the hospital after leaving the operating room	1
• outside the hospital within the recovery period of six months (no accident!)	2
Patient who remained alive for six months	
• yet required - not pre-operatively scheduled – extensive care in an ICU after operation (more than 20 TISS-28 points on a single day or more than 3 ICU days)	4
• yet required - not pre-operatively scheduled - a moderate amount of care in an ICU after operation (not more than 20 TISS-28 points at a single day or less than 3 ICU days)	5
Patient who underwent routine recovery on a normal ward with a postoperative hospitalisation	
• ≥ 10 days longer than clinic standard	7
• < 10 days longer than clinical standard	8
• no longer than clinical standard for the particular operation	9

(Reproduced with permission form Ref. 3).

However, its closeness to real-life made specifications and tailoring to cultural and social conditions necessary, as pointed out in the concept of outcome:

- Since the **mortality** was assessed over a period of six months, a different weight should be given to different times of survival (Table 6). Dying in the operation theatre is much more adverse than in the 6 month follow up period.
- **Intensive care** was considered to represent difficulties in recovery which were more severe than those managed in a normal ward. However, the principle of observed versus expected (see above) can be determined only if the scheduled care is subtracted from that actually given as a consequence of the patient's status and progress after operation. In the centers of this trial and many other German centers one day in an ICU with moderate amount of care was scheduled for ASA 3 and 4 patients after operations for colorectal cancer. Thus extensive care in an ICU still earns a score of 4, whether it was on day one or later, but moderate care of up to three additional days added to day one after operation was moderate care (5 points).
  The amount of care was hitherto measured by the TISS-score [147] in the modified version of Keene and Cullen [148]. This was applied to postoperative outcome analysis using the McPeek index [34,132,149,150]. Quite recently the classical TISS-76 index (76 items) was replaced by TISS-28 [151]. TISS-28 was superior to TISS-76 in several criteria of validation [146], and was also superior to TISS-9 (Nursing manpower use score) [152] due to more experience with validation [153]. TISS-28 was therefore used in this study.

Based on the large data pool from the surgical ICU of Cologne [153], the critical problem for the modified McPeek index of differentiating between moderate and extensive care can be solved. More than 20 TISS-28 points during a single day denotes extensive care.

- **Postoperative hospitalization** was considered as the third component in the first step of recovery after operation. The second component was recovery at home or a mixture of care in ambulatory services and re-hospitalization depending on "late" complications such as pulmonary infections or thromboembolism after discharge from the hospital [149]. Increased hospitalization time was correlated with rate and severity of complications [154]. However, a meta-analysis of randomized trials in cholecystectomy had shown [149] that standard hospitalization time/hospital varies considerably, so that four days for a conventional cholecystectomy in one study were considerably shorter than eight days for laparoscopic cholecystectomy in another trial. This difficulty should be solved again by the principle of observed versus expected, defining a standardized hospitalization time for recovery without complications by all primary surgeons in this trial for each type of operation. This principle was successfully applied in the 1994 Mainz-Marburg trial [35]. An undesirable recovery scoring 7 points (Table 6) was then more than half of the standard hospitalization time, or $\geq$ 10 days longer than the clinical standard. Less than 10 days scores 8 points and the optimum was a stay not longer than the clinical standard for the particular operation (Table 6). Optimum recovery, which avoided the 14 types of postoperative complications listed did not lead to exceeding the standard hospitalization time, but was usually shorter than the expected standard.
- **Assessment of the McPeek index points** of each patient will be performed after conducting the trial by a clinician and a methodologist.

Analysis of Clinical Relevance: The True Endpoint Measured by the Methodology of Qualitative Research

Novel ways to analyze effectiveness and outcome are plagued by the problem that the present scientific medical community is not yet familiar with such new concepts and methodologies. Certain items of this study protocol must therefore be explained in some detail to be acceptable, especially the clinically relevant endpoint [64] which is the central part of evidence-based medicine and hence of this protocol and trial.

The methodology needed for answering the question of the true endpoint in this study is qualitative research [155,156]. It has been defined as an "interdisciplinary, interpretative field of inquiry. The qualitative researcher uses predominantly non-statistical analytic procedures to generate information from data gathered from field observations, structured interviews, focus groups, case studies, document analyses and other sources that describe routine and problematic moments and meanings in individual lives" [157].

It was important to emphasize that academic surgeons (Troidl [64], McKneally in Ref. [1]) identified this very practical problem, not basic scientists or philosophers. The classical endpoint in surgical trials, "return to work," was a complex endpoint where motivation confounds analysis (McKneally in Ref. [1], p. 643). In the six month period of recovery in this trial overcoming incontinence and dysuria, coming home, involvement in social events or returning to work is the true endpoint, and their relation to the primary statistical endpoints is completely unknown.

After the practical experience of the field study on tumor follow-up in the county of Marburg-Biedenkopf [138], in which quality of life assessment with the EORTC index in almost 400 patients with breast cancer was compared with qualitative analysis, a similar structured interview had been developed. Six months after operation the patient and the research clinician spend about 20 minutes, not only asking questions of the structured interview like: "What did you find worst? What did you find best? What was most important to you in the last six months?", but the clinician also listens to the patient and records all spontaneous comments. These interviews were taped and analyzed at the end of the study, not only by descriptive statistics but also by concepts of social psychology [157].

Further Endpoints

The many endpoints (Table 7) which will be analyzed with descriptive and explorative statistics are not a serious problem. The variables in the two primary outcome constructs must be assessed and the events in the true endpoint analysis were part of the structured interview.

On the basis of recent studies [158-160] the immune status was assessed preoperatively in the morning before operation, in the morning of day one, three and day six.

Sub-optimum recovery as an outcome construct played a considerable role as an endpoint in previous studies [35,149,150]. It was defined as a McPeek index of less than optimum (< 9 scoring points) and/or with at least one postoperative complication within 30 days after operation. In this study, a period of six months for the primary endpoints had been established and thus the results obtained from a corresponding definition of sub-optimum recovery cannot be predicted, but will be calculated.

4.6 Statistical Analysis and Sample Size

Primary Endpoints for Statistical Analysis

The estimation of sample size in the randomized trial was based on the first primary endpoint, global quality of life, which was self-assessed by the patient.

For the patient's assessment of postoperative recovery, a speedy return of quality of life (QoL) to an acceptable level of 80 points was decisive. A good QoL with 80 points was normally not the case before operation. It was expected from the statistical model that patients with G-CSF will achieve a high quality of life earlier (Figure 5). This improvement was most pronounced at hospital discharge and decreases over time, although with the present clinical knowledge, no data are available which support whether patients with G-CSF had higher scores for QoL even six months after operation. However, according to Fairclough [161], the Area Under the Curve (AUC) as a measure of postoperative gain of quality of life up to the pre-disease, not pre-operative level, of about 80 points was an acceptable expectation and was used in this study (Figure 5). The QoL-index was determined for each patient at discharge from hospital, two months later and six months later. These QoL-values were plotted on the time axis and the AUC under these three points was the primary endpoint.

Table 7. Secondary endpoints of the G-CSF prophylaxis trial (Reproduced with permission form Ref. 3).

Groups of variables in relation to design	Specifications
(1) Parts of McPeek index and of the outcome analysis of laparoscopic versus conventional surgery	• Mortality rate/6 months • Complication rate/6 months – anastomotic leakage – wound infection – pneumonia – peritonitis, sepsis – postoperative bleeding – reoperation – cardiovascular disturbances – stress ulceration – urinary tract infection – thromboembolism – pulmonary embolism • Hospital stay (absolute days) • Re-admission rate/6 months • Re-operation rate/6 months • Rate of non-optimum recovery
(2) Parts of the EORTC index of quality of life	• Somatic symptoms and functioning • Duration and severity of pain • Psychological distress • Fatigue syndrome • Impairment of social encounters • Return to work – change of working position – change of working status – amount of disability
(3) Events in true endpoint analysis	• Duration of intestinal atony • Cessation of incontinence (rate and time) • Cessation of involuntary urination • Coming home after chemotherapy, radiotherapy and rehabilitation • Return to work • Changes in weight over 6 months
(4) Measures of immuno-insufficiency before and after operation	• Complete blood count at various times • Granulocyte phagocytic activity • HLA-DR expression on monocytes • LPS induced release of TNF-α from whole blood • G-CSF levels in plasma • Procalcitonin levels in plasma • IL-6, IL-8, IL18 levels in plasma

Definitions of complications taken from two studies on perioperative risks (72, 121).

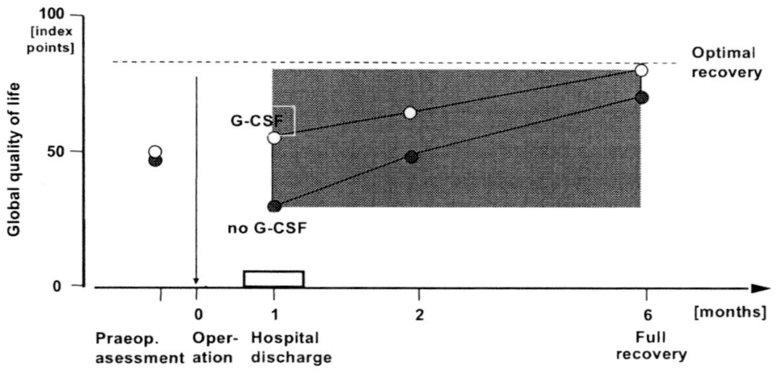

Figure 5. Expected development of global quality of life in colorectal cancer patients with and without G-CSF prophylaxis. Assessment of preoperative and postoperative recovery (EORTC-QLQ-C30 and QLQ C38 index): expected influence of G-CSF (o — o) following the analysis of a control group with rectal cancer (n=119) without G-CSF (• — •) in the field study in Marburg-Biedenkopf [119]. A maximum of about 80 index points in global quality of life is considered as an acceptable quality of life due to the coping effect (132). (Reproduced with permission form Ref. 3).

Let Q_1 be the QoL-index postoperatively, Q_2 the QoL after two months and Q_3 the QoL after 6 months.

Then the AUC was calculated using the following equation:

$$AUC = Q_1 + 3Q_2 + 2Q_3).$$

The second primary endpoint, the McPeek recovery index, was not used to calculate the sample size.

Sample Size

The estimates of the mean and standard deviation of the area under the curve for the control group were taken from a trial with 47 cancer patients in all of whom quality of life had been determined in exactly the same way at three different time points with a follow-up duration of six months. The mean AUC was 350 points and the standard deviation 99 points. Expecting an increase to 430 points for the AUC of the G-CSF group, we need according to the Friedman-formula [84] a sample size of 32 patients per group. Including a safety margin we fix our sample size at 40 patients for the G-CSF group and 40 patients for the control group. According to an analysis of patient recruitment for two consecutive years [162], the duration of the trial was anticipated to be about two years.

Statistical Hypotheses

The two null hypotheses will be simultaneously tested in the study:

H_0^{QoL} : $\mu_{(GCSF,QoL)} = \mu_{(C,QoL)}$ is tested against the alternative H_1^{QoL} : $\mu_{(GCSF,QoL)} \neq \mu_{(C,QoL)}$.
H_0^{McPeek} : $\mu_{(GCSF,McPeek)} = \mu_{(C,McPeek)}$ is tested against the alternative H_1^{McPeek} : $\mu_{(GCSF,McPeek)} \neq \mu_{(C,McPeek)}$.

μ_{GCSF}, is the expected value of the AUCs for all patients in the G-CSF group and μ_C for the control group, respectively.

Confirmatory Analysis

The conventional two-sample two-sided t-test with a nominal significance level of $\alpha = 0.05$; $\beta = 0.2$ will be used to test the single hypothesis. To adjust for multiple testing, a hierarchical testing procedure will be used:

First, the null-hypothesis H_0^{QoL} will be tested at nominal $\alpha = 0.05$.

If the null-hypothesis H_0^{QoL} was rejected, then the null-hypothesis H_0^{McPeek} will be tested at nominal $\alpha = 0.05$. According to the principle of closed testing [163], this procedure maintains the simultaneous type I error of 0.05.

In addition to the two-sample, two-sided t-test the conventional 95 % confidence interval for the difference of the means will also be determined. For safety reasons mortality rates of both groups will be published.

If the null-hypothesis H_0^{QoL} was rejected, we will recommend:

- The use of a G-CSF prophylaxis in colorectal cancer patients with high perioperative risk for an adverse postoperative outcome.
- The analysis of immune modifiers in smaller trials and not in large multi-center trials. Clinical standardization is more important than a high number of patients.
- The use of CMRTs to test clinical conditions and interactions with the study drug before the definite clinical trial is set up.

If the null-hypothesis H_0^{QoL} cannot be rejected, both null-hypotheses will be maintained with the interpretation: it could not be shown that G-CSF prophylaxis had an effect on global QoL, and it could not be shown that G-CSF had an effect on the modified McPeek index in the patients under study. The superiority of smaller trials with standardized clinical management as compared to multi-center trials could not be shown.

4.7. Center Based Clinical Guideline for Postoperative Anastomotic Leakage

The need for reducing the variability of clinical decisions within complex treatment processes reveals a lack of high level evidence (Table 8) for most medical measures [164]. Without sound scientific evidence, marked variations may exist in diagnosis and management [165], leading to considerable and unjustifiable heterogeneity in clinical treatment modalities [166]. While these variations may not disadvantage the patient, they could impair medical and economic planning [167] and hamper the design and clinical conduct of complex clinical randomized trials. In the design of our trial, the treatment of postoperative anastomotic leakage was an important point of heterogeneity.

Table 8. Level of Evidence

I:	Evidence obtained from at least one properly randomised controlled trial
II-1:	Evidence obtained from well-designed controlled trials without randomisation
II-2.:	Evidence obtained from well-designed cohort of case control analytic studies, preferably from more than one center or research group
II-3:	Evidence obtained from multiple time series with or without intervention. Dramatic results in uncontrolled experiments (such as the results of the introduction of penicillin treatment in the 1940s) could also be regarded as this type of evidence
III:	Opinions of respected authorities, based on clinical experience; descriptive studies and case reports; or reports of expert committees

Reprinted from the US Preventive Service Task Force. Guide to clinical preventive services. In: Margolis C and Cretin S. (eds.) Implementing clinical practice guidelines. Chicago: AHA Press p 61, 1998 (166). Differing from prior tables ranking evidence, case reports with important findings were defined as evidence level II-3.

Clinical guidelines are effective in reducing arbitrariness and thus improving medical care, provided the components of development, dissemination and implementation are all equally appropriate [168].

When developing a guideline, one must gather information, find consensus and present the formal work-up of the decision and treatment alternatives with a particular logic 'clarity'. Consensus can be achieved by several methods, but it should be a formal, well-structured process. Here the method of a Nominal Group Process (NGP) was chosen [169]. Methodologically, the NGP was started with the production of a seed algorithm. A bottom up approach was chosen by the steering group of the Lucerne Study Group: each center presented a 'typical' case of anastomotic leakage from its own patients. The discharge summary of each case was entered into an action-time table that was then transformed into a torso algorithm without other options at the decision nodes, and was completed to give a full case-based algorithm [66,170]. Abstracting from these algorithms produced a "seed algorithm", forming the basis of the NGP for consensus finding of the Lucerne Study Group [171].

Throughout the NGP, comments of each group member were collected and grouped together into similar issues by the meeting leader who was professionally familiar with this technique [171]. The ongoing process, however, did not reach a consensus; it was the most difficult NGP the meeting leader had ever done [171]. Voting and an extensive discussion did not lead to a revised seed algorithm that could serve as adequate proposal for a second nominal group round [65]. Another approach was therefore chosen to solve the problem of heterogeneity: the creation of a small multicenter instead of a large multicenter trial. The current study protocol is therefore limited to three centers, restricting the problems of dissemination and implementation to a local level and, in this way, strongly facilitating them.

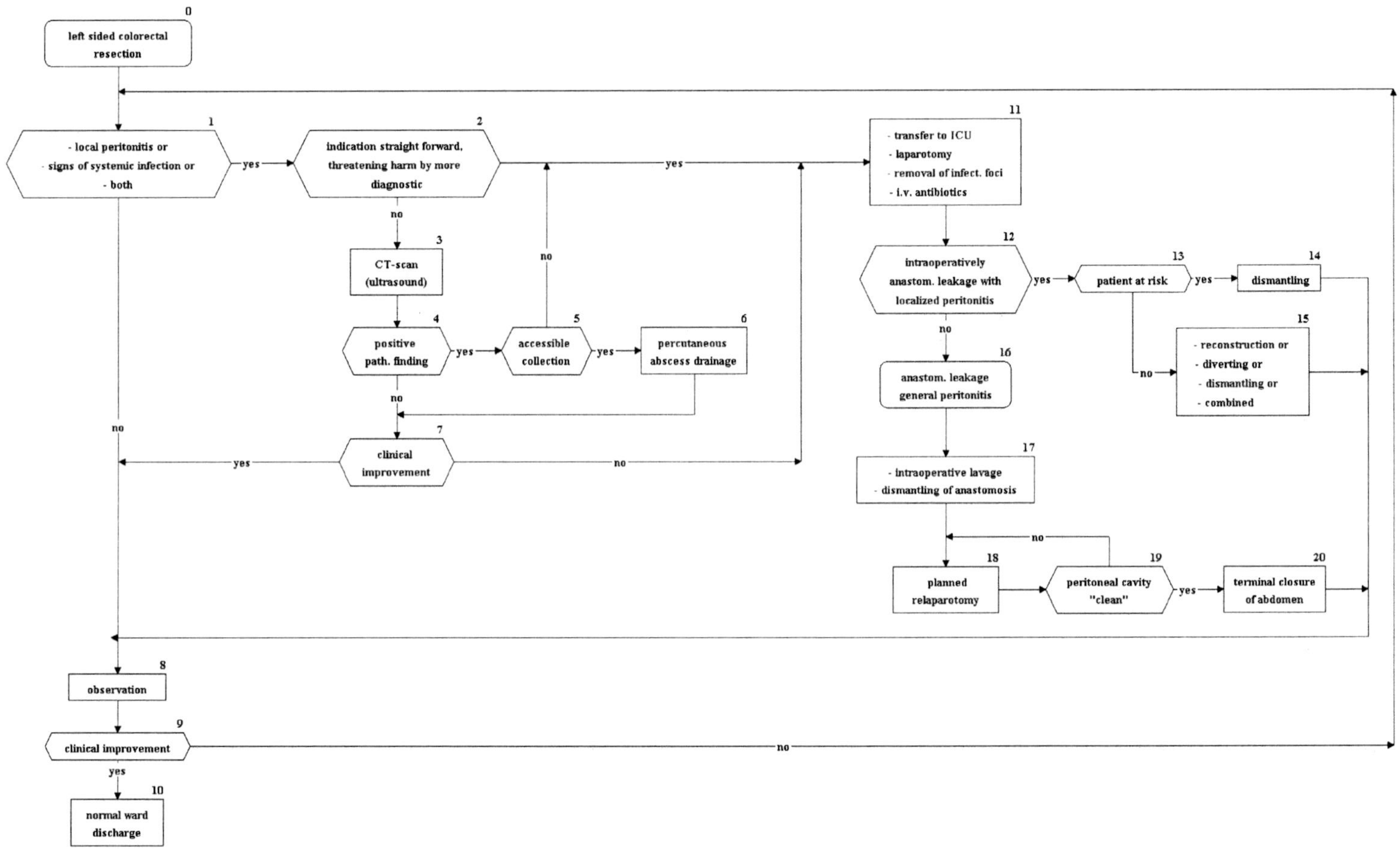

Figure 6. Center based algorithm for the treatment of septic complications following anastomotic leakage in colorectal surgery (Reproduced with permission form Ref. 4).

Levels of evidence were applied to all decisions in the algorithm (Figure 6) from best evidence (I = metaanalysis or randomized trials) to lowest (III = opinion of experts) as suggested by the US-Department of Health and Human Services [172], (Table 8).

The methodological approach was:

- To raise a question for each clinical problem in the algorithm. (e.g.: what sign or symptom justify a re-operation after left-sided colorectal resection?)
- A Medline and Cochrane library search with the relevant keywords was performed. (e.g.: colon resection, rectal resection, re-operation, peritonitis and complication).
- The papers were gathered, ranked in evidence, and summarized in a statement on the particular problem of the clinical algorithm. This process was performed by two clinical and one methodological study leader.

Several trials with high levels of evidence in investigating methods to prevent anastomotic leakage were detected, but no benefit could be identified for any of the surgical strategies compared. Stapled anastomosis is as safe as hand sewn [173] (level of evidence I). Mechanical bowl preparation (high volumes of solvents used in bowl cleaning) does not promote a suspected bacterial translocation [174] (level of evidence I) but evidence for its preventing anastomotic leakage is lacking [175] (level of evidence I). The technique of omentoplasty was not shown to prevent anastomotic leakage [176] (level of evidence I), nor did drainage of pelvic anastomosis reduce the risk of anastomotic leakage [177,178] (level of evidence I).

Evidence for each decision node and action box of the algorithm (Figure 6) was identified and demonstrated in detail in part three of the study protocol [4]. In general in most cases only evidence for a specific treatments on level III exists. Non the less, the clinical algorithm (Figure 6) was accepted as a guideline by all three participating centers for the treatment of anastomotic leakage in the trial. Fulfillment and deviations from the guideline will be analyzed at the end of the trial.

5. DISCUSSION

Clinical trial protocols often lack necessary details and, in particular, explanations why one option was chosen instead of several others which were open for discussion and may had been chosen by another group. The protocol of the Mainz-Marburg trial [34], however did not have this weakness and had found many followers since its publication in 1988. Pilz et al. [179] followed this prototype in a sepsis trial. Together with Altman and Chalmers in Oxford, study protocols published before this trial were collected in order to improve the reporting of methodological details of randomized clinical trials in the future [19,20,180,181].

Several prospective studies (including separately published protocols) had been necessary to confirm the conditions fixed in this study protocol. Pre-testing of trial conditions was a new, necessary component in future trial development - but it was usually not funded [180,181]. There were too many failed trials in the treatment with cytokines especially in sepsis, and we believe that most failure was caused by quick and superficial study designs and protocols which were formally and legally correct, but not scientifically sound for such complex clinical issues. Industrial speakers unfortunately claim too often: We had no time! But failures take more time to correct than careful planning and are combined with enormous costs as demonstrated recently in a trial with anti-thrombin III [182]. Only one large company initiated sepsis trial, with activated protein, was successive in the reduction of the 28 day mortality rate [183].

Beside some methodological failures of previous trials such as patient heterogeneity and others listed by Bone [184], two additional important points had to be considered:

- The clinical complexity was not adequately tested in animals before the studies were conducted. For this reason the model of clinic modeling randomized trials (CMRTs) was developed [31] to analyze the complex interaction of clinical interventions.
- A standardization of the anesthetic and surgical management was not performed prospectively. This includes specific treatment before operation (prophylaxis with heparin, antibiotics, antihistamines, pre-medication), on the day of operation (anesthesia, operative procedures, one scheduled ICU day), and in the postoperative course (management of pain and a guideline for the treatment of anastomotic leakage). Without standardizing these clinical interventions, all of which may influence the immune system, benefits of an immune modifier such as G-CSF will not be detectable. This is a major problem of large multicenter trials. Neither a standardization of antibiotic prophylaxis (simple to perform) e.g. [21,185], nor a guideline for the operative intervention (not easy to perform) was included in any study protocol. Progress in sepsis therapy or in surgical outcome research will not be obtained by un-standardized multicenter trials. For this reason, some smaller studies (50-100 patients) may be superior to large multicenter trials if they assess many details. Standardization of the surgical management is hardly possible in large multicenter trials, as our results of the nominal group process with the Lucerne Study Group have shown.

In the meantime our trial was conducted in three centers in two years with an additional half year for the follow up of the last randomized patients. From the whole trial only one patient was withdrawn, because the operation of the assigned patient was not performed at the day scheduled. The trial concept demonstrated feasibility and utility and can be used for other cytokines. Analysis of the results will show whether a G-CSF prophylaxis will be effective for one of the primary endpoints (global quality of life, health status or the true endpoint) and which antibiotic combination with G-CSF is most effective. The effects on other endpoints in mechanistic and patient defined domains will guide the direction of further clinical trials with G-CSF.

Acknowledgements

This development of the study protocol was supported by grants from the Deutsche Forschungsgemeinschaft (Ba 1560/2-2 and 2-3), the German Ministry of Health (FB2-43332-

70/6), the Deutsche Forschungsgemeinschaft (SFB 297) and AMGEN Europe. The second meeting of the Consensus Group (January 1997 in Marburg /Lahn) (Germany)) was supported by grants from Hoffmann La Roche AG (Germany, Switzerland), Aventis-Behring GmbH (Germany, USA), Thomae GmbH, Boehringer Ingelheim KG (Germany), Schwabe Arzneimittel (Germany), Grünenthal GmbH (Germany), Fresenius AG (Germany) and by the University of Marburg (Germany).

REFERENCES

[1] Lorenz W, McKneally M, Troidl H, Banerjee JK, Benbasset J, Dziri C, Fagniez P-L, Little JM, Wong J, Wulff HR: Surgical research around the world, in Troidl H, McKneally MF, Mulder DS, Wechsler AS, McPeek B, Spitzer WO (eds): *Surgical research: basic principles and clinical practice*. ed.3rd. New York, Springer, pp 637-654, 1998.

[2] Lorenz W, Stinner B, Bauhofer A, Rothmund M, Celik I, Fingerhut A, Koller M, Lorijn RHW, Nyström P-O, Sitter H, Schäfer H, Schein M, Solomkin JS, Troidl H, Wyatt J, Wittmann DH, Lucerne Group for Consensus-assisted Development of the Study Protocol on Prevention of Abdominal Sepsis: Example G-CSF: Granulocyte-colony stimulating factor in the prevention of postoperative infectious complications and sub-optimum recovery from operation in patients with colorectal cancer and increased preoperative risk (ASA 3 and 4). Protocol of a controlled clinical trial developed by consensus of an international study group. Part one: Rationale and hypothesis. *Inflamm.Res.* 50:115-122, 2001.

[3] Bauhofer A, Lorenz W, Stinner B, Rothmund M, Koller M, Sitter H, Celik I, Farndon JR, Fingerhut A, Hay J-M, Lefering R, Lorijn R, Nyström P-O, Schäfer H, Schein M, Solomkin J, Troidl H, Volk H-D, Wittmann DH, Wyatt J, Lucerne Group for Consensus-assisted Development of the Study Protocol on Prevention of Abdominal Sepsis: Example G-CSF.: Granulocyte-colony stimulating factor in the prevention of postoperative infectious complications and sub-optimum recovery from operation in patients with colorectal cancer and increased preoperative risk (ASA 3 and 4). Protocol of a controlled clinical trial developed by consensus of an international study group. Part two: design of the study. *Inflamm.Res.* 50:187-205, 2001.

[4] Stinner B, Bauhofer A, Lorenz W, Rothmund M, Plaul U, Torossian A, Celik I, Sitter H, Koller M, Black A, Encke A, Greger B, van Goor H, Hanisch E, Hesterberg R, Klose KJ, Lacaine F, Lorijn RHW, Solovera J, Margolis C, Neugebauer E, Nyström P-O, Reemst PHM, Schein M, Solovera J, Lucerne Group for Consensus-assisted Development of the Study Protocol on Prevention of Abdominal Sepsis: Example G-CSF: Granulocyte-colony stimulating factor in the prevention of postoperative infectious complications and sub-optimum recovery from operation in patients with colorectal cancer and increased preoperative risk (ASA 3 and 4). Protocol of a controlled clinical trial developed by consensus of an international study group. Part

three: individual patient, complication algorithm and quality management. *Inflamm.Res* 50:233-248, 2001.

[5] Solomkin JS, Meakins JL, Allo MD, Dellinger EP, Simmons RL: Antibiotic trials in intra-abdominal infections: a critical evaluation of study design and outcome reporting. *Ann.Surg.* 200:29-39, 1984.

[6] Nyström P-O, Bax R, Dellinger EP, Dominioni L, Knaus WA, Meakins JL, Ohmann C, Solomkin JS, Wacha H, Wittmann DH: Proposed definitions for diagnosis, severity scoring, stratification, and outcome for trials in intra-abdominal infection. *World J.Surg.* 14:148-158, 1990.

[7] Gorbach SL, Condon RE, Conte JE, Kaiser AB, Ledger WJ, Nichols RL: General guidelines for the evaluation of new anti-infective drugs for the prophylaxis of surgical infections: evaluation of new anti-infective drugs for surgical prophylaxis. *CID* 15 (Suppl 1):S313-S338, 1992.

[8] Members of the ACCP/SCCM consensus conference committee, Bone RC, et al: American College of Chest Physicians/Society of Critical Care Medicine Consensus Conference: Definitions for sepsis and organ failure and guidelines for the use of innovative therapies in sepsis. *Crit.Care Med.* 20:864-874, 1992.

[9] Lorenz W, Neugebauer E, Pilz G, Werdan K, Lorenz M, et al: Methodology of clinical trials in sepsis: discussion about the trial protocol of supplemental immunoglobulin therapy in sepsis and septic shock. *Theor.Surg.* 9:10-67, 1994.

[10] Bone RC: Sepsis, sepsis syndrome, and the systemic inflammatory response syndrome (SIRS). *JAMA* 273:155-156, 1995.

[11] Petros AJ, Marshall JC, van Saene HKF: Should morbidity replace mortality as an endpoint for clinical trials in intensive care? *Lancet* 345:369-371, 1995.

[12] Dellinger RP, Truman HS: Post hoc analyses in sepsis trials: a formula for disappointment? *Crit.Care Med.* 24:727-729, 1996.

[13] Zeni F, Freeman B, Natanson C: Anti-inflammatory therapies to treat sepsis and septic shock: a reassessment. *Crit.Care Med.* 25:1095-1100, 1997.

[14] Vincent J-L: Search for effective immunomodulating strategies against sepsis. *Lancet* 351:922-923, 1998.

[15] Lorenz W, Troidl H, Solomkin JS, Nies C, Sitter H, Koller M, Krack W, Roizen MF: Second step: testing - outcome measurements. *World J.Surg.* 23:768-780, 1999.

[16] Graf J, Doig GS, Cook DJ, Vincent JL, Sibbald WJ: Randomized, controlled clinical trials in sepsis: has methodological quality improved over time? *Crit care med* 30:461-472, 2002.

[17] Balk RA, Bone RC: Methodological issues in the design and implementation of controlled clinical trials in severe sepsis and septic shock. *Theor.Surg.* 9:32-37, 1994.

[18] McPeek B, Mosteller F, McKneally MF, Neugebauer E: Experimental methods: clinical trials, in Troidl H, Spitzer WO, Mulder DS, Wechsler AS, McPeek B, McKneally MF, Balch CM (eds): *Principles and practice of research.* ed.2nd. New York, Springer, pp 114-125, 1991.

[19] Altman DG: Better reporting of randomised controlled trials: the CONSORT statement. *Br.Med.J.* 313:570-571, 1996.

[20] Moher D, Schulz KF, Altman D: The CONSORT statement: revised recommendations for improving the quality of reports of parallel-group randomized trials. *JAMA* 285:1987-1991, 2001.

[21] Fisher CJ, Dhainaut JA, Opal SM, Pribble JP, Balk RA, Slotman GJ, Iberti TJ, Rackow EC, Shapiro MJ, Greeman RL, Reines DH, Shelly MP, Thompson BW, LaBrecque JF, Catalano MA, Knaus WA, Sadoff JC: Recombinant human interleukin-1 receptor antagonist in the treatment of patients with sepsis syndrome. *JAMA* 271:1836-1843, 1994.

[22] Ziegler EJ, Fisher CJ, Sprung CL, Straube RC, Sadoff JC, Foulke GE, Wortel CH, Fink MP, Dellinger RP, Teng NNH, Allen IE, Berger HJ, Knatterud GL, LoBuglio AF, Smith CR, HA-1A Sepsis Study Group: Treatment of Gram-negative bacteriemia and septic shock with HA- 1A human monoclonal antibody against endotoxin. *N.Engl.J.Med.* 324:429-436, 1991.

[23] Goergen I, Hartung T, Leist M, Niehoerster M, Tiegs G, Uhlig S, Weitzel F, Wendel A: Granulocyte colony-stimulating factor treatment protects rodents against lipopolysaccharide-induced toxicity via suppression of systemic tumor necrosis factor alpha. *J.Immunol.* 149:918-924, 1994.

[24] Lorenz W, Reimund K-P, Weitzel F, Celik I, Kurnatowski M, Schneider C, Mannheim W, Heiske A, Neumann K, Sitter H, Rothmund M: Granulocyte colony-stimulating factor prophylaxis before operation protects against lethal consequences of postoperative peritonitis. *Surgery* 116:925-934, 1994.

[25] Hartung T, Döcke W-D, Gantner F, Krieger G, Sauer A, Stevens P, Volk HD, Wendel A: Effect of granulocyte colony-stimulating factor treatment on ex vivo blood cytokine response in human volunteers. *Blood* 85:2492-2489, 1995.

[26] Nelson S: Role of granulocyte colony-stimulating factor in the immune response to acute bacterial infection in the nonneutropenic host: an overview. *Clin.Infect.Dis.* 18:197-204, 1994.

[27] Dale DC, Liles WC, Summer WR, Nelson S: Granulocyte colony-stimulating factor: role and relationships in infectious diseases. *J.Infect.Dis.* 172:1061-1075, 1995.

[28] Bauhofer A, Huttel M, Reimund K-P, Celik I, Greger B, Lorenz W: Effective prophylaxis with rhG-CSF in abdominal sepsis: a new mechanism improving the antimicrobial functions of granulocytes (Wirksame Prophylaxe mit rhG-CSF bei abdomineller Sepsis: Verbesserung der antimikrobiellen Funktion von Granulozyten als neuer Mechanismus in vivo). *Langenbecks Arch.Chir.Forum* 593-596, 1997.

[29] Ertel W, Keel M, Buergi U, Hartung T, Imhof HG, Trentz O: Granulocyte colony-stimulating factor inhibits neutrophil apoptosis at the local site after severe head and thoracic injury. *J.Trauma.* 46:784-792, 1999.

[30] Feterowski C, Weighardt H, Emmanuilidis K, Hartung T, Holzmann B: Immune protection against septic peritonitis in endotoxin-primed mice is related to reduced neutrophil apoptosis. *Eur.J Immunol.* 31:1268-1277, 2001.

[31] Bauhofer A, Lorenz W, Celik I, Stinner B, Solovera J, Lorijn R: Haematopoetic cytokines, G-CSF and abdominal surgery, in Schein M, Wise L (eds): *Cytokines and the abdominal surgeon*. Austin, Texas, Landes Bioscience, pp 117-141, 1998.

[32] Celik I, Lorenz W, Stinner B, Duda D, Sitter H, Sauer S, Junge A, Hoppe M: Clinical modelling randomised trials (CMRT) in animals as a new intermediate between biological experiments and randomised clinical trials: application to antihistamine prophylaxis in anaesthesia and surgery. *Inflamm.Res.* 47 Suppl 1:S66-S68, 1998.

[33] Bauhofer A, Stinner B, Kohlert F, Reckzeh B, Lorenz W, Celik I: Granulocyte colony-stimulating factor but not peritoneal lavage increases survival rate after experimental abdominal contamination and infection. *Br.J Surg* 89:1457-1463, 2002.

[34] Lorenz W, Dick W, Junginger T, Ohman C, Ennis M, Immich H, McPeek B, Dietz W, Weber D: Induction of anaesthesia and perioperative risk: influence of antihistamine H1 + H2-prophylaxis and volume substitution with Haemaccel-35 on cardiovascular and respiratory disturbances and histamine release. Protocol of a controlled clinical trial. *Theor.Surg.* 3:55-77, 1988.

[35] Lorenz W, Duda D, Dick W, Sitter H, Doenicke A, Black A, Weber D, Menke H, Stinner B, Junginger T, Rothmund M, Ohmann C, Healy MJR, the trial group Mainz/Marburg: Incidence and clinical importance of perioperative histamine release: randomised study of volume loading and antihistamines after induction of anaesthesia. *Lancet* 343:933-940, 1994.

[36] Bauhofer A, Reimund K-P, Schütz P, Huttel M, Celik I: G-CSF increases PMN functions in rats with abdominal infection and sepsis (AIS). *Shock Suppl.* 5:10, 1996.

[37] Bauhofer A, Witte K, Lemmer B, Middeke M, Lorenz W, Celik I: Quality of life in animals as a new outcome for surgical research: G-CSF as a quality of life improving factor. *Eur.Surg Res.* 34:22-29, 2002.

[38] Bauhofer A, Witte K, Celik I, Pummer S, Lemmer B, Lorenz W: Sickness behavior, an animal equivalent to quality of life, is improved in septic rats by G-CSF and antibiotic prophylaxis. *Langenbeck's Arch.Surg.* 386:132-140, 2001.

[39] Gough A, Clapperton M, Rolando N, Foster AVM: Granulocyte-colony-stimulating factor in diabetic foot infection. *Lancet* 351:370, 1998.

[40] de Lalla F, Pellizzer G, Strazzabosco M, Martini Z, Du JG, Lora L, Fabris P, Benedetti P, Erle G: Randomized prospective controlled trial of recombinant granulocyte colony-stimulating factor as adjunctive therapy for limb-threatening diabetic foot infection. *Antimicrob.Agents Chemother.* 45:1094-1098, 2001.

[41] Yonem A, Cakir B, Guler S, Azal OO, Corakci A: Effects of granulocyte-colony stimulating factor in the treatment of diabetic foot infection. *Diabetes Obes.Metab* 3:332-337, 2001.

[42] Pajkrt D, Manten A, van der Poll T, Tiel van Buul MM, Jansen J, Wouter ten Cate J, Van Deventer SJ: Modulation of cytokine release and neutrophil function by granulocyte colony-stimulating factor during endotoxemia in humans. *Blood* 90:1415-1424, 1997.

[43] Frumkin LR: Role of granulocyte colony stimulating factor and granulocyte-macrophage colony-stimulating factor in the treatment of patients with HIV infection. *Curr.Opin.Hematol.* 4:200-206, 1997.

[44] Kuritzkes DR, Parenti D, Ward DJ, Rachlis A, Wong RJ, Mallon KP, Rich WJ, Jacobson MA: Filgrastim prevents severe neutropenia and reduces infective morbidity

in patients with advanced HIV infection: results of a randomized, multicenter, controlled trial. G-CSF 930101 Study Group. *AIDS* 12:65-74, 1998.

[45] Kuritzkes DR: Neutropenia, neutrophil dysfunction, and bacterial infection in patients with human immunodeficiency virus disease: the role of granulocyte colony-stimulating factor. *Clin.Infect.Dis.* 30:256-260, 2000.

[46] Weiss M, Gross-Weege W, Schneider M, Neidhardt H, Liebert S, Mirow N, Wernet P: Enhancement of neutrophil function by in vivo filgrastim treatment for prophylaxis of sepsis in surgical intensive care patients. *J.Crit.Care* 10:21-26, 1995.

[47] Weiss M, Gross-Weege W, Harms B, Schneider EM: Filgrastim (RHG-CSF) related modulation of the inflammatory response in patients at risk of sepsis or with sepsis. *Cytokine.* 8:260-265, 1996.

[48] Hartung T, von Aulock S, Schneider C, Faist E: How to leverage an endogenous immune defense mechanism: the example of granulocyte colony-stimulating factor. *Crit Care Med.* 31:S65-S75, 2003.

[49] Stephens DP, Fisher DA, Currie BJ: An audit of the use of granulocyte colony-stimulating factor in septic shock. *Intern.Med J* 32:143-148, 2002.

[50] Nelson S, Belknap SM, Carlson RW, Dale D, DeBoisblanc B, Farkas S, Fotheringham N, Ho H, Marrie T, Movahhed H, Root R, Wilson J: A randomized controlled trial of filgrastim as an adjunct to antibiotics for treatment of hospitalized patients with community- acquired pneumonia. CAP Study Group. *J.Infect.Dis.* 178:1075-1080, 1998.

[51] Nelson S, Heyder AM, Stone J, Bergeron MG, Daugherty S, Peterson G, Fotheringham N, Welch W, Milwee S, Root R: A randomized controlled trial of filgrastim for the treatment of hospitalized patients with multilobar pneumonia. *J Infect.Dis.* 182:970-973, 2000.

[52] Hartmann LC, Tschetter LK, Habermann TM, Ebbert LP, Johnson PS, Mailliard JA, Levitt R, Suman VJ, Witzig TE, Wieand HS, Miller LL, Moertel CG: Granulocyte colony-stimulating factor in severe chemotherapy- induced afebrile neutropenia. *N.Engl.J.Med.* 336:1776-1780, 1997.

[53] Bohlius J, Reiser M, Schwarzer G, Engert A: Impact of granulocyte colony-stimulating factor (CSF) and granulocyte-macrophage CSF in patients with malignant lymphoma: a systematic review. *Br.J.Haematol.* 122:413-423, 2003.

[54] Dudley HAF: Extracranial-intracranial bypass, one; clinical trials, nil. *Br.Med.J.* 294:1501-1502, 1998.

[55] Torossian A, Rühlmann S, Middeke M, Lorenz W, Wulf H, Bauhofer A: Deleterious effects of mild hypothermia in septic rats are ameliorated by granulocyte-colony stimulating factor. *Anesthesiology* (in press):2003.

[56] Hill AB: The philosophy of clinical trial, in Hill AB, Platt R (eds): *Statistical methods in clinical and preventive medicine*. Edinburg, Livingstone, pp 13, 1962.

[57] Turner JA, Deyo RA, Loeser JD, von Korff M, Fordyce WE: The importence of placebo effects in pain treatment and research. *JAMA* 271:1609-1614, 1994.

[58] Koller M, Lorenz W: Threats to double-blinding in sepsis trials: role of expectancies toward treatment outcome, in Faist E, Baue AE, Schildberg FW (eds): *The immune*

consequences of trauma, shock and sepsis - mechanisms and therapeutic approaches. Lengerich, Pabst Scienc Publishers, pp 640-645, 1996.

[59] Koller M, Lorenz W: Quality of life: a deconstruction for clinicians. *J.R.Soc.Med.* 95:481-488, 2002.

[60] Lorenz W, Koller M: Empirically-based concepts of outcome and quality of life in medicine, in Gimmler A, Lenk Ch, Aumüller G (eds): *Health and quality of life. Philosophical, medical and cultural aspects*. Münster, LIT-Verlag, pp 123-136, 2002.

[61] Koller M, Kussmann J, Lorenz W, Jenkins M, Voss M, Arens E, Richter E, Rothmund M: Symptom reporting in cancer patients - the role of negative affect and experienced social stigma. *Cancer* 77:983-995, 1996.

[62] McPeek B, Gasko M, Mosteller F: Measuring outcome from anesthesia and operation. *Theor.Surg.* 1:2-9, 1986.

[63] Bauhofer A, Menke H, Koller M, Sitter H, Torossian A, Nies C, Celik I, Lorenz W: Postoperative outcome assessed by the McPeek recovery score - validation in three trials. *Br.J.Surg.* (in press):2003.

[64] Troidl H, Wechsler AS, McKneally M: How to choose a relevant end point, in Troidl H, Spitzer WO, McPeek B, Mulder DS, McKneally MF, Wechsler AS (eds): *Basic principles and clinical practice*. ed.3rd. New York, Springer, pp 303-320, 1998.

[65] Encke A, Hanisch E, Sitter H, Greger B, Bauhofer A, Margolis C, Lorenz W: Models of evaluation in planning and standardization of surgical treatment: sepsis as an example. *Langenbecks Arch.Chir.* Suppl 2:323-329, 1997.

[66] Sitter H, Dietz W, Stinner B, Geks J, Bauhofer A, Celik I, Prünte H, Lorenz W: Klinische Leitlinien als Teil eines umfassenden Qualitätsmanagement (Clinical guidelines as part of a concept for total quality management). *Zentralbl.Chir.* 124:318-326, 1999.

[67] Matthews DE, Farewell VT: *Using and understanding medical statistics*, ed.3rd, Basel, S. Karger, 1996.

[68] Eidelman LA, Sprung CL: Why have new effective therapies for sepsis not developed? *Crit.Care Med.* 22:1330-1334, 1995.

[69] Solomkin JS, Fink MP: Very large-scale, randomized, clinical trials in sepsis and septic shock. *Crit.Care Med.* 22:1-2, 1994.

[70] Bernard GR: Sepsis trials - intersection of investigation, regulation, funding and practice. *Am.J.Respir.Crit.Care Med.* 152:4-10, 1995.

[71] Sibbald WJ, Vincent J-L: Round table conference on clinical trials for the treatment of sepsis. *Crit.Care Med.* 23:394-399, 1995.

[72] Fink MP: Another negative clinical trial of a new agent for the treatment of sepsis: rethinking the process of developing adjuvant treatments for serious infections. *Crit.Care Med.* 23:989-991, 1995.

[73] Reimund K-P, Lorenz W, Celik I, Bauhofer A, Greger B, Seitz R, Rothmund M: Management of leucopenic sepsis. *Lancet* 346:382-383, 1995.

[74] Wunderink RG, Leeper KV, Schein RMH, Nelson S, DeBoisblanc B, Backer B, Fotheringham N, Logan E: Clinical response to filgrastim (r-metHuG-CSF) in pneumonia with severe sepsis. *Am.J.Respir.Crit.Care Med.* 153:A123,1996.

[75] Menke H, John KD, Klein A, Lorenz W, Junginger T: Preoperative risk assessment with the ASA-score: a prospective trial for evaluation of mortality and morbidity in different ASA-classes of 2937 patients with general surgery. *Chirurg* 63:1029-1034, 1992.

[76] Lorenz W, Dick W, Junginger T, Ohmann C, Doenicke A, Rothmund M: Biomedical and clinimetric approaches in the cause assessment of perioperative risk: establishment of a German ASA-classification. *Langenbecks Arch.Chir.* 372:199-209, 1987.

[77] Pollock AV, Evans M: Writing a scientific paper, in Troidl H, McKneally MF, Mulder DS, Wechsler AS, McPeek B, Spitzer WO (eds): *Surgical research - Basic Principles and Clinical Practice*. ed.3rd. New York, Springer, pp 111-117, 1998.

[78] Rhode H, Heistermann S, Viehoff G: Systematic documentation of postoperative complications (Systematische Eerfassung postoperativer Komplikationen). *Chirurg* 60:49-54, 1989.

[79] Krack W, Nies C, Sitter H, Celik I, Kaufmann T, Kraus M, Lorenz W: Prediction of postoperative outcome from perioperative changes of mediators in cholecystectomy - an application of Bayes'Theorem. *Inflamm.Res.* 48 Suppl. 1:S49-S50, 1999.

[80] Celik I, Hoppe M, Lorenz W, Sitter H, Isahaque N, Jungraithmayr W, Kapp B, Schmiedel E, Klose KJ: Randomised study comparing a non-ionic with an ionic contrast medium in patients with malignancies: first answer with a new diagnostic approach. *Inflamm.Res.* 48,Suppl.1:S47-S48, 1999.

[81] Jones S, Schechter CB, Smith C, Rose DN: Is HIV infection a risk factor for complications of surgery? *Mt.Sinai J.Med.* 69:329-333, 2002.

[82] Cheung RC, Hsieh F, Wang Y, Pollard JB: The impact of hepatitis C status on postoperative outcome. *Anesth.Analg.* 97:550-4, table, 2003.

[83] Newman GW, Guarnaccia JR, Remold HG, Kazanjian PH, Jr.: Cytokines enhance neutrophils from human immunodeficiency virus- negative donors and AIDS patients to inhibit the growth of Mycobacterium avium in vitro. *J.Infect.Dis.* 175:891-900, 1997.

[84] Friedman LM, Furberg CD, DeMets DL: *Fundamentals of clinical trials*, ed.2nd, Littelton, Massachusetts, PSG publishing Company Inc., pp 1-302, 1985.

[85] Vose JM, Armitage JO: Clinical applications of hematopoetic growth factors. *J.Clin.Oncol.* 13:1023-1035, 1995.

[86] Miller JA, Beveridge RA: A comparison of efficacy of GM-CSF and G-CSF in the therapeutic setting of chemotherapy induced neutropenia. *Blood* 84 suppl. 1:78a, 1994.

[87] Smith WS, Sumnicht GE, Sharpe RW, Samuelson D, Millard FE: Granulocyte colony-stimulating factor versus placebo in addition to penicillin G in a randomized blinded study of gram-negative pneumonia sepsis: analysis of survival and multisystem organ failure. *Blood* 86:1301-1309, 1995.

[88] American Society of Clinical Oncology: Update of recommendations for the use of hematopoietic colony-stimulating factors. Evidence-based clinical practice guidelines. *J.Clin.Oncol.* 14:1957-1960, 1996.

[89] Grigg AP, Roberts AW, Raunow H, Houghton S, Layton JE, Boyd AW, McGrath KM, Mahr D: Optimizing dose and scheduling of Filgrastim (granulocyte colony-stimulating

factor) for mobilization and collection of peripheral blood progenitor cells in normal volunteers. *Blood* 86:4437-4445, 1998.

[90] Tanaka H, Kaneko T: Pharmacokinetics of recombinant human granulocyte colony-stimulating factor in the rat. *Drug Metabolism and Disposition* 19:200-204, 1991.

[91] Heard SO, Fink MP, Gamelli RL, Solomkin JS, Joshi M, Trask AL, Fabian TC, Hudson LD, Gerold KB, Logan ED: Effect of prophylactic administration of recombinant human granulocyte colony-stimulating factor (filgrastim) on the frequency of nosocomial infections in patients with acute traumatic brain injury or cerebral hemorrhage. The Filgrastim Study Group. *Crit.Care Med.* 26:748-754, 1998.

[92] Nelson S, Farkas S, Fotheringham N, Ho H, Marrie T, Movahhed H: Filgrastim in the treatment of hospitalized patients with community acquired pneumonia (CAP). *Am.J.Respir.Crit.Care Med.* 153:A536,1996.

[93] Gough A, Clapperton M, Rolando N, Foster AVM, Philpott-Howard J, Edmonds ME: Randomised placebo controlled trial of granulocyte colony-stimulating factor in diabetic foot infection. *Lancet* 350:855-859, 1997.

[94] Lord BI, Bronchud MH, Owens S, Chang J, Howell A, Souza L, Dexter TM: The kinetics of human granulopoiesis following treatment with granulocyte colony-stimulating factor in vivo. *Proc.Natl.Acad.Sci.USA* 86:9499-9503, 1989.

[95] Repp R, Valerius T, Sendler A, Gramatzki M, Iro H, Kalden JR, Platzer E: Neutrophils express the high affinity receptor for IgG (Fc gamma RI,CD64) after in vivo application of recombinant human granulocyte colony-stimulating factor. *Blood* 7:885-889, 1991.

[96] Valerius T, Repp R, de Wit TPM, Dexter TM, Platzer E, Kalden JR, Gramatzki M, van de Winkel JGJ: Involvement of the high-affinity receptor for IgG (Fc gamma RI; CD64) in enhanced tumor cell cytotoxicity of neutrophils during granulocyte colony-stimulating factor therapy. *Blood* 82:931-939, 1993.

[97] McKenna PJ, Nelson S, Andresen J: Filgrastim (rhuG-CSF) enhances ciprofloxacin uptake and bactericidal activity of human neutrophils in vitro. *Am.J.Respir.Crit.Care Med.* 153:A535,1996.

[98] Fink MP, O`Sullivan PO, Menconi MJ, Wollert SP, Wang H, Youssef ME, Bellelsls JM: Effect of granulocyte colony-stimulating factor on systemic and pulmonary responses to endotoxin. *J.Trauma* 34:571-578, 1993.

[99] Shimoda K, Okamura S, Inaba S, Okamura T, Ohga S, Ueda K, Niho Y: Granulocyte colony-stimulating factor and platelet aggregation. *Lancet* 341:633, 1993.

[100] Welte K, Grabrilove J, Bronchud MH, Platzer E, Morstyn G: Filgrastim (r-metHuG-CSF): the first 10 years. *Blood* 88:1907-1929, 1996.

[101] Wagner K, Koller M, Keil A, Trott D, Engenhart-Cabillic R, Pfab R, Lorenz W: Radiotherapy in surgical and nonsurgical patients: therapy related expectations, quality of life and physician ratings. *Chirurg* 69:252-258, 1998.

[102] Pocock SJ: Methods of randomization, in Pocock SJ (ed): *Clinical trials*. Chichester, Wiley & Sons Ltd., pp 79-80, 1983.

[103] Kingston RD, Walsh S, Robinson C, Jeacock J, Keeling F: Significant risk factors in elective colorectal surgery. *Ann.R.Coll.Surg.Engl.* 77:369-371, 1995.

[104] McLauchlan GJ, Anderson ID, Grant IS, Fearon KCH: Outcome of patients with abdominal sepsis treated in an intensive care unit. *Br.J.Surg.* 82:524-529, 1995.

[105] Bokey EL, Chapuis PH, Fung C, Hughes WJ, Koorey SG, Brewer D, Newland RC: Postoperative morbidity and mortality following resection of the colon and rectum for cancer. *Dis.Colon Rectum* 38:480-486, 1995.

[106] Hermanek P, Mansmann U, Staimmer DS, Riedl S, Hermanek P: The German experience: the surgeon as a prognostic factor in colon and rectal cancer surgery. *Surg.Oncol.Clin.N.Am.* 9:33-49, 2000.

[107] Knaus WA, Draper EA, Wagner DP, Zimmerman JE: APACHE II: a severity of disease classification system. *Crit Care Med.* 13:818-829, 1985.

[108] Knaus WA, Wagner DP, Harrell FE, Draper EA: What determines prognosis in sepsis? Evidence for a comprehensive individual patient risk assessment approach to the design and analysis of clinical trials. *Theor.Surg.* 9:20-27, 1994.

[109] Meakins JL: Surgeons, surgery and immunomodulation. *Arch.Surg.* 126:494-498, 1991.

[110] Christensen C, Cottrell JJ, Murakami J, Mackesy ME, Fetzer B, Elstein AS: Forecasting survival in the medical intensive care unit: a comparison of clinical prognoses with formal estimates. *Meth.Inform.Med.* 32:302-308, 1993.

[111] Shortell SM, Zimmerman JE, Rousseau DM, Gillies RR, Wagner DP, Draper EA, Knaus WA, Duffy J: The performance of intensive care units: does good management make a difference? *Med.Care* 32:508-525, 1994.

[112] Hays WL: The analysis of covariance, in Hays WL (ed): *Statistics*. ed.4th. Orlando, Holt, Rinehart and Winston Inc. The Dryden Press, Saunders College Publishing, pp 734-767, 1988.

[113] Kaptchuk TJ: Powerful placebo: the dark side of the randomised trial. *Lancet* 351:1722-1725, 1998.

[114] Lienert GA: *Distribution free methods in biostatistics II*, Meisenheim am Glan, Hain, pp 320-332 and 527-530, 1978.

[115] Lorenz W: Outcome: definition and methods of evaluation, in Troidl H, McKneally MF, Mulder DS, Wechsler AS, McPeek B, Spitzer WO (eds): *Surgical research: basic principals and clinical practice*. ed.3rd. New-York, Springer, pp 513-520, 1998.

[116] Bühl A, Zöfel P: *SPSS for windows, release 10*, ed.7, München, Addison-Wesley, pp 1-734, 2000.

[117] Rangel-Frausto MS, Pittet D, Costigan M, Hwang T, Davis CS, Wenzel RP: The natural history of the systemic inflammatory response syndrome (SIRS). A prospective study. *JAMA* 273:117-123, 1995.

[118] Zimmerman JE, Shortell SM, Rousseau DM, Duffy J, Gillies RR, Knaus WA, Devers K, Wagner DP, Draper EA: Improving intensive care: observations based on organizational case studies in nine intensive care units: a prospective, multicentre study. *Crit.Care Med.* 21:1443-1451, 1993.

[119] Deans G, Odling-Smee W, Parks GT, Roy DA: Auditing perioperative mortality. *Ann.Royal Coll.Surg.Engl* 69:185-187, 1998.

[120] Rosenberg J, Pedersen MH, Ramsing T, Kehlet H: Circadian variation in unexpected postoperative death. *Br.J.Surg.* 79:1300-1302, 1992.

[121] Mangano DT: Anesthetics, coronary artery disease and outcome: unresolved controversies. *Anesthesiology* 70:175-178, 1989.

[122] Mangano DT: Perioperative cardiac morbidity. *Anesthesiology* 72:153-184, 1990.

[123] Mangano DT, Browner WS, Hollenberg M, Li J, Tadeo IM, and the Study of Perioperative Ischemia (SIP) Research Group: Long-term cardiac prognosis following noncardiac surgery. *JAMA* 268:233-239, 1992.

[124] Mangano DT: Prospective risk assessment: many studies, few solutions. Is a cardiac risk assessment paradigm possible? *Anesthesiology* 83:897-901, 1995.

[125] Prause G, Ratzenhofer-Comenda B, Pierer G, Smolle-Jüttner F, Glanzer H, Smolle J: Can ASA grade or Goldman's cardiac risk index predict peri-operative mortality? A study of 16,227 patients. *Anaesthesia* 52:203-206, 1997.

[126] Howell SJ, Sear YM, Yeates D, Goldacre M, Sear JW, Foex P: Risk factors for cardiovascular death after elective surgery under general anaesthesia. *Br.J.Anaesth.* 80:14-19, 1998.

[127] Menke H, Klein A, Böttger Th, Bahr W, Junginger T: Pulmonale Komplikationen nach abdominalchirurgischen Eingriffen. Identifizierung unterschiedlicher Risikogruppen. (Pulmonary complications after abdominal surgical interventions. Identification of different risk groups). *Chirurg* 63:548-554, 1992.

[128] Dawes LG, Aprahamian C, Condon RE, Malangoni MA: The risk of infection after colon injury. *Surgery* 100:796-803, 1986.

[129] Bone RC: Immunological dissonance: a continuing evolution in our understanding of the systemic inflammatory response syndrome (SIRS) and the multiple organ dysfunction syndrome (MODS). *Annu.Internal Med.* 125:680-687, 1996.

[130] Jimenez MF, Watson WG, Parodo J, Evans D, Foster D, Steinberg M, Rotstein OD, Marshall JC: Dysregulated expression of neutrophil apoptosis in the systemic inflammatory response syndrome. *Arch.Surg.* 132:1263-1270, 1997.

[131] Williams JF, Zimmerman JE, Wagner DP, Hawkins M, Knaus WA: African-American and white patients admitted to the intensive care unit: is there a diffenence in the therapy and outcome? *Crit.Care Med.* 23:626-636, 1995.

[132] Bass EB, Steinberg EP, Pitt HA, Griffiths RI, Lillemoe KD, Saba GP, Jones C: Comparison of the rating scale and the standard gamble in measuring patient preferences for outcomes of gallstone disease. *Med.Decis.Making* 14:307-314, 1994.

[133] Menke H, Graf C, Lorenz W, Lang E, Junginger T: Einflußgrößen der postoperativen Wiederherstellung nach Kolon- und Rektumoperationen. (Parameters modulating the postoperative recovery after colon and rectum operations). *Acta Chir.Austriaca* 23:62-63, 1991.

[134] Camilleri-Brennan J, Steele RJC: Quality of life after treatment for rectal cancer. *Br.J.Surg.* 85:1036-1043, 1998.

[135] Aaronson NK, Ahmedzai S, Bergmann B, Bullinger M, Cull A, Duez NJ: The european organisation for research and tratment of cancer QLQ-C30: a quality of life insturment fore use in international clincal trialsin oncology. *J.Natl.Cancer Inst.* 85:356-376, 1993.

[136] Sprangers MA, Groenvold M, Bjordal K, Blazeby J, Aaronson NK: The European Organization for Research on Treatment of Cancer approach to developing

questionnaire modules. An update and overview. EORTC Quality of Life Study Group. *Qual.Life Res.* 7:291-300, 1998.

[137] Koller M, Lorenz W: Quality of life research in patients with rectal cancer: traditional approaches versus a problem-solving oriented perspective. *Langenbeck's Arch.Surg.* 383:427-436, 1998.

[138] Lorenz, W., Schulz, K.-D., Rothmund, M., Bastian, U., Kopp, I., and Koller, M.Report to the German Federal Ministry of Health: field study on supply of tumor patients with breast and rectal cancer under special consideration of quality of life pp 1-52, 1998.

[139] Troidl H: Lebensqualität: Ein relevanter Endpunkt in der Chirurgie (Quality of life: a relevant endpoint in surgery). *Chirurg* 60:445-449, 1989.

[140] Slevin ML, Plant H, Lynch D, Drinkwater J, Gregory WM: Who should measure quality of life, the doctor or the patient? *Br.J.Cancer* 57:109-112, 1988.

[141] Boorse C: Health as a theoretical concept. *Phil.Science* 44:542-573, 1977.

[142] Hare RM: Health. *J.Med.Ethics* 12:174-181, 1986.

[143] Koller M, Lorenz W, Wagner K, Keil A, Trott D, Engenhart-Cabillic R, Nies C: Expectations and quality of life of cancer patients undergoing radiotherapy. *J.R.Soc.Med.* 93:621-628, 2000.

[144] Koller M, Kussmann J, Lorenz W, Rothmund M: Die Erfassung und Dokumentation der Lebensqualität nach Tumortherpie (The registration and documentation of quality of life after cancer therapy), in Wagner G, Hermanek P (eds): *Organ specific tumor documentation.* Berlin, Heidelberg, Springer-Verlag, pp A2.1-A2.12, 1995.

[145] Pennebaker JW: *The psychology of physical symptoms*, New York, Springer-Verlag, pp 1-197, 1982.

[146] Lawton MP: Quality of life and affect in later life, in Magai C, Mc Fadden S (eds): *Handbook of emotion, adult development and aging.* Academic Press, pp 327-348, 1996.

[147] Cullen DJ, Civetta JM, Briggs BA, Ferrara L: Therapeutic Intervention Scoring System: a method for quantitative comparison of patient care. *Crit.Care Med.* 2:57-60, 1974.

[148] Keene AR, Cullen DJ: Therapeutic Intervention Scoring System: update 1983. *Crit.Care Med.* 11:1-3, 1983.

[149] Nies, C.Non-optimum results in recovery from biliary surgery: a result of interaction between strain of the neuroendocrine system, mast cell activation and modulation of the immune system Habilitation Thesis, Philipps-University, Marburg pp 1-179, 1997.

[150] Klag, J.*Conventional cholecystectomy in the higher age - alters the mediator histamine the outcome?* Thesis, Philipps-University, Marburg pp 1-101, 1994.

[151] Reis Miranda D, de Rijk A, Schaufelin W: Simplified Therapeutic Intervention Scoring System: the TISS-28 items - results from a multicenter study. *Crit.Care Med.* 24:64-73, 1996.

[152] Reis Miranda D, Moreno R, Iapichino G: Nine equivalents of nursing manpower use score (NEWS). *Intens.Care Med.* 23:760-765, 1997.

[153] Lefering R: Biostatistical aspects of outcome evaluation using TISS-28. *Eur.J.Surg.* 584 (suppl.):56-61, 1999.

[154] Feldman L, Barkun J, Barkun A, Samalis J, Rosenberg L: Measuring postoperative complications in general surgery patients using an outcomes-based strategy; comparison with complications presented at morbidity and mortality rounds. *Surgery* 122:711-720, 1997.

[155] Martin DK, McKneally MF: Qualitative research, in Troidl H, McKneally MF, Mulder DS, Wechsler AS, McPeek B, Spitzer WO (eds): *Surgical research. Basic principles and clinical practice*. ed.3rd. New York, Springer, pp 235-241, 1998.

[156] Denzin NK, Lincoln YS: *Handbook of qualitative research*, Thousend Oaks, Sage Publications, pp 1-643, 1994.

[157] West SG, Wicklund RA: *A primer of social psychological theories*, Monterey, Brooks/Cole, pp 6-331, 1980.

[158] Döcke WD, Randow F, Syrbe U, Krausch D, Asadullah K, Reinke P, Volk H-D, Kox W: Monocyte deactivation in septic patients: restoration by IFN-gamma treatment. *Nature Med.* 3:678-681, 1997.

[159] Nyström P-O: The systemic inflammatory response syndrome: definitions and aetiology. *J.Antimicrobial.Chemother.* 41:1-7, 1998.

[160] Lin RY, Astiz ME, Saxon JS, Saha DC, Rackow EC: Relationships between plasma cytokine concentrations and leukocyte functional antigen expression on patients with sepsis. *Crit.Care Med.* 22:1595-1602, 1994.

[161] Fairclough DL: Summary measures and statistics for comparison of quality of life in a clinical trial of cancer therapy. *Stat.Med.* 16:1197-1209, 1997.

[162] Rothmund M, Lorenz W: *Annual report 1996 and 1997 of the Clinic of General Surgery and the Institute of Theoretical Surgery*, Marburg, Clinic of the Philipps-University, 1997.

[163] Marcus R, Peritz E, Gabriel K: On closed testing procedures with special reference to ordered analysis of variance. *Biometrika* 63:655-660, 1976.

[164] Smith R: Where is the wisdom...? The poverty of medical evidence. *Br.Med.J.* 303:798-799, 1991.

[165] Feinstein AR: A bibliography of publications on observer variability. *J.Chronic.Dis.* 38:619-632, 1985.

[166] Chassin MR, Brook RH, Park RE, Keesey J, Fink A, Kosecoff J, Kahn K, Merrick N, Solomon DH: Variations in the use of medical and surgical services by the Medicare population. *N.Engl.J.Med.* 314:285-290, 1986.

[167] Jenkins D: Investigations: how to get from guidelines to protocols. *BMJ* 303:323-324, 1991.

[168] Grimshaw JM, Russell IT: Effect of clinical guidelines on medical practice: a systematic review of rigorous evaluations. *Lancet* 342:1317-1321, 1993.

[169] Delbecq AL, van de Ven C: A group process model for problem identification and program planning. *J.Appl.Biol.Behav.Sci-* 7:466-492, 1971.

[170] Margolis CZ, Society for mdeical decision making committee on standardization of clinical algorithms: Proposal for clinical algorithm standards. *Med.Dec.Making* 12:149-154, 1992.

[171] Margolis C, Cretin S: *Implementing clinical practice guidelines*, Chicago, AHA press, pp 1-223, 1999.

[172] US Preventive Service Task Force.: Guide to clinical preventive services., in Margolis C, Cretin S (eds): *Implementing clinical practice guidelines*. pp 1-123, 1998.

[173] Docherty JG, McGregor JR, Akyol AM, Murray GD, Galloway DJ: Comparison of manually constructed and stapled anastomoses in colorectal surgery. West of Scotland and Highland Anastomosis Study Group. *Ann.Surg.* 221:176-184, 1995.

[174] Kale TI, Kuzu MA, Tekeli A, Tanik A, Aksoy M, Cete M: Aggressive bowel preparation does not enhance bacterial translocation, provided the mucosal barrier is not disrupted: a prospective, randomized study. *Dis.Colon Rectum* 41:636-641, 1998.

[175] Burke P, Mealy K, Gillen P, Joyce W, Traynor O, Hyland J: Requirement for bowel preparation in colorectal surgery. *Br.J.Surg.* 81:907-910, 1994.

[176] Merad F, Hay JM, Fingerhut A, Flamant Y, Molkhou JM, Laborde Y: Omentoplasty in the prevention of anastomotic leakage after colonic or rectal resection: a prospective randomized study in 712 patients. French Associations for Surgical Research. *Ann.Surg.* 227:179-186, 1998.

[177] Sagar PM, Hartley MN, Macfie J, Mancey-Jones B, Sedman P, May J: Randomized trial of pelvic drainage after rectal resection. *Dis.Colon Rectum* 38:254-258, 1995.

[178] Merad F, Yahchouchi E, Hay JM, Fingerhut A, Laborde Y, Langlois-Zantain O: Prophylactic abdominal drainage after elective colonic resection and suprapromontory anastomosis: a multicenter study controlled by randomization. French Associations for Surgical Research. *Arch.Surg.* 133:309-314, 1998.

[179] Pilz G, Fateh-Moghadam S, Viell B, Bujdoso O, Döring G, Marget W, Neumann R, Werdan K: Supplemental immunoglobulin therapy in sepsis and septic shock - comparison of mortality under treatment with polyvalent i.v. immunoglobulin versus placebo. *Theor.Surg.* 8:61-83, 1993.

[180] Chalmers I, Altman DG: How can medical journals help prevent poor medical research? Some opportunities presented by electronic publishing. *Lancet* 353:490-493, 1999.

[181] Lorenz W: Bias in reporting of trials. *Lancet* 353:1277, 1999.

[182] Warren BL, Eid A, Singer P, Pillay SS, Carl P, Novak I, Chalupa P, Atherstone A, Penzes I, Kubler A, Knaub S, Keinecke HO, Heinrichs H, Schindel F, Juers M, Bone RC, Opal SM: Caring for the critically ill patient. High-dose antithrombin III in severe sepsis: a randomized controlled trial. *JAMA* 286:1869-1878, 2001.

[183] Bernard GR, Vincent JL, Laterre PF, LaRosa SP, Dhainaut JF, Lopez-Rodriguez A, Steingrub JS, Garber GE, Helterbrand JD, Ely EW, Fisher CJJr: Efficacy and safety of recombinant human activated protein C for severe sepsis. *N.Engl.J.Med* 344:699-709, 2001.

[184] Bone RC: Why sepsis trials fail. *JAMA* 276:565-566, 1996.

[185] Baumgartner J-D, Glauser MP, McCutchan JA, Ziegler EJ, van Melle G, Klauber MR, Vogt M, Muehlen E, Luethy R, Chiolero R, Geroulanos S: Prevention of Gram-negative shock and death in surgical patients by antibody to endotoxin core glycolipid. *Lancet* 13 July:59-63, 1985.

In: Focus on Colorectal Cancer Research
Editor: Julia D. Martinez, pp. 287-322

ISBN #1-59454-101-9

Chapter XI

HEREDITARY COLORECTAL CANCER

Piercarlo Saletti
Division of Oncology, Institute of Oncology of Southern Switzerland,
Ospedale S Giovanni, 6500 Bellinzona, Switzerland
E-mail: pcsaletti@bluewin.ch

ABSTRACT

Cancer is a genetic disease. Most cancer-causing mutations are somatic, occurring in the affected tissue during the course of carcinogenesis. However, most cancers also have an hereditary component that is caused by predisposing mutations that affect the germline, are heritable and contribute to the initiation of carcinogenesis. Colorectal cancer is probably the condition for which the most is known about the genes affected by cancer-causing mutations, their normal functions and their carcinogenic effects when mutated. Hereditary colorectal cancer syndromes are classified according to the presence of unusually large number of adenomatous or hamartomatous polyps. The polyposis syndromes include Familial Adenomatous Polyposis and its variants. The hamartomatous polyposis syndromes include juvenile polyposis, Peutz-Jeghers syndrome, and Cowden syndrome. More common than any of the polyposis syndromes is the Hereditary Non-Polyposis Colorectal Cancer.

This chapter addresses the molecular basis of these syndromes with particular emphasis to the recent advances in this rapidly progressive field and the applications of such knowledge in developing new diagnostic, preventive and therapeutic strategies.

INTRODUCTION

Colorectal cancer (CRC) represents the third most common cause of malignant death in developed countries after lung and breast cancer for women, and after lung and prostate cancer for men in the US [1].The incidence of disease varies widely between countries. The incidence is highest in Australia, New Zealand, North America, Western Europe and Japan, where it approximates or exceeds 40 cases per 100,000 males and about 30 cases per 100,000 females [2]. The risk of CRC increases with age, with an approximate doubling of the incidence for each decade from 40 to 80 years. About 90% of colonic tumours are diagnosed after the 5th decade, and 60% of them are located in the distal colon [3,4].

CRC is one of the human cancers which most clusters in families, even when inherited syndromes are excluded. Immediate relatives of individuals with CRC have an approximate two-fold increased risk of developing large bowel neoplasms and adenomatous polyps compared to average-risk population. CRC risk is three-fold or even higher if two or more first-degree relatives have CRC or a single first-degree relative with CRC is diagnosed before 5th decade. A second-degree relative (grandparent, aunt or uncle) with intestinal cancer increases a person's risk by 50%. The average age of CRC increases the person's risk by about 50%, and the average age of CRC in relatives is about 10 years less than in average risk individuals [5-9]. A recent study on twin individuals estimated that 34% of all CRC are related to predisposing genetic factors [10]. A small percentage of cases of CRC diagnosed each year are accounted for by rare inherited CRC syndromes, as less than 10% of CRC neoplasms arise from hereditary major susceptibility genes. Inherited syndromes (Table 1) include those in which colonic polyps are a major manifestation of disease (subdivised into familial adenomatous polyposis and the hamartomatous polyposis syndromes) and those in which they are not (Hereditary Non-Polyposis Colorectal Cancer, HNPCC).

Table 1: Conditions associated with gastrointestinal polyps

Syndrome	Genes
Adenomatous polyposis syndromes	
Familial adenomatous polyposis	*APC* (chrom 5q21), *MYH*
Attenuated adenomatous polyposis	
Gardner syndrome	
Turcot syndrome	
Hamartomatous syndromes	
Peutz-Jeghers syndrome	*STK11* (chrom. 19p)
Familial juvenile polyposis	*SMAD4* (chrom 18q), *PTEN* (chrom 10), *BMPRIA*
Cowden's syndrome	*PTEN* (chrom 10q)
Bannayan-Ruvalcaba-Riley syndrome	*PTEN*
Cronkhite-Canada syndrome	
Gorlin's syndrome	*PTCH* (chrom. 9q)
McCune-Albright syndrome	*Gs proteins*
Familial hyperplastic polyposis	
Hereditary Non-Polyposis Colorectal Cancer	*hMSH2, hMLH1, hMSH6, hMSH3, hPMS1, hPMS2*
Muir-Torre syndrome	
Turcot syndrome	

This chapter deals with the genetic aspects of CRC. The first part summarizes the clinical features of the well-recognized polyposis syndromes, and the related aspects of management.

The second part is devoted to the molecular/genetic aspects of cancer susceptibility and their use in clinical practice, with special emphasis on HNPCC.

PART 1. POLYPOSIS SYNDROMES

Familial Adenomatous Polyposis (FAP)

Clinico-Pathological Features

FAP is an autosomal dominantly inherited syndrome, which was first described in detail by Bussey in 1975 at London St Mark's Registry. The penetrance of mutation typically approaches 100%, although in Ashkenazi Jews it is approximately 10% to 20% as a consequence of the I1307K *APC* polymorphism [11, 12]. FAP is responsible for less than 1% of all CRCs [13], and its prevalence is about 1 in 8,000-10,000. This condition is defined by evidence of more than 100 adenomas, which are in practice counted through an endoscope. Because adenomas are generally less than 1 cm, it is likely that colonoscopy can understimate the number of polyps present. This means that if 50 or even fewer polyps are seen, the individual may still have FAP. Consequently, affected individuals develop from hundreds to thousands of colorectal adenomas by the age of 40 [14] (Fig 1). Adenomas are uniformly distributed in any part of the colon, mostly of tubular histologic appearance; villous adenomas have been reported, although rare. In addition, biopsies of flat mucosa may also show adenomatous changes. In certain patients, the colonic polyp phenotype is greatly reduced, adenomas are predominantly or exclusively located in the right colon and occur later than in classical FAP. This variant is called attenuated FAP (AFAP) [15]. In FAP, adenomas are so numerous that CRC is virtually inevitable. In the absence of prophylactic colectomy, death from CRC occurs in all of patients by age 50, with the majority of individuals affected by colonic malignancy within the 4th decade [16].

Malignant and Non-Malignant Extracolonic Manifestations

Classical FAP is associated with several extracolonic manifestations. Adenomas frequently involve the small bowel, particularly the duodenum, and the region of the ampulla of Vater is the predilection site [17]. The prevalence of duodenal adenomas varies from 50% to 90%, and the risk of small intestine cancer ranges from 4% to 12% [18]. Thus, periampullary adenocarcinoma represents the second most common neoplasm in FAP. A recent report suggests that AFAP should also be included in the differential diagnosis of patients with ampullary/duodenal tumours [19]. Gastric polyps are common findings in FAP. Most of them are fundic gland polyps, traditionally thought not to carry malignant potential, although it is controversial [20]. Gastric adenomas may also occur in FAP, and they are considered as precursors of gastric cancer, although the risk of gastric cancer is not markedly increased in most studies involving FAP families. Additional malignancies such as sarcomas, hepatoblastoma, pancreatic carcinoma, medulloblastomas (as in the Turcot's syndrome) and papillary thyroid carcinoma may also develop, although less frequent [21].

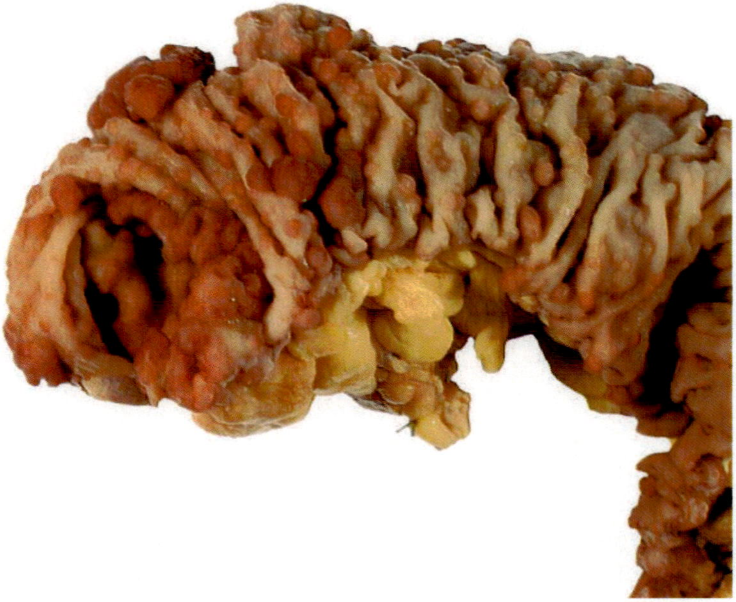

Fig 1. Colon resection specimen from a patient with Familial Adenomatous Polyposis. The mucosa is carpeted with multiple adenomas.

Desmoid tumours are slow-growing tumours that consist of proliferations of well-differentiated fibroblasts, and they occur predominantly in the small bowel, mesentery, peritoneum or abdominal wall (Fig 2). Although distant metastases are absent, desmoids are locally aggressive and grow into neighbouring structures. The prevalence of desmoid tumours in patients with FAP is about 10% [22]. The lifetime risk of developing desmoid tumours is about 20%. In FAP, most tumours are intra-abdominal or located in the abdominal wall. Next to colorectal cancer, desmoid tumours are the most frequent cause of death in FAP. Risk factors for the development of desmoid tumours are previous surgical procedures [23], pregnancy, female sex (> 70% in women aged 20 to 40), and a family history of desmoid tumours. Other benign conditions are related to FAP, such as osteoma, fibroma, diffuse fibrose of the mesentery, exostosis, odontoma and other dental abnormalities. The association of florid adenomatous polyposis, desmoids, multiple osteomas, skin tumours and epidermoid cysts is connected to Gardner's syndrome [24].

Congenital hypertrophy of the retinal pigment epithelium (CHRPE) is the most frequent extraintestinal manifestation of FAP. Present in about 80% of families with FAP, CHRPE is a highly reliable and early marker of the disease, and ophtalmoscopic examination represents a simple, non-invasive, unexpensive tool to allow early detection of gene carriers. Studies over the past years have addressed the histologic characteristics of the pigmented fundus lesions and the definition of universal criteria. Features usually consist of variable large (from 0.1 to greater than 1.0 optic disk diameter), darkly pigmented, ovalar lesions, with surrounding halo. Most FAP patients have four or more CHRPE areas, often bilateral [25]. CHRPE is regarded as a benign non-progressive condition, however recently a case of adenocarcinoma apparently arising from retinal pigment epithelium has been reported [26].

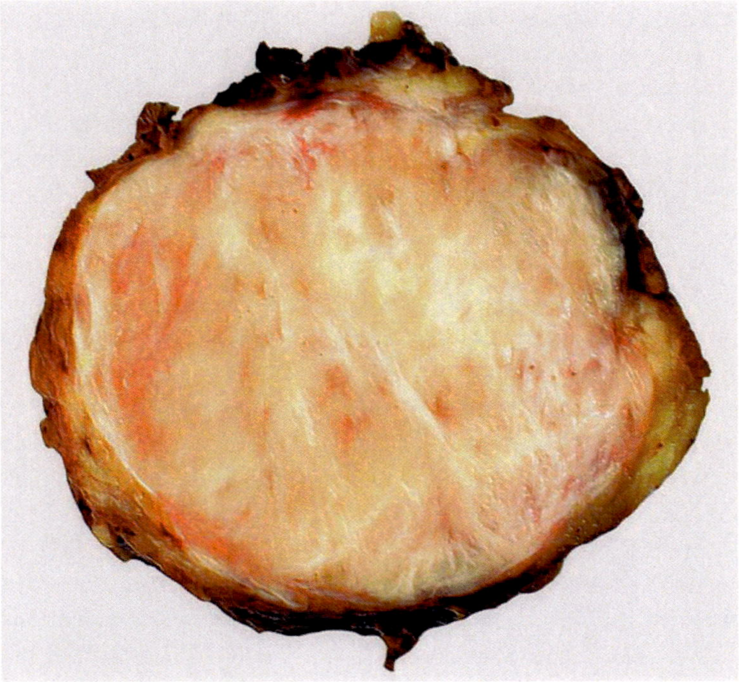

Fig 2. Ten centimeters, well circumscribed mesenteric desmoid (a).

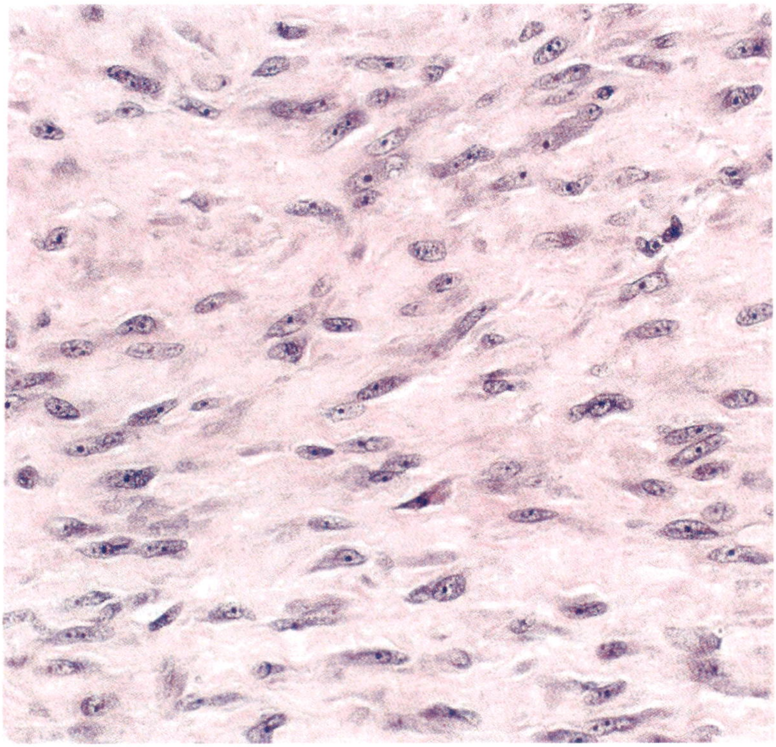

Fig 2. Microscopically, desmoids are composed of fibroblastic cells in a collagenous stroma (b).

From Genetics to Genotype-Phenotype Correlations

Germline mutations in the *APC* (*A*denomatous *P*olyposis *C*oli) gene is the initiating event for the development of FAP. This large gene is located on chromosome 5q21 [27-30], and consists of 15 exons, of which exon 15 is the largest (6.5 kb). The *APC* gene acts as a tumour suppressor gene, which mediates growth regulation signals between the cadherin-catenin complex, that is active in cell adhesion, and cytoskeletal tubules [31]. The observation that the large majority of mutations in the *APC* gene result in a truncated protein allowed for the development of an *in vitro* synthesis protein assay (protein truncation test), which is a sensitive method for detecting these truncated gene products from patient blood samples. Using these methods, mutations of *APC* gene could be identified in up to 80% of families [32,33].

The position of the mutation along the *APC* gene has been correlated with the disease phenotype. Chain-terminating mutations located within the first six exons are usually associated with milder forms of the disease, including AFAP; a similar mild clinical course is related to mutations of the *APC* gene both at the 5' end or in the 3' half, or in case of mutations at codon 1597 [34,35]. On the other hand, patients with codon 1309 deletion or mutations at codon 1323, 1407, and 233 are associated with large numbers of polyps or earlier diagnosis of FAP [36,37]. CHRPE has been found to be dependent on the position of the mutation in the *APC* gene. Originally it was thought that CHRPE did not occur in association with FAP if the germline mutation occurred before exon 9 [38,39]. Additional evidence indicates that there is a 3' boundary occurring after codon 1444 [40,41]. Individuals with *APC* mutation beyond codon 1444 have been found to carry a 12-fold increased risk of developing desmoids, compared with patients in which the mutation is located upstream. There is in addition a 17-fold higher risk of developing desmoids if the mutation is located beyond codon 1309, compared with mutations upstream of codon 452 [23]. In a very recent publication, the cumulative frequency of extracolonic manifestations was highest for mutations between codons 976 and 1067 [42]. Recently, biallelic germ-line *MYH* mutations have been demonstrated in approximately 8% of patients with classical adenomatous polyposis and no *APC* mutation [43].

In conclusion, consistent relationships between genotype and phenotype have been established for the clinical course of the disease and for some extracolonic manifestations. However, these correlations are not clear-cut, since there are considerable intrafamilial variations [44] that may be explained by the possible influence of modifier genes [45]. Consequently, the clinical manifestations of FAP and the prognosis in a given individual gene carrier cannot be predicted based on the knowledge of the germline mutation alone.

Managament of Patients

If FAP is left untreated, the lifetime risk of developing CRC is virtually 100%. Consequently, once the diagnosis is established, the proband and the relatives should be referred to genetic counselling in order to discuss in depth the indications for genetic testing, which will have an impact on clinical management of at risk individuals, but also raise ethical, legal and psychosocial issues. If the mutation can be identified in an individual, non-affected members should undergo presymptomatic testing. Family members proven not to be mutation carriers can be discharged from mental distress and the economical burden of annual surveillance.

Since the risk of developing CRC is irrespective of adenoma density, patients with FAP should be offered total colectomy with ileorectal anastomosis or proctocolectomy with restorative ileoanal anastomosis once colonic polyps have developed [46], especially if larger than 5 mm or showing villous or high-grade dysplasia features. If rectum sparing surgery is performed, endoscopic lifelong surveillance of the rectal stump is recommended every 6 to 12 months to remove any adenomas [47], as there is a 3.5% risk of CRC in it after 5 years, rising to 10% at 10 years. Such prophylactic screening and surgery have been demonstrated to significantly improve survival of FAP patients [48]. Upper endoscopy is also needed, since upper GI cancers develop in 5% of patients, with an estimated prevalence of duodenal dysplasia of up to 90%. Upper endoscopy, including duodenoscopy and biopsy of the ampulla of Vater, should be performed by the age 25 [49], and subsequent exams should be repeated depending upon the severity of polyp burden, empirically every 1 to 3 years. If adenomas are encountered, they should be biopsied and, if possible, removed. If adenomas are not endoscopically manageable, surgical resection is indicated.

Screening of at-risk relatives usually begins by the age of 10-12 years with annual flexible sigmoidoscopy, although it should be emphasized that colonic adenomas can be detected in very young children [50]. Once adenomas are identified, with or without a verified *APC* mutation, annual colonoscopy is required [51]. As the disease advances, which is often the case in the late 10s and early 20s, too many adenomas may be present for adequate and safe colonoscopic polypectomy, consequently prophylactic subtotal colectomy followed by annual surveillance endoscopy of the remaining rectum should be offered. On the other hand, in the absence of positive findings, sigmoidoscopy should be continued at least until the fourth decade, although very variable age of onset has been reported, even beyond this age [52]. If AFAP is suspected, complete colonoscopy should be preferred as adenomas develop predominantly in the right colon. Ophthalmoscopic examination and DNA testing can contribute to the definition of risk in relatives with negative bowel examinations. Thus, family members with negative mutation analysis may be reassured and discharged from intensive surveillance. In contrast, in individuals with positive phenotype and negative mutation analysis FAP cannot be excluded, and test should be considered as non-informative.

Chemoprevention aims either to block the initiation of tumorigenic process or to arrest or reverse the progression of premalignant cells to cancer. In FAP, two early positive studies investigated the activity of ascorbic acid with or without vitamin E and fiber [53,54], whereas no benefit was noted using calcium supplementation [55]. An attractive approach is the prophylactic use of non steroidal anti-inflammatory drugs such as sulindac and celecoxib, although results of published trials are conflicting. FAP patients experienced approximately 30% reduction of colorectal adenomas when treated with celecoxib 400 mg twice a day for six months [56]. A recent trial showed standard doses of sulindac can not prevent the development of adenomas/cancer in FAP patients [57]. An additional study shows that a statistically significant reduction of polyp burden occured after six months of treatment with sulindac 200 mg daily. However, polyp burden increased in median after approximately 49 months, and no benefit was observed in terms of inhibition of progression of adenomas to carcinoma [58]. Interestingly, a recent study showed a significant reduction in duodenal polyposis after six months of treatment with celecoxib 400 mg twice daily [59].

In conclusion, chemopreventive agents do not replace the need for prophylactic surgery and cannot be recommended for primary treatment of FAP, even if they might induce adenoma regression. These medications are consequently still an investigational approach, although they may delay surgical procedures or prevent the need for a re-intervention in patients who undergo sparing rectum surgery.

Inherited Hamartoma Polyposis Syndromes

The other category of hereditary polyposis conditions are the hamartomatous syndromes, characterized by hamartomatous polyps constituted of normal elements indigenous to the site in which polyps arise. These syndromes are much rarer than other CRC predispositions, and do not confer as high a risk for CRC as the polyposis syndromes. Phenotype distinctions between various entities is often not easy, as many clinical features are common in several hamartoma syndromes. Nevertheless, the exact classification of these syndromes is important since cancer risk may vary among them, and progress in molecular genetic evaluation play a role for this purpose. Peutz-Jeghers syndrome (PJS) and familial juvenile polyposis (FJP) represent the two major entities associated with hamartomatous polyps. Because both syndromes are rare, there are no reliable estimates of their frequency, which probably approximates to 1 in 100000 births.

Peutz-Jeghers Syndrome

The syndrome, which is transmitted in an autosomal dominant fashion with high penetrance, is characterized by the presence of diffuse hamartomatous polyps of the gastrointestinal tract and pigmented macules, often seen from birth or early age, involving buccal mucosa, lips and digits but frequently fading during adulthood. Polyps occur at very young age, and most patients experienced symptoms (bleeding and obstruction often due to intussusception) before age 20. Polyps are typically benign and most commonly located in jejunum and ileum, although stomach and colon are frequently involved (40% of cases) [60], and their size can vary from a few millimetres to "giant" polyps. A histologic feature of PJS polyps is an arborizing pattern of smooth muscle supporting normal lamina propria and glands (Fig 3). Affected patients carry a very high cumulative risk of developing gastrointestinal cancers (colorectal 39%, pancreas 36%, stomach 29%, small bowel 13% and oesophagus < 1%) and other cancers, such as breast (54%), ovary (21%), uterus (19%), lung (15%) and testis (9%) [61].

Due to the rarity of syndrome, the efficacy of intensive surveillance remains unproven. Nonetheless the increased risk of CRC makes large bowel surveillance reasonable, and colonoscopy is recommended at three year intervals starting from age 15. When encountered, polyps should be removed by endoscopy or laparotomy, especially if greater than 1 cm. Upper endoscopy is also reasonable starting from age 20 at three year intervals in view of the age of distribution of published cases of gastroduodenal cancers [62]. Some authors recommend surveillance for extraintestinal malignancies including yearly mammography, gynaecological evaluation and pelvic ultrasound, and three-yearly cervical smears starting age 20-25 [63]. Early testicular ultrasound screening is also recommended because of the risk of testicular cancer of Sertoli cell type, especially if a feminizing phenotype develops.

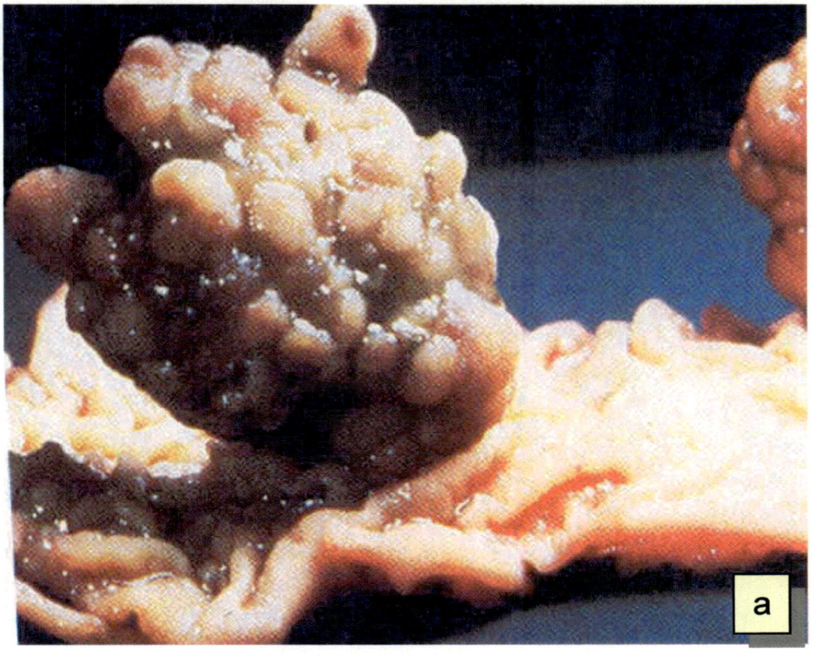

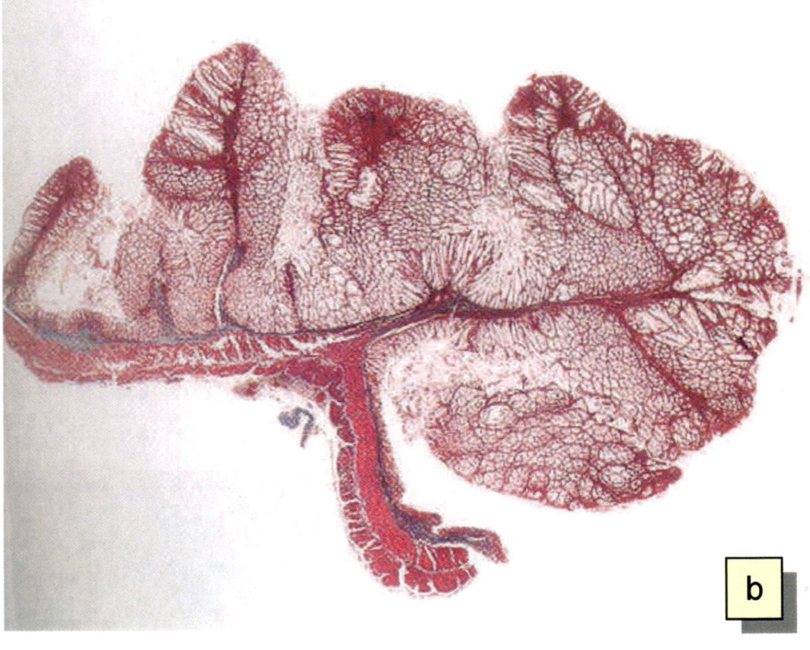

Fig 3. Macroscopic appearance of a Peutz-Jeghers polyp (a). Microscopic features include atypical branching of the muscularis separating and surrounding islands of variable size glands lined by normal colonic epithelium (b).

Germline mutation of the tumour suppressor gene *STK11* (or *LBK1*), which encodes a serine threonine kinase involved in transduction signals, have been found to cause 40% cases of PJS [64,65]. However, significant genetic heterogeneity has been shown in PJS, suggesting that other loci may be involved in the molecular basis of the syndrome [66].

Familial Juvenile Polyposis

Individuals with familial juvenile polyposis (FJP) usually present few to several hundred hamartomatous polyps mostly located in the colon and rectum, nonetheless they may be also encountered in stomach and small bowel. Some of these polyps may co-exist with some adenomatous polyps [67]. Polyps typically have round contours and a smooth surface, are more often pedunculated, and vary from a few millimeters to several centimetres. Histologically hamartomatous polyps are characterized by dilated glands in an abundant stroma, although dysplastic and adenomatous transformation has been observed [68]. Affected individuals will continue to form polyps throughout their life and carry an increased risk for CRC and other digestive tumours arising in duodenum, stomach and pancreas. One study reported that 38% of patients develop CRC, whereas extracolonic cancers have been found in approximately 20% of individuals [69]. In an additional study only 18 of 87 affected patients developed CRC, on average diagnosed in the third decade [67].

FJP is rare and consequently evidence based management is limited. However, in asymptomatic children from affected families, entire large bowel surveillance is generally recommended from early teen years at intervals of one to two years and, when found, polyps should be removed. Since polyps recur throughout lifetime, durable surveillance is indicated in proven gene carriers or affected individuals. In case of multiple polyps, especially if dysplastic or adenomatous, prophylactic colectomy should be offered. Due to the additional risk of digestive malignancies, upper endoscopy with small bowel contrast X-rays seem to be reasonable at one to two year intervals starting from age 20-25, although there is no data to support this approach.

FJP is an autosomal dominant condition, in which 50% of mutations have been found in *SMAD4*, a tumour suppressor gene located on chromosome 18q [70]. Much rarer, mutations have also been described in the *PTEN* gene, and this seems to correlate with an increased risk of thyroid and breast cancer [71]. Finally, germline mutations in the bone morphogenetic protein receptor *BMPR1A* are thought to cause a minority of cases of FJP [72].

It should be stressed that isolated juvenile type intestinal polyps can occur in about 1-2% of children, however this does not seem to be associated with an excess of cancer risk.

Part 2. Clinical Correlations and Genetics: The Hereditary Non-Polyposis Colorectal Cancer as a Model of Application

Clinical Features

HNPCC (Lynch syndrome) is inherited in an autosomal dominant fashion. It is characterized by development of CRCs at an early age (median age 46 years), an excess of synchronous and metachronous tumours, and a predominance (approximately 70%) of cancers proximal to the splenic flexure [73-75]. In gene carriers, the lifetime risk of developing CRC approaches 80% [76]. Affected individuals have an increased risk of developing carcinomas at other sites, including the endometrium, stomach (particularly in Asian countries), pancreas, biliary tract, small intestine, urothelium and ovary [77,78].

In female gene carriers, the cumulative risk of endometrial cancer is 42% by age 70 versus 3% in the general population, and is in fact greater than the risk of CRC (30%) [73,79-81]. Lung, hematopoetic and breast cancers appear to be less common in HNPCC [73,79,82]. One study reported that the relative risk of cancer for women is significantly greater than for men, specifically for cancers of the stomach, pancreas and lung [83]. This observation has not been confirmed in subsequent reports [73,84,85].

Patients with Muir-Torre syndrome, a variant of HNPCC, also develop adenomas and carcinomas of the sebaceous glands, basal cell carcinoma and multiple keratoacanthomas of the skin [86]. Some cases of Turcot's syndrome, which is characterized by an excess of central nervous system cancers (glioblastoma multiforme) are also thought to represent a variant of HNPCC.

Clinical Diagnostic Criteria

The Amsterdam criteria were established by the International Collaborative Group for HNPCC (ICG-HNPCC) to identify likely gene carriers for research purposes at the time when the genetic cause of HNPCC was unknown. The Amsterdam criteria are as follows: 1) histologically verified CRC in three or more relatives, one of whom is a first-degree relative of the other two, 2) CRC involving at least two successive generations, and 3) one or more CRC cases diagnosed before age 50. All the criteria must be met, and for all FAP should be excluded [87]. Epidemiologic studies have demonstrated that approximately 1% to 5% of all colorectal malignancies satisfy these strict criteria for defining HNPCC [88-92].

The Amsterdam criteria were never intended to be a clinical definition, and their weaknesses in a clinical setting have been identified: 1) the importance of familial lifestyle/environmental factors inducing chance of familial aggregations for a frequent tumour such as bowel cancer; 2) the failure to consider family size in pedigree assessment (the relative probability of diagnosis increases by about 25% with each additional first-degree relative) [93]; 3) the often insufficient documentation of disease and cause of death prevents identification of individuals satisfying the criteria; and 4) the failure to recognise the contribution of endometrial [94] and other extracolonic cancers to the HNPCC diagnosis.

Since a large number of individuals who may still have HNPCC do not fullfil the Amsterdam criteria, less stringent clinical scenarios have been promulgated including other associated HNPCC-cancers as proposed in Amsterdam II criteria [95] (Table 2). Other diagnostic criteria such as the Bethesda guidelines (Table 3) were established with the aim of identifying individuals with CRC on whom MSI testing should be considered, based on clinical and pathological features [96].

Table 2: Amsterdam criteria I and II

Amsterdam I

At least three relatives with CRC, all the following criteria should be present:

- one should be a first-degree relative of the other two
- at least two successive generations should be affected
- at least one CRC should be diagnosed before the age of 50
- FAP must be excluded

Amsterdam II

At least three relatives with an HNPCC-associated cancer (CRC, endometrium, small bowel, ureter, or renal pelvis):

- one should be a first-degree relative of the other two
- at least two successive generations should be affected
- at least one of cancer of the HNPCC spectrum should be diagnosed before the age of 50
- FAP should be excluded

Table 3: Bethesda guidelines for HNPCC*

- individuals with cancer in families that meet the Amsterdam criteria
- individuals with two HNPCC-related cancers, including
  - synchronous and metachronous CRC or
  - associated extracolonic cancers (endometrial, ovarian, gastric,
  - hepato-biliary, small intestinal, renal pelvis and ureteral)
- individuals with CRC and a first-degree relative with CRC and/or HNPCC-related extracolonic cancer and/or a colorectal adenoma, in which one of the cancers was diagnosed at age < 45, and the adenoma was diagnosed at age < 40
- individuals with CRC or endometrial cancer diagnosed at age < 45
- individuals with right-sided CRC with an undifferentiated pattern (solid/cribriform, defined as poorly differentiated or undifferentiated carcinoma composed of irregular, solid sheets of large eosinophilic cells and containing small gland-like spaces; medullary carcinoma) on histopathology diagnosed at age < 45
- individuals with signet ring cell-type CRC (composed of > 50% signet ring cells) diagnosed at age < 45
- individuals with adenomas diagnosed at age < 40

* Meeting all features listed under any numbered criteria is sufficient

Pathological Features

Typical features of CRC in HNPCC include diploidy, an excess of extracellular mucin, heavy lymphoid infiltration, a large number of signet cells, and poor differentiation with areas of necrosis [82,97-99]. Despite the presence of these pathological features, patients with HNPCC tumours of the bowel seem to have a better prognosis than sporadic CRC of a similar stage [100,101]. This may be due to the high mutation load in these tumours, resulting from the defective MMR system, which may be disadvantageous for tumour survival [102]. Moreover, cancers with high mutational activity may trigger a stronger localised antitumour immune response [103-105]. Finally, the predominant diploid status correlates with lower biological aggressiveness and represents an independent prognostic variable [100,106].

Adenoma: Precursor of Malignancy in HNPCC

In the general population there is evidence that CRCs arise from adenomatous polyps, with a transition time on average of 10 years [107]. The term dysplasia-carcinoma sequence is probably more accurate than the adenoma-carcinoma sequence, as cells may acquire genetic mutations necessary for malignant transformation prior to the development of a detectable adenoma. Aberrant crypt foci, particularly if large and dysplastic, may represent the earliest identifiable precursors of adenoma [108,109].

The misleading term "non-polyposis" is used to distinguish HNPCC from FAP, which is characterized by hundreds to thousands of colonic adenomas. The frequency of adenomas in HNPCC patients is not significantly increased compared with the general population [95,110]. There is, however, evidence suggesting that CRC in HNPCC does develop from pre-existing adenomatous polyps [75,111], which appear to show an accelerated propensity for malignant transformation (within 2 to 3 years) with respect to those of the general population [110,112] and which are more likely to be large, villous and severely dysplastic. Early studies suggested that adenomas in HNPCC are more proximally located, corresponding to the site of cancer distribution [113,114], but more recently a similar distribution of adenomas in the general population has been suggested [115].

Microsatellite Instability, the Hallmark of the Defective DNA Mismatch Repair System

Microsatellite sequences (MSs) are stretches of DNA, which are highly polymorphic within a population, they are inherited and conserved from one generation to the next [116], and can be identified in normal or tumour tissue. The length of these repetitive sequences ranges from 1 to 6 nucleotides (for instance, single base: $(A)_n$, two bases: $(CA)_n$, etc), where n ranges from 10 to 60 [117,118]. The exact function of MSs remains unknown. They may act directly in gene regulation in the recombination processes. The repair of errors that occur during DNA replication is a highly conserved cellular function. MMR is carried out by proteins which recognize and excise mismatched base pairs and replace them with the correct bases. In bacteria, the MMR system safeguards the genome by both protecting against mutation during DNA replication and preventing recombination between non-homologous regions of DNA. Studies performed in *E. Coli* and yeast first revealed that deficiences in the MMR system result in the instability of DNA repeat sequences [119,120]. Although studies in mammalian cells are limited, it has been assumed that the human MMR system is analogous to that in lower organisms [121,122].

MSI (formerly known as replication error phenotype or ubiquitous somatic mutations) is the hallmark of MMR deficiency. It is defined as an alteration in the length of an MS sequence within tumour DNA when compared with normal DNA from an individual. As a consequence of mispairings, insertions or deletions, MSI arises from changes in the number of units of mono-, di-, and trinucleotide DNA repeats, which due to their repetitive nature are prone to errors during replication [123-125]. Both alleles of a MMR gene need to be inactivated to cause MMR deficiency. The latter results in susceptibility to tumour formation as errors which accumulate in genes responsible for growth regulation are not repaired [126-128]. MMR mutations may be inherited or acquired as result of exposure to environmental agents e.g. carcinogens like heterocyclic amines [129]. MSI can also be seen in non-malignant conditions such as ulcerative colitis and chronic pancreatitis, both inflammatory diseases that may predispose to cancer. In this setting, it has been suggested that chronic inflammation can lead to the saturation and subsequent failure of the MMR system, increasing the mutation rate [130,131].

MSI analysis is technically not difficult, since DNA from tumour and normal tissue can be tested by genotyping fluorescently labeled polymerase chain reaction primers using an automated sequencer [116,132,133] (Fig 4). The short mononucleotide (A) or (T) repeats and dinucleotide sequences are used more frequently as markers of instability than larger repeat sequences, as they are the most sensitive markers. Unified diagnostic criteria for MSI in CRC have been proposed using a reference panel of 5 markers (mononucleotides: BAT25, BAT26; dinucleotides: D5S346, D2S123, D17S250) [113]. Tumours are classified as MSI-H (high-frequency MSI: 2 or more of the 5 markers show instability), MSI-L (low-frequency MSI: only 1 of the 5 markers shows instability), and MSS (stable tumours with no markers showing instability). Several criticisms of the use of these guidelines have been raised. Some investigators feel that the use of a mononucleotide marker exhibiting high sensitivity such as BAT26 alone would be sufficient for MSI identification [134]. In addition, by using 5 markers there is a risk of overestimating MSI as the demonstration of mutations in MS sequences does not necessarily mean MMR deficiency, since mutations can be also due to spontaneous errors of replication of these highly unstable sequences [135].

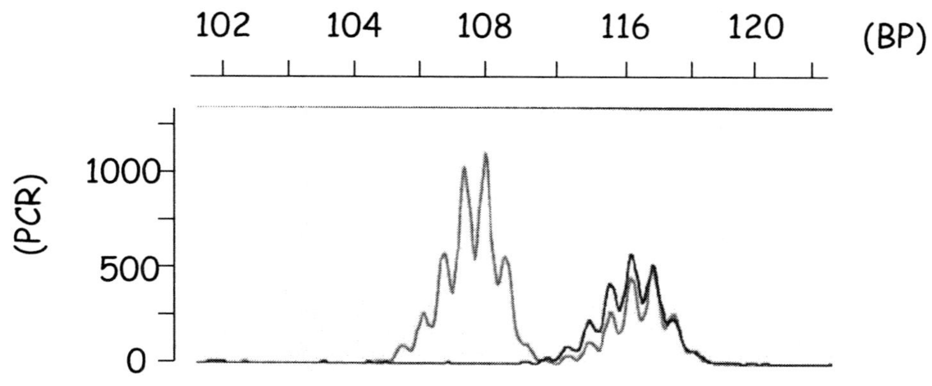

Fig 4. Microsatellite analysis. A cross sectional image of the products of a polymerase chain reaction using the fluorescently labelled marker Bat-26.

Molecular Features: HNPCC versus Sporadic Colorectal Tumours

HNPCC

In HNPCC, MSI is the hallmark of defective MMR. The resulting mutator phenotype predisposes genes which regulate cell proliferation and apoptosis to an increased mutation rate [125,136]. In 1993, MSI was observed in CRCs arising from not only patients with HNPCC but also sporadic tumours [123,125]. Six MMR genes have been characterized, namely *hMSH2, hMLH1, hMSH6, hMSH3, hPMS1* and *hPMS2* [137-146]. Tumorigenesis in HNPCC occurs as a result of germline mutation in one of the MMR genes (*hMSH2* and *hMLH1* account for 70-90%), followed by a somatic mutation of the wild-type allele. Germline alterations in HNPCC genes by themselves do not lead to an increased mutation burden in colonic mucosa [147]. Another gene carrying MSs in their own coding sequences involved in the mutator pathway is the *Transforming Growth Factor-ß type II* (*TGF-ßII*) receptor, which behaves like a tumour suppressor gene during CRC development and represents a critical target of inactivation in MMR deficient tumours [148,149]. Other regulating genes such as the *BAX* gene [150] and *Insulin-like Growth Factor II* receptor [151] have also been identified, and when mutated they play a direct role in tumorigenesis as growth-promotors. When mutated, *TGF-ßII* receptor and *BAX* genes do not have significant prognostic impact on colon cancer exhibiting MSI [152].

In HNPCC tumours exhibiting MSI, mutations of *APC, p53,* K-*ras* and loss of heterozygosity on tumour suppressor genes occurs less frequently than in sporadic tumours [149], suggesting that HNPCC CRCs develop via a different pathway from their sporadic counterpart.

Genotype-phenotype correlations in HNPCC have been reported with mutations of *hMSH2* associated with cancers of the endometrium (not significantly), renal pelvis, ureter, stomach, and ovary more often than *hMLH1* mutations [153], while individuals carrying mutations of *hMSH6* have an atypical HNPCC syndrome, characterized by a late onset of cancer [154]. Mutations of *hMSH6* have been analyzed in kindreds in which no *hMLH1* and *hMSH2* were expressed. Mutations of *hMSH6* in these kindreds are associated to an atypical HNPPC syndrome, characterized by a very high rate of of hyperplastic lesions or carcinomas of the endometrium (73% in female *hMSH6* carriers *vs* 29%-31% in *hMLH1/hMSH2* carriers). Again, these *hMSH6* mutated kindreds show a delayed age of cancer onset [155]. Mutations in nucleases such as *hEXO1* are less frequent and are sometimes associated with atypical HNPCC tumour phenotypes [156].

Sporadic colorectal tumours exhibiting MSI show a striking similarity to HNPCC CRCs, suggesting a possible common pathway of these tumours [157]. MSI has been also demonstrated in a subgroup of tumours of the Muir-Torre syndrome, which implies that these tumours may also arise via a similar pathway [158]. MSI, shown in 86% to 95% of CRCs in HNPCC patients, is also demonstrated in 57% of their colonic polyps (versus only 3% for sporadic adenomas), which is indirect evidence that adenomas are precursors of cancer in HNPCC. Indeed MSI has been detected in all histopathological stages of HNPCC tumours, suggesting that loss of MMR occurs at an early stage in carcinogenesis [149].

Sporadic Colorectal Cancers

About 15% of sporadic CRCs display MSI [110,123,124,154,159-161], but for affected individuals less than 35 years old the frequency increases to 58% [162]. In common with HNPCC, sporadic CRCs exhibiting MSI are almost always situated in the proximal colon, occur in younger people, tend to be of large size and with an exophytic growth pattern, and show in general a tendency towards better prognosis compared to MSI negative sporadic tumours [160,163-166], although there is no definitive consensus for the latter observation [167-169]. However, only a minority of sporadic tumours exhibiting MSI have mutations in hMSH2 or hMLH1 [128,148,160]. In fact, in MSI-sporadic tumours MMR is generally inactivated by epigenetic gene silencing via methylation of the hMLH1 gene promoter rather than by mutation [170-172]. There are conflicting reports about the prevalence of hMSH3 and hMSH6 in sporadic MSI positive sporadic CRCs. One study suggested they account for 36% [173], but this was not supported in a subsequent report [174]. It is possible that MSI in sporadic tumours is caused by factors other than defects in known MMR genes. The exonucleases of DNA polymerases participate in correcting errors of DNA replication in unicellular organisms, and similar mutations may account for some of the sporadic cancers exhibiting MSI [175].

Molecular Assessment and Clinical Management

Identification of Patients

Controversies

The clinical identification of HNPCC gene carriers can be difficult as there is no identifiable phenotype. Accurate documentation of the family history of malignancy combined with clinical observation remains the first step in identifying individuals at increased risk for the disorder. Subsequent molecular testing for MSI of tumours from affected family members may be helpful in the diagnosis, particularly in identifying HNPCC patients who might otherwise have been excluded by the "Amsterdam criteria" alone [176]. Some studies have shown that MSI is not by itself a reliable marker of familial predisposition for CRC, and so should not be considered as sole evidence for an inherited MMR syndrome [177,178]. In one study, only 50% of families meeting "Amsterdam criteria" for HNPCC had tumours exhibiting MSI [179]. Conversely, relying solely on the family history without inclusion of the MSI status, may lead to the overdiagnosis of MMR deficiency [180]. Other authors have shown that the extension of "Amsterdam criteria" to extracolonic tumours of HNPCC spectrum results in a very low mutation detection rate for *hMSH2* and *hMLH1* [181]. Recently, a study has shown that a large-scale molecular screening could be feasible through MSI assessment followed by mutation analysis. Using three clinical criteria (young age, previous tumours and positive family history), 94% of patients exhibiting mutations of *hMLH1/hMSH2* had at least one of these features, detected in 22% of the studied group [182]. As noted, MSI prevalence is higher among younger patients exhibiting "sporadic" tumours [162]. This subset of patients may have an inherited predisposition towards developing CRCs, emphasising the need for an accurate review of their family histories.

Who to Test for Microsatellite Instability?

The high proportion of MSI observed in HNPCC tumours has led to the suggestion that the syndrome could be diagnosed by testing tumours for MSI, although it is known that about 15% of sporadic cancers exhibit MSI. The relatively high rate of MSI in adenomas of HNPCC patients (57%) compared with sporadic cases (3%) may prove to be a better predictor of HNPCC, and has the advantage of being helpful before diagnosis of any carcinoma [111,183]. This analysis would be particularly useful in cases where the family history is incomplete.

A theoretical positive predictive value (PPV) of 6% for HNPCC has been estimated in finding MSI in individuals with a single CRC, and this rises to 30% for individuals with a single adenoma. These percentages increase substantially in the case of individuals exhibiting multiple tumours carrying MSI (PPV for CRCs and adenomas of 29% and 95%, respectively) [184]. The Bethesda guidelines have been developed to assist in the selection of tumours for MSI analysis, in an attempt to identify more HNPCC kindreds. The objective of a recent study was to validate these guidelines in a small group of patients with apparently sporadic CRCs. Sensitivity and PPV were 43% and 27%, respectively. However, an increase in discriminative power was observed using two criteria alone, i.e. testing proximal located CRC with mucinous histology and/or age < 45 years (sensitivity and PPV were 85% and 46%, respectively) [185].

Endoscopic Surveillance

HNPCC family members with confirmed genetic mutation or for individuals with a significant clinical risk for the syndrome require careful endoscopic surveillance. Since up to 70% of the cancers occur proximally to the splenic flexure, colonoscopy is mandatory when screening individuals from HNPCC families. Recommendations for endoscopic surveillance have been proposed by the ICG-HNPCC [115]. It has been arbitrarily suggested [75,84,186] endoscopic examination should start at 25 years (or 5 years earlier than the earliest onset of CRC in the family), but there is less clear guidance on when to stop surveillance [91,186]. In proven gene carriers, an argument supporting life-long endoscopic follow-up is that > 80% of HNPCC patients continue to have recurrent adenomas on successive colonoscopies [75]. The optimal interval between endoscopic exams is undetermined. Nonetheless, most authors recommend a total colonoscopy every one to three years depending on findings at the initial examination [82,84,186-188], with more frequent examinations in proven gene carriers or in those presenting with adenomas, on the basis of the accelerated progression to carcinoma.

To date, there are no reported controlled trials evaluating the impact of screening on the other cancers of HNPCC spectrum. In families with cases of gastric cancer, upper endoscopy is recommended at age 50 years or five years less than the first gastric cancer case, although no studies in this setting have been reported. Concerning endometrial and ovarian cancer, a yearly surveillance program including curettage for cytologic analysis combined with transvaginal ultrasound imaging and CA 125 screening have been proposed starting from 25 years [82]. Among families with urinary tract cancers, annual urine cytology should be considered.

Role of Surgery

Because the entire colonic mucosa is susceptible to development of synchronous and metachronous cancers, partial resection is not an adequate procedure in HNPCC patients affected with CRC. A subtotal colectomy with an ileorectal anastomosis (STC) represents the surgical approach of choice.

As a prophylactic measure, colectomy is recommended for preventing CRC in FAP. This can be justified as the gene penetrance is near 100% and adenomas are so numerous that malignancy is virtually certain to occur. Prophylactic colectomy in HNPCC patients is controversial. The unexpectedly high occurrence of interval cancers in patients undergoing surveillance at two to three yearly intervals has prompted some to argue for prophylactic surgery as an alternative to even more aggressive endoscopic screening in gene carriers [189]. However, penetrance is incomplete and about 20% of gene carriers do not develop CRCs [190]. Furthermore, in one study, structured endoscopic surveillance reduces by 62% the CRC incidence in at-risk members of families with HNPCC [191]. There are several points to consider about prophylactic colectomy. The rectum remains at risk of cancer (so surveillance using rigid or flexible sigmoidoscopy is essential), and STC does not modify the risk of cancer in the other target organs of the HNPCC spectrum. The surgical morbidity and mortality rate of approximately 10% and 1% respectively (data obtained from FAP patients registries) must be weighed against the benefit of the procedure. Major complications include anastomotic leak, subphrenic abscesses, late bowel obstruction and increased defecation frequency. The best time for surgery can only be guessed at the median age at diagnosis of cancer within a family. Finally, the psychosocial impact of a surgery needs to be considered. Prophylactic surgery has been considered as an alternative to endoscopic polypectomy in: 1) patients with proven germline mutation who develop adenomas (because of their high lifetime risk for CRC and on the basis of accelerated progression to malignancy) [189,190], or 2) individuals of highly suspected HNPCC families without proven germline mutations but having adenomas exhibiting MSI [192]. In conclusion, at present there is insufficient data to recommend for or against primary prophylactic surgery in mutation carriers, and this option must be discussed with a fully informed patient.

The option of preventive hysterectomy and bilateral salpingo-ovariectomy has been advocated in women gene carriers having completed their family planning [82].

Prognostic Importance

It has been suggested that evaluation of the MSI status of colorectal tumours might be an important predictor of prognosis. Several descriptive studies have suggested better survival among patients whose CRCs show two or more altered MSs compared with MS stable tumours [124,159,179], matched for stage and grade. The impression of a generally more favourable outcome is supported by further publication showing a 5-year survival rate of 65% for HNPCC patients with *hMLH1* mutation compared with 44% for those with sporadic CRCs [193]. Similar better outcome has been reported in Danish and Japanese HNPCC patients [194,195]. However, no significant (or only limited for node-positive CRCs) survival advantage has been shown in additional two series of HNPCC patients [196,197]. Moreover, in tumours occurring at very early age (within 3th decade) MSI seems also not to correlate with favourable prognosis [198]. In another study, positive MSI status correlates with improved prognosis only in cases of a proximally located cancer [199]. As previously mentioned there is no significant difference in survival for tumours exhibiting MSI compared with MS stable cancers in a setting of sporadic cases [167].

Testing for MSI in patients with a primary CRC may be a useful tool to predict an increased risk for developing additional colonic and non-colonic malignancies [200]. These conclusions have been substantiated in a subset of nonfamilial CRCs, with mainly left-sided cancers (89% patients with sporadic metachronous multiple cancers displayed MSI, compared with 14% for those with single tumour) [201].

Drug Resistance

Studies *in vitro* and *in vivo* have shown that MMR modulates the response to the cytotoxic effects of some DNA damaging drugs. Although the underlying mechanism is not clearly understood (the defective MMR may impair cell cycle arrest and apoptosis induced by DNA damage), it is well recognized that loss of functional MMR in tumour cell lines confers variable resistance to several chemotherapeutics drugs, such as alkylating agents, cisplatin, procarbazine, etoposide, doxorubicin and busulfan [202-206].

5-Fluorouracil (5-FU) based regimens are currently widely employed in adjuvant and palliative setting for bowel cancer treatment. The choice of 5-FU reflects the generally high sensivity of CRC tumour cell lines to 5-FU and its deoxynucleoside, 5-fluorodeoxyuridine (5-FdUrd). Cytotoxic activity is mediated by incorporation of 5-fluorouridine monophosphate into RNA and inhibition of DNA synthesis.

In vitro analysis on CRC cell lines has shown that 5-FU treatment provides a growth advantage for MMR deficient cells, suggesting a possible pathway for tumour resistance to this agent. In particular, increased resistance to 5-FU and 5-FdUrd has been observed in *hMLH1, hMSH2,* and *hMSH6* defective cell lines [207-209]. Nonetheless, two additional reports are in disagreement with these findings [205,210], which suggests that other factors may play a major role in fluoropyrimidine sensitivity, for instance the *p53* status [212]. Is MSI indeed a favourable parameter of response to chemotherapy? Some series support this hypothesis [164,212,213]. Patients with mutated or overexpressed *p53* seem not to have a survival benefit from adjuvant chemotherapy, and in addition a strong inverse correlation between *p53* alterations and MSI status has been shown [213]. In view of the latter observation, the better therapeutic response generally associated with MSI may be counterbalanced by the *p53* status, which does not necessarily result in improvement of patient survival. Interestingly, a decrease of expression of MMR proteins, especially *hMLH1*, has been observed at least in ovarian cancer after several courses of cisplatin based chemotherapy. Nonetheless, this finding does not always underlie a reduced clinical response to treatment [214].

In breast cancer cell lines, low level resistance to topoisomerase I inhibitors camptothecin has been associated with loss of *hMLH1* function [215]. In colon cancer, investigations *in vitro* have shown high sensitivity of MMR defective cell lines to the topoisomerase I inhibitors, camptothecin and irinotecan [216-218]. Again *p53* status influences cytotoxicity of these drugs, producing a sensitization to irinotecan when inactivated [216,219]. Taken together, similar observation could have a clinical relevance, since an appropriate choice of drugs might influence the outcome for patient with tumours exhibiting MSI.

Since patients with tumours showing MSI may have a survival advantage, it may also be of interest to evaluate whether this is related to the response of tumours carrying MSI to chemotherapeutic agents, as this could have implications for innovative therapeutic approaches. For example, an interesting report has pointed out that the reintroduction of a normal copy of *hMLH1* gene in human colon tumour cell lines exhibiting MSI restores MMR activity and reverses tolerance to alkylating agents [220].

5-Iodo-2'-deoxyuridine (IdUrd) and bromodeoxyuridine (BrdUrd) are halogenated thymidine analogues (HTD) effective *in vivo* and *in vitro* as radiosensitizer in human cancers. Recently it has been shown that MMR-deficient, drug-resistant cells can be targeted for radiosensitization by IdUrd and BrdUrd. These thymidine (dThd) analogs become incorporated into DNA and form reactive uracil radicals after ionizing radiation, increasing strand breaks. IdUrd and BrdUrd appear to be removed from DNA in MMR-proficient cells with limited toxicity or disruption of the cell cycle, while accumulating at much higher levels in MMR-deficient cells. MMR proteins may participate in the recognition and removal of HTD from DNA. Consequently, whereas MMR-deficient cell and tumour xenograft have shown intrinsic resistance to several antiblastic agents, the HTD appears to selectively target such cells for potential enhanced radiation sensitivity. In another words, a combined approach of IdUrd or BrdUrd with radiation therapy may be effective in killing MMR-deficient tumours in patients which are resistant to many cancer chemotherapy agents commonly used in the clinic [221,222]. More recently, functional MMR has been shown to be required for activation of the S-phase checkpoint in response to ionizing radiation [223].

Chemoprevention

By interfering with the molecular events, chemoprevention could inhibit or reverse the development of adenomas or the progression from adenoma to carcinoma. Therefore, there is an increasing interest in the use of drugs to prevent the development of colorectal adenomas and carcinomas, especially in high risk individuals. The most attractive proposition for chemoprevention remains the non-steroidal anti-inflammatory drugs (NSAIDs). NSAIDs exert their effect by inhibition of both cyclooxygenase (COX) 1 and 2, catalytic enzymes involved in prostaglandin synthesis [224]. COX-1 is expressed constitutively and plays an important role in protecting gastroduodenal mucosa, whereas COX-2 gene is rapidly induced in response to tumour promoters, cytokines, and growth factors. The analysis of COX-2 expression, but not COX-1, has shown that it is elevated in up to 90% of sporadic CRCs and 40% of adenomas, but not in normal colonic epithelium. NSAIDs may achieve different degrees of inhibition of COX-1 and COX-2 genes. The mechanisms by which the inhibition of COX-2 leads to decreased colon carcinogenesis are not fully understood, but they may involve an increase in apoptosis, the regulation of angiogenesis, or both [225,226]. In experimental models, treatment with a NSAID like sulindac induces a decrease of the number of intestinal adenomas by more than 90% and total volume of colon tumours by more 52%, respectively [227,228]. Non selective COX-1 inhibitor sulindac has been shown to reduce polyp number and size in FAP patients [229], although a recent study suggests that standard doses of sulindac did not slow the development of adenomas in this setting [57]. Variable doses of aspirin have been tested in two important randomized placebo-controlled trials, showing a significant reduction of adenomas in patients with previous history of adenoma or colorectal cancer [230,231]. Nonetheless, large-scale use of prophylactic aspirine cannot be recommended, since potential benefit must be balanced with toxicity in further trials. In addition, it is unlikely that aspirin can replace colonoscopic surveillance, as the protective effect of aspirin seems not complete. Aspirin is thought to act via both suppression of expression of COX-2 [232] or prostaglandin-independent pathway [233]. Of particular interest are COX-2 inhibitors like celecoxib and rofecoxib, since anti-inflammatory properties are maintained while carrying lower gastrointestinal toxicity when compared with COX-1 inhibitors. In a study, celecoxib was administered for six months of twice-daily treatment with 400 mg, resulting in significant decrease of polyp burden in FAP patients [56]. Similarly, an high significant reduction in polyp formation was observed in patients with FAP with rofecoxib 25 mg/daily [234].

In a recent publication, the administration of aspirin or sulindac resulted in a suppression of MSI phenotype in MMR (hMSH2, hMLH1, hMSH6) deficient CRC cell lines. It is this time- and dose-dependent reversible effect on the induction of apoptosis that results in genetic selection for cells that retain stable MSs rather than the antiproliferative properties of NSAIDs [235]. The pharmacological prevention of CRC in HNPCC carriers is currently being evaluated in clinical trials. Patients eligible for the CAPP (Concerted Action Polyp Prevention) 2 trial are randomized in a factorial design to receive 600 mg aspirin and/or 30 mg corn starch with placebo control. The primary endpoint is the incidence of bowel neoplasia, and the secondary endpoint is the incidence of associated extracolonic malignancies [236]. Another randomized placebo-controlled study compared celecoxib at different doses (200 mg bid vs 400 mg bid) versus placebo bid for 12 months. The results of this trial are pending.

Final Remarks

The essential step for diagnosing a hereditary cancer syndrome is the construction and evaluation of the pedigree, which first provides information about empirical inherited risk. The careful compilation of family history is the most valuable component for the diagnosis, even if, often, limited information is available. Detailed information should include type and site of all cancers, age of onset of tumours, presence of multiple synchronous or metachronous cancers, and association with other clinical features that may be related to cancer (for instance, presence of intestinal adenomas). All clinical details should be supported by pathological findings. This workup is often sufficient to identify a hereditary colorectal cancer syndrome, although a convincing diagnosis of cancer susceptibility cannot always be made. The exclusion of a particular high-risk condition contributes to reassuring the family members, conversely, the pedigree analysis may suggest a defined inheritance, even in the absence of molecular confirmation. Genetic counselling is a broad spectrum process involving diagnosis, risk assessment, explanation of medical and genetic facts and possible options of therapeutic/prophylactic interventions. The process includes pre-test evaluation, genetic testing (when indicated, it may contribute to confirmation of diagnosis), post-test counselling and evaluation of surveillance and prevention strategies that reflect the natural history of the disorder. Special attention should be paid to the need for continuous support for high-risk patients and relatives in order to prevent anxiety during counselling sessions as well as for cancer prevention by regular screening and early diagnosis. Once an inherited syndrome is established, counselling should be extended to the consenting family members in a face to face modality, although sessions may include multiple family individuals. Presymptomatic testing must be offered after obtaining of an informed consent. Information about potential risks of discomfort including psychological harm and socio-familial consequences should be elucidated in details prior to genetic testing.

Advances in the field of molecular genetics of CRC are in continuous expansion. The application of these discoveries to hereditary CRC has important implications in understanding the development of CRC. The application of these discoveries 1) to screening and detection of the disease at earlier and more curable stages; 2) to more accurate prognosis, complementary to clinical staging and histopathological analysis; and 3) to identifying treatment options (in predicting response or even as a tool for selecting specific therapeutic approaches) remains an important challenge for the future.

Acknowledgments

The author would like to thank Prof Hansjakob Müller (Labor Humangenetik, Abt. Medizinische Genetik, Dept. Klinische-Biologische Wissenschaften, Basel, Switzerland) for the highly appreciated advice and for his enthusiastic collaboration.

REFERENCES

[1] Jemal A, Murray T, Samuels A et al. Cancer statistics, 2003. *CA Cancer J Clin* 2003; 53:5-26

[2] Parkin DM, Pisani P, Ferlay J. Global cancer statistics. *CA Cancer J Clin* 1999; 49:33-64

[3] No author listed. Stat bite: Incidence of colon and rectum cancer by age and ethnicity, 1992-1999. *J Natl Cancer Inst* 2003; 95:349

[4] Austoker J. Screening for colorectal cancer. *BMJ* 1994; 309:382-6

[5] St. John DJB, Mc Dermott FT, Hopper JL et al. Cancer risk in relatives of patients with common colorectal cancer. *Ann Intern Med* 1993; 118:785-90

[6] Houlston RS, Murday V, Harocopos C et al. Screening and genetics counselling for relatives of patients with colorectal cancer in a family cancer clinic. *Br Med J* 1990; 301:366-8

[7] Fuchs CS, Giovanucci EL, Colditz GA et al. A prospective study of family history and the risk of colorectal cancer. *N Engl J Med* 1994; 331:1669-74

[8] Burt RW. Colon cancer screening for colorectal cancer. *Gastroenterology* 2000; 119:837-53

[9] Slattery ML, Kerber RA. Family history of cancer and colon cancer risk: the Utah Population Database. *J Natl Cancer Inst* 1994; 86:1618-26

[10] Lichtenstein P, Holm NV, Verkasaio PK et al. Environmental and heritable factors in the causation of cancer-analysis of cohorts of twins from Sweden, Denmark, and Finland. *N Engl J Med* 2000; 343:78-85

[11] Drucker L, Shpilberg O, Neumann A et al. Adenomatous polyposis coli I1307K mutation in Jewish patients with different ethnicity: prevalence and phenotype. *Cancer* 2000; 88:755-60

[12] Strul H, Baremboim E, Leshno M et al. The I1307K adenomatous polyposis coli gene variant does not contribute in the assessment of the risk for colorectal cancer in Ashkenazi Jews. *Cancer Epidemiol Biomarkers Prev* 2003; 12:1012-5

[13] Bulow S. Results of national registration of familial adenomatous polyposis. *Gut* 2003; 52:742-6

[14] Petersen GM, Slack J, Nakamura Y. Screening guidelines and premorbid diagnosis of familial adenomatous polyposis using linkage. *Gastroenterology* 1991; 100:1658-64

[15] Lynch HT, Smyrk HT, McGinn T et al. Attenuated familial adenomatous polyposis (AFAP). A phenotypically and genotypically distinctive variant of FAP. *Cancer* 1995; 76:2427-33

[16] Lindor NM, Greene MH. The concise handbook of family cancer syndromes. Mayo Familial Cancer Program. *J Natl Cancer Inst* 1998; 90:1039-71

[17] Bjork J, Akerbrant H, Iselius L et al. Periampullary adenomas and adenocarcinomas in familial adenomatous polyposis: cumulative risks and APC gene mutations. *Gastroenterology* 2001; 121:1127-35

[18] Kadmon M, Tandara A, Herfarth C. Duodenal adenomatosis in familial adenomatous polyposis coli. A review of the literature and results from the Heidelberg Polyposis Register. *Int J Colorectal Dis* 2001; 16:63-75

[19] Trimbath JD, Griffin C, Romans K et al. Attenuated familial adenomatous polyposis presenting as ampullary adenocarcinoma. *Gut* 2003; 52:903-4

[20] Hofgartner WT, Thorp M, Ramus MW et al. Gastric adenocarcinoma associated with fundic gland polyps in a patient with attenuated familial adenomatous polyposis. *Am J Gastroenterol* 1999; 94:2275-81

[21] Giardiello FM, Offerhaus GJ, Lee DH et al. Increased risk of thyroid and pancreatic carcinoma in familial adenomatous polyposis. *Gut* 1993; 34:1394-6

[22] Bertario L, Russo A, Sala P et al. Genotype and phenotype factors as determinants of desmoid tumors in patients with familial adenomatous polyposis. *Int J Cancer* 2001; 95:102-7

[23] Heiskanen I, Jarvinen HJ. Occurrence of desmoid tumours in familial adenomatous polyposis and results of treatment. *Int J Colorectal Dis* 1996; 11:157-62

[24] Gardner EJ. A genetic and clinical study of intestinal polyposis, a predisposing factor for carcinoma of the colon and rectum. *Am J Hum Genet* 1951; 3:167-76

[25] Ruhswurm I, Zehetmayer M, Dejaco C et al. Ophtalmic and genetic screening in pedigrees with familial adenomatous polyposis. *Am J Opthalmol* 1998; 125:680-6

[26] Shields JA, Shields CL, Eagle RC et al. Adenocarcinoma arising from congenital hypertrophy of the retinal pigment epithelium. *Arch Ophtalmol* 2001; 119:597-602

[27] Bodmer WF, Baily CJ, Bodmer J et al. Localisation of the gene for familial adenomatous polyposis on chromosome 5. *Nature* 1987; 328:614-6

[28] Leppert M, Dobbs M, Scambler P et al. The gene for in familial polyposis coli maps to the long arm of chromosome 5. *Science* 1987; 238:1411-3

[29] Kinzler KW, Nilbert MC, Su L et al. Identification of FAP locus genes from chromosome 5q21. *Science* 1991; 253:661-5

[30] Groden J, Thliveris A, Samowitz W et al. Identification and characterization of the in familial adenomatous polyposis coli gene. *Cell* 1991; 66:589-600

[31] Munemitsu S, Albert I, Souza B et al. Regulation of intracellular ß-catenin levels by the adenomatous polyposis coli (APC) tumour-suppressor protein. *Proc Natl Acad Sci* USA 1995; 92:3046-50

[32] Giardiello FM, Petersen GM, Piantadosi S et al. APC gene mutations and extraintestinal phenotype of familial adenomatous polyposis. *Gut* 1997; 40:521-5

[33] Giardiello FM. Genetic testing in hereditary colorectal cancer. *JAMA* 1997; 278:1278-81

[34] Spirio L, Olschwang S, Groden Jet al. Alleles of the APC gene: an attenuated form of familial polyposis. *Cell* 1993; 75:951-7

[35] Friedl W, Meuschel S, Caspari R et al. Attenuated familial adenomatous polyposis due to a mutation in the 3' part of the APC gene. A clue for understanding the function of the APC protein. *Hum Genet* 1996; 97:579-84

[36] Nugent KP, Phillips RK, Hodgson SV et al. Phenotypic expression in familial adenomatous polyposis: partial prediction by mutation analysis. *Gut* 1994; 35:1622-3

[37] Caspari R, Friedl W, Mandl M et al. Familial adenomatous polyposis: mutation at codon 1309 and early onset of colon cancer. *Lancet* 1994; 343:629-32

[38] Olschwang S, Tiret E, Laurent-Puig P et al. Restriction of ocular fundus lesions to a specific subgroup of *APC* mutations in adennomatous polyposis coli patients. *Cell* 1993; 75:959-68

[39] Wallis YL, Macdonald F, Hulten M et al. Genotype-phenotype correlation between position of constitutional *APC* gene mutation and CHRPE expression in familial adenomatous polyposis. *Hum Genet* 1994; 94:543-8

[40] Caspari R, Olschwang S, Friedl W et al. Desmoid tumors and lack of ophtalmic lesions (CHRPE) associated with *APC* mutations beyond codon 1444. *Hum Mut Genet* 1995; 4:337-40

[41] Scott RJ, van der Luijt R, Spycher M et al. Novel germline *APC* gene mutation in a large familial adenomatous polyposis kindred displying variable phenotype. *Gut* 1995; 36:731-6

[42] Bertario L, Russo A, Sala P et al. Multiple approach to the exploration of genotype-phenotype correlations in familial adenomatous polyposis. *J Clin Oncol* 2003; 21:1698-707

[43] Sieber OM, Lipton L, Crabtree M et al. Multiple colorectal adenomas, classic adenomatous polyposis, and germ-line mutations in MYH. *N Engl J Med* 2003; 348:791-9

[44] Bunyan DJ, Shea-Simmonds J, Reck AC et al. Genotype/phenotype correlations of new causative *APC* gene mutations in patients with familial adenomatous polyposis. *J Med Genet* 1995; 32:728-31

[45] Crabtree MD, Tomlinson IP, Hughes SV et al. Explaining variation in familial adenomatous polyposis: relationship between genotype and phenotype and evidence for modifier genes. *Gut* 2002; 51:420-3

[46] Phillips RKS, Spigelman AD. Can we safely delay or avoid prophylactic colectomy in familial adenomatous polyposis (FAP)? *Br J Surg* 1996; 83:769-70

[47] Giardiello FM, Brensinger JD, Petersen GM. AGA technical review on hereditary colorectal cancer and genetic testing. *Gastroenterology* 2001; 121:198-213

[48] Heiskanen I, Luostarinen T, Järvinen HJ. Impact of screening examinations on survival in familial adenomatous polyposis. *Scand J Gastroenterol* 2000; 35:1284-7

[49] Debinski HS, Spigelman AD, Hatfield A et al. Upper intestinal surveillance in familial adenomatous polyposis. *Eur J Cancer* 1995; 31A:1149-53

[50] Distante S, Nasoulias S, Somers GR et al. Familial adenomatous polyposis in a 5 year old child: a clinical pathological and molecular genetic study. *J Med Genet* 1996; 33:157-60

[51] Rex DK, Johnson DA, Lieberman DA et al. Colorectal cancer prevention 2000: screening recommendations of the American college of gastroenterology. *Am J Gastroenterol* 2000; 95:868-77

[52] Evans DGR, Guy SP, Thakker N et al. Non-penetrance and late appearance of polyps in families with familial adenomatous polyposis. *Gut* 1993; 34:1389-93

[53] Bussey HJR, De Cosse JJ, Deschner EE et al. A randomised trial of ascorbic acid in polyposis coli. *Cancer* 1982; 50:1434-9

[54] De Cosse JJ, Miller HH, Lesser ML. Effect of wheat fiber and vitamin C and E on rectal polyps in patients with familial adenomatous polyposis. *J Natl Cancer Inst* 1989; 91:1290-7

[55] Stern HS, Gregorie RC, Koshtan H. Long-term effects of dietary calcium on risk markers for colon cancer in patients with familial polyposis. *Surgery* 1990; 108:528-33

[56] Steinbach G, Lynch PM, Phillips RKS et al. The effect of celecoxib, a cyclooxygenase-2 inhibitor, in familial adenomatous polyposis. *N Engl J Med* 2000; 342:1946-52

[57] Giardiello FM, Yang VW, Hylind ML et al. Primary chemoprevention of familial adenomatous polyposis. *New Engl J Med* 2002; 346:1054-9

[58] Tonelli F, Valanzano R, Masserini L et al. Long-term treatment with sulindac in familial adenomatous polyposis: is there an actual efficacy in prevention of rectal cancer? *J Surg Oncol* 2000; 74:15-20

[59] Phillips RK, Wallace MH, Lynch PM et al. A randomised, double blind, placebo controlled study of celecoxib, a selective cyclooxygenase 2 inhibitor, on duodenal polyposis in familial adenomatous polyposis. *Gut* 2002; 50:857-60

[60] Hyer W. *Polyposis syndromes: pediatric implications*. Gastrointestinal Endoscopy Clinics of North America 2001; 11:659-82

[61] Giardiello FM, Brensinger JD, Tersmette AC et al. Very high risk of cancer in familial Peutz-Jeghers syndrome. *Gastroenterology* 2000; 119:1447-53

[62] Tomlinson IP, Houlston RS. Peutz-Jeghers syndrome. *J Med Genet* 1997; 34:1007-11

[63] Spigelman AD, Arese P, Phillips RK. Polyposis: the Peutz-Jeghers syndrome. *Br J Surg* 1995; 82:1311-4

[64] Jenne DE, Reimann N, Nezu J et al. Peutz-Jeghers syndrome is caused by mutations in a novel serine threonine kinase. *Nat Genet* 1998; 18:38-43

[65] Hemminki A, Markie D, Tomlinson I et al. A serine/threonine kinase gene defective in Peutz-Jeghers syndrome. *Nature* 1998; 391:184-7

[66] Boardman LA, Couch FJ, Burgart LJ et al. Genetic heterogeneity in Peutz-Jeghers syndrome. *Hum Mutat* 2000; 16:23-30

[67] Jass JR, Williams CB, Bussey HJR et al. Juvenile polyposis -a precancerous condition. *Histopathology* 1988; 13:619-30

[68] Jarvinen H, Franssila KO. Familial juvenile polyposis coli: increased risk of colorectal cancer. *Gut* 1984; 25:792-800

[69] Howe JR, Mitros FA, Summers RW. The risk of gastrointestinal carcinoma in familial juvenile polyposis. *Ann Surg Oncol* 1998; 5:751-6

[70] Howe JR, Roth S, Ringold JC et al. Mutations in the SMAD4/DPC4 gene in juvenile polyposis. *Science* 1998; 280:1086-88

[71] Olschwang S, Serova-Sinilnikova OM, Lenoir GM et al. PTEN germ-line mutations in juvenile polyposis coli. *Nat Genet* 1998; 18:12-4

[72] Zhou XP, Woodford-Richens K, Lehtonen R et al. Germline mutations in BMPR1A/ALK3 cause a subset of cases of juvenile polyposis syndrome and of Cowden and Bannayan-Riley-Ruvalcaba syndromes. *Am J Hum Genet* 2001; 69:704-11

[73] Watson P, Lynch HT. Extracolonic cancer in hereditary nonpolyposis colorectal cancer. *Cancer* 1993; 71:677-85

[74] Lynch HT, Watson P, Lanspa SJ et al. Natural history of colorectal cancer in hereditary nonpolyposis colorectal cancer (Lynch syndromes I and II). *Dis Colon Rectum* 1988; 31:439-44

[75] Lanspa SJ, Lynch HT, Smyrk TC et al. Colorectal adenomas in the Lynch syndromes. Results of a colonoscopy screening program. *Gastroenterology* 1990; 98:1117-22

[76] Watson P, Lynch HT. The tumour spectrum in HNPCC. *Anticancer Res* 1994; 14:1635-9

[77] Park YJ, Shin K-H, Park J-G. Risk of gastric cancer in hereditary non-polyposis colorectal cancer in Korea. *Clin Cancer Res* 2000; 6:2994-8

[78] Aarnio M, Sankila R, Pukkala E et al. Cancer risk in mutation carriers of DNA-mismatch–repair genes. *Int J Cancer* 1999; 81:214-8

[79] Vasen HFA, Offerhaus GJA, den Hartog Jager FCA et al. The tumour spectrum in hereditary non-polyposis colorectal cancer: a study of 24 kindreds in the Netherland. *Int J Cancer* 1990; 46:31-4

[80] Watson P, Vasen HFA, Mecklin JP et al. The risk of endometrial cancer in hereditary nonpolyposis colorectal cancer. *Am J Med* 1994; 96:516-20

[81] Dunlop MG, Farrington SM, Carothers AD et al. Cancer risk associated with germline DNA mismatch repair gene mutations. *Hum Mol Genet* 1997, 6:105-10

[82] Lynch HT, Smyrk TC, Watson P et al. Genetics, natural history, tumour spectrum, and pathology of hereditary nonpolyposis colorectal cancer: an updated review. *Gastroenterology* 1993; 104:1535-49

[83] Itoh H, Houlston RS, Harocopos C et al. Risk of cancer death in first-degree relatives of patients with hereditary non-polyposis cancer syndrome (Lynch type II): a study of 130 kindreds in United Kingdom. *Br J Surg* 1990; 77:1367-70

[84] Lynch HT, Smyrk T, Watson P et al. Hereditary colorectal cancer. *Semin Oncol* 1991; 18:337-66

[85] Lynch HT, Watson P, Smyrk T et al. Colon cancer genetics. *Cancer* 1992; 70:1300-12

[86] Lynch HT, Fusaro RM, Roberts L et al. Muir-Torre syndrome in several members of a family with a variant of cancer family syndrome. *Br J Dermatol* 1985; 113:295-301

[87] Vasen HFA, Mecklin JP, Meera Khan P et al. The International Collaborative Group on Hereditary Non-Polyposis Colorectal Cancer (ICG-HNPCC). *Dis Colon Rectum* 1991; 34:424-5

[88] Ponz de Leon M, Pedroni M, Benatti P et al. Hereditary colorectal cancer in the general population: from cancer registration to molecular diagnosis. *Gut* 1999; 45:32-8

[89] Mecklin JP. Frequency of hereditary colorectal carcinoma. *Gastroenterology* 1987; 93:1021-5

[90] Kee F, Collins BJ. How prevalent is cancer family syndrome? *Gut* 1991; 32:509-12

[91] Aaltonen LA, Salovaara R, Kristo P et al. Incidence of hereditary nonpolyposis colorectal cancer and the feasibility of molecular screening for the disease. *N Engl J Med* 1998; 338:1481-7

[92] Kee F, Collins BJ. Families at risk of colorectal cancer: who are they? *Gut* 1992; 33:787-90

[93] Percesepe A, Anti M, Roncucci L et al. The effect of family size on estimates of the frequency of hereditary non-polyposis colorectal cancer. *Br J Cancer* 1995; 72:1320-3

[94] Hakala T, Mecklin JP, Forss M et al. Endometrial carcinoma in the cancer family syndrome. *Cancer* 1991; 68:1656-9

[95] Vasen HF, Watson P, Mecklin JP et al. New clinical criteria for of hereditary nonpolyposis colorectal cancer (HNPCC, Lynch syndrome) proposed by the International Collaborative group on HNPCC. *Gastroenterology* 1999; 116:1453-6

[96] Rodriguez-Bigas MA, Boland CR, Hamilton SR et al. A National Cancer Institute Workshop on Hereditary Nonpolyposis Colorectal Cancer Syndrome: meeting highlights and Bethesda guidelines. *J Natl Cancer Inst* 1997; 89:1758-62

[97] Mecklin JP, Sipponen P, Järvinen HJ. Histopathology of colorectal carcinomas and adenomas in cancer family syndrome. *Dis Colon Rect* 1986; 29:849-53

[98] Kouri M, Laasonen A, Mecklin JP et al. Diploid predominance in hereditary nonpolyposis colorectal carcinoma evaluated by flow cytometry. *Cancer* 1990; 65:1825-9

[99] Frei JV. Hereditary nonpolypsis colorectal cancer (Lynch syndrome II). Diploid malignancies with prolonged survival. *Cancer* 1992; 69:1108-11

[100] Lynch HT, Lynch PM, Albano WA et al. The cancer syndrome: a status report. *Dis Colon Rectum* 1981; 24:311-22

[101] Albano WA, Recabaren JA, Lynch HT et al. Natural history of hereditary cancer of the breast and colon. *Cancer* 1982; 50:360-3

[102] Shibata D, Peinado MA, Ionov Y et al. Genomic instability in repeated sequences is an early somatic event in colorectal tumourigenesis that persists after transformation. *Nature Genet* 1994; 6:273-81

[103] Bodmer W, Bishop T, Karran P. Genetic steps in colorectal cancer. *Nature Genet* 1994; 6:217-9

[104] Naito Y, Saito K, Shiiba K et al. CD8+ T cells infiltrated within cancer cell nests as a prognostic factor in human colorectal cancer. *Cancer Res* 1998; 58:3491-4

[105] Guidoboni F, Gafa R, Viel A et al. Microsatellite instability and high content of activated cytotoxic lymphocytes identify colon cancer patients with a favorable prognosis. *Am J Pathol* 2001; 159:297-304

[106] Rognum TO, Lund E, Meling GI et al. Near diploid large bowel carcinomas have better five-year survival than aneuploid ones. *Cancer* 1991; 68:1077-81

[107] Morson BC. Evolution of cancer of the colon and rectum. *Cancer* 1974; 34:845-9

[108] Pretlow TP, Barrow BJ, Ashton WS et al. Aberrant crypts: putative preneoplastic foci in human colonic mucosa. *Cancer Res* 1991; 51:1564-7

[109] Takayama T, Katsuki S, Takahashi Y et al. Aberrant crypt foci of thr colon as precursors of adenoma and cancer. *N Engl J Med* 1998; 339:1277-84

[110] Jass JR, Stewart SM. Evolution of hereditary non-polyposis colorectal cancer. *Gut* 1992; 33:783-6

[111] Aaltonen LA, Peltomäki P, Mecklin JP et al. Replications errors in benign and malignant tumours hereditary nonpolyposis cancer patients. *Cancer Res* 1994; 54:1645-8

[112] Jass JR. Colorectal adenomas in surgical specimens from subjects with hereditary non-polyposis colorectal cancer. *Histopathology* 1995; 27:263-7

[113] Boland CR, Thibodeau SN, Hamilton SR et al. A national cancer institute workshop on microsatellite instability for cancer detection and familial predisposition: develpment of international criteria for the determination of microsatellite instability in colorectal cancer. *Cancer Res* 1998; 58:5248-57

[114] Hodgson SV, Harocopos C, Gaglia P. Screening results in a family cancer clinic: five years experience. *Anticancer Res* 1993; 13:2581-5

[115] Jass JR. Diagnosis of hereditary non-polyposis colorectal cancer. *Histopathology* 1998; 32:491-7

[116] Weber JL, May PE. Abundant class of human DNA polymorphism which can be typed using the polymerase chain reaction. *Am J Hum Genet* 1989; 44:388-96

[117] Beckmann JS, Weber JL. Survey of human and rat MS. *Genomics* 1992; 12:627-31

[118] Litt M, Luty JA. A hypervariable microsatellite revealed by in vitro amplification of a dinucleotide repeat within the cardiac muscle actin gene. *Am J Hum Genet* 1989; 44:397-401

[119] Levinson G, Gutman GA. High frequencies of short frameshifts in poly-CA/TG tandem repeats borne by bacteriophage M13 in Escherichia Coli K-12. *Nucleic Acids Res* 1987; 15:5323-38

[120] Strand M, Prolla TA, Liskay RM et al. Destabilization of tracts of simple repetitive DNA in yeast by mutations affecting DNA mismatch repair. *Nature* 1993; 365:274-6

[121] Prolla TA, Pang Q, Alani E et al. MLH1, PMS1, and MSH2 interactions during the initiation of DNA mismatch repair in yeast. *Science* 1994; 265:1091-3

[122] Fishel R, Ewel A, Lee S et al. Binding of mismatched microsatellite DNA sequences by the human MSH2 protein. *Science* 1994; 266:1403-5

[123] Aaltonen LA, Peltomäki P, Leach FS et al. Clues to the pathogenesis of familial colorectal cancer. *Science* 1993; 260:812-6

[124] Thibodeau SN, Bren G, Schaid D. Microsatellite instability in cancer of the proximal colon. *Science* 1993; 260:816-9

[125] Ionov Y, Peinado MA, Malkhosyan S et al. Ubiquitous somatic mutations in simple repeated sequences reveal a new mechanism for colonic carcinogenesis. *Nature* 1993; 363:558-61

[126] Parsons R, Li GM, Longley MJ et al. Hypermutability and mismatch repair deficiency in RER^+ tumour cells. *Cell* 1993; 75:1227-36

[127] Hemminki A, Peltomäki P, Mecklin JP et al. Loss of the wild type MLH1 gene is a feature of hereditary nonpolyposis colorectal cancer. *Nature Genet* 1994; 8:405-410

[128] Liu B, Nicolaides N, Markowitz S et al. Mismatch repair gene defects in sporadic colorectal cancers with microsatellite instability. *Nat Genet* 1995; 9:48-55

[129] Nagao M, Ushijima T, Toyota M et al. Genetic changes induced by heterocyclic amines. *Mutat Res* 1997; 376:161-7

[130] Brentnall TA, Crispin DA, Bronner MP et al. Microsatellite instability in nonneoplastic mucosa from patients with chronic ulcerative colitis. *Cancer Res* 1996; 56:1237-40

[131] Brentnall TA, Chen R, Lee JG et al. Microsatellite instability and K-ras mutations associated with pancreatic adenocarcinoma and pancreatitis. *Cancer Res* 1995; 55:4264-7

[132] Gruis NA, Abeln ECA, Bardoel AFJ et al. PCR-based microsatellite polymorphisms in the detection of loss of heterozygosity in fresh and archival tumour tissue. *Br J Cancer* 1993; 68:308-13
[133] Toh Y, Oki E, Oda S et al. An integrated microsatellite length analysis using an automated fluorescent DNA sequencer. *Cancer Res* 1996; 56:2688-91
[134] de la Chapelle A. Testing tumors for microsatellite instability. *Eur J Hum Genet* 1999; 7:407-8
[135] Perucho M. Correspondence re: Boland CR et al. A national cancer institute workshop on microsatellite instability for cancer detection and familial predisposition: develpment of international criteria for the determination of microsatellite instability in colorectal cancer. Cancer Res 1998; 58:5248-5257. *Cancer Res* 1999; 59:249-56
[136] Loeb A. Microsatellite instability: marker of a mutator phenotype in cancer. *Cancer Res* 1994; 54:5059-63
[137] Fishel R, Lescoe MK, Rao MRS et al. The human mutator homolog MSH2 and its association with hereditary non-polyposis colon cancer. *Cell* 1993; 75:1027-38
[138] Bronner CE, Baker SM, Morrison PT et al. Mutation in the DNA mismatch repair gene homologue hMLH1 is associated with hereditary non-polyposis colon cancer. *Nature* 1994; 368:258-61
[139] Nicolaides NC, Papadopoulos N, Liu B et al. Mutations of two PMS homologues in hereditary nonpolyposis colon cancer. *Nature* 1994; 371:75-80
[140] Leach FS, Nicolaides NC, Papadopoulos N et al. Mutations of a mutS homolog in hereditary non-polyposis colorectal cancer. *Cell* 1993; 75:1215-25
[141] Kolodner RD, Hall NR, Lipford J et al. Structure of the human MSH2 locus and analysis of two Muir-Torre kindreds for MSH2 mutations. *Genomics* 1994; 24:516-26
[142] Kolodner RD, Hall NR, Lipford J et al. Structure of the human MLH1 locus and analysis of a large hereditary nonpolyposis colorectal carcinoma kindred for MLH1 mutations. *Cancer Res* 1995; 55:242-8
[143] Liu B, Parsons RE, Hamilton SR et al. hMSH2 mutations in hereditary non-polyposis colorectal cancer kindreds. *Cancer Res* 1994; 54:4590-4
[144] Papadopoulos N, Nicolaides NC, Wei YF et al. Mutation of a mutL homolog in hereditary colon cancer. *Science* 1994; 263:1625-9
[145] Akiyama Y, Sato H, Yamada T et al. Germ-line mutation of the hMSH6/GTBP gene in an atypical hereditary nonpolyposis colorectal cancer kindred. *Cancer Res* 1997; 57:3920-3
[146] Miyaki M, Konishi M, Tanaka K et al. Germline mutation of MSH6 as the cause of hereditary nonpolyposis colorectal cancer. *Nature Genet* 1997; 17:271-2
[147] Williams GT, Geraghty JM, Campbell F et al. Normal colonic mucosa in hereditary non-polyposis colorectal cancer shows no generalized increase in somatic mutations. *Br J Cancer* 1995; 71:1077-80
[148] Parsons R, Myeroff LL, Liu B et al. Microsatellite instability and mutations of the transforming growth factor beta type II receptor gene in colorectal cancer. *Cancer Res* 1995; 55:5548-50

[149] Konishi M, Kikuchi-Yanoshita R, Tanaka K et al. Molecular nature of colon tumours in hereditary nonpolyposis colon cancer, familial polyposis, and sporadic colon cancer. *Gastroenterology* 1996; 111:307-17

[150] Rampino N, Yamamoto H, Yonov Y et al. Somatic frameshift mutations in the BAX gene in colon cancers of microsatellite mutator phenotype. *Science* 1997; 275:967-9

[151] Souza RF, Appel R, Yin J et al. Microsatellite instability in the insulin-like growth factor II receptor gene in gastrointestinal tumours. *Nature Genet* 1996; 14:255-7

[152] Samowitz WS, Curtin K, Neuhausen S et al. Prognostic implications of BAX and TGFßRII mutations in colon cancer with microsatellite instability. Genes Chromosomes *Cancer* 2002; 35:368-71

[153] Vasen HF, Wijnen JT, Menko FH et al. Cancer risk in families with hereditary nonpolyposis colorectal cancer diagnosed by mutation analysis. *Gastroenterology* 1996; 110:1020-7

[154] Akiyama Y, Sato H, Yamada T et al. Germ-line mutation of the hMSH6/GTBP gene in an atypical hereditary nonpolyposis colorectal cancer kindred. *Cancer Res* 1997; 57:3920-3

[155] Wijnen J, de Leeuw W, Vasen H et al. Familial endometrial cancer in female carriers of hMSH6 germline mutations. *Nat Genet* 1999; 23:142-4

[156] Genschel J, Bazamore LR, Modrich P. Human exonuclease I is required for 5' and 3' mismatch repair. *J Biol Chem* 2002; 277:13302-11

[157] Peltomäki P, Lothe RA, Aaltonen LA et al. Microsatellite instability is associated with tumours that characterize the hereditary non-polyposis colorectal carcinoma syndrome. *Cancer Res* 1993; 53:5853-5

[158] Honchel R, Halling KC, Schaid DJ et al. Microsatellite instability in Muir-Torre syndrome. *Cancer Res* 1994; 54:1159-63

[159] Lothe RA, Peltomäki P, Meling GI et al. Genomic instability in colorectal cancer: relationship to clinicopathological variables and family history. *Cancer Res* 1993; 53:5849-52

[160] Kim H, Jen J, Vogelstein B et al. Clinical and pathological characteristics of sporadic colorectal carcinomas with DNA replication errors in microsatellite sequences. *Am J Pathol* 1994; 145:148-56

[161] Senba S, Konishi F, Okamoto T et al. Clinicopathologic and genetic features of nonfamilial colorectal carcinomas with DNA replication errors. *Cancer* 1998; 82:279-85

[162] Liu B, Farrington SM, Petersen GM et al. Genetic instability occurs in the majority of young patients with colorectal cancer. *Nat Med* 1995; 1:348-52

[163] Gryfe R, Kim H, Hsieh ET et al. Tumor microsatellite instability and clinical outcome in young patients with colorectal cancer. *N Engl J Med* 2000; 342:69-77

[164] Elsaleh H, Joseph D, Grieu F et al. Association of tumour site and sex with survival benefit from adjuvant chemotherapy in colorectal cancer. *Lancet* 2000; 355:1745-50

[165] Elsaleh H, Iacopetta B. Microsatellite instability is a predictive marker for survival benefit from adjuvant chemotherapy in a population-based series of stage III colorectal carcinoma. *Clin Colorectal Cancer* 2001; 1:104-9

[166] Samowitz WS, Curtin K, Ma KN et al. Microsatellite instability in sporadic colon cancer is associated with an improved prognosis at the population level. *Cancer Epidemiol Biomarkers Prev* 2001; 10: 917-23

[167] Feeley KM, Fullard JF, Heneghan MA et al. Microsatellite instability in sporadic colorectal carcinoma is not an indicator of prognosis. *J Pathol* 1999; 188:14-7

[168] Salahshor S, Kressner U, Fisher H et al. Microsatellite instability in sporadic colorectal cancer is not an independent prognostic factor. *Br J Cancer* 1999; 81:190-3

[169] Barratt PL, Seymour MT, Stenning SP et al. DNA markers predicting benefit from adjuvant fluorouracil in patients with colon cancer. *Lancet* 2002; 360:1381-91

[170] Cunningham JM, Christensen ER, Tester DJ et al. Hypermethylation of the hMLH1 promoter in colon cancer with microsatellite instability. *Cancer Res* 1998; 58:3455-60

[171] Veigl ML, Kasturi L, Olechnowicz J et al. Biallelic inactivation of hMLH1 by epigenetic gene silencing, a novel mechanism causing human MSI cancers. *Proc Natl Acad Sci* USA 1998; 95:8698-702

[172] Nakagawa H, Chadwick RB, Peltomäki P et al. Loss of imprinting of the insulin-like growth factor II gene occurs by biallelic methylation in a core region of H19-associated CTCF-binding sites in colorectal cancer. *Proc Natl Acad Sci* USA 2001; 98:591-6

[173] Yin J, Kong D, Wang S et al. Mutation of hMSH3 and hMSH6 mismatch repair genes in genetically unstable human colorectal and gastric carcinomas. *Hum Mutat* 1997; 10:474-8

[174] Benachenhou N, Guiral S, Gorska-Flipot I et al. Allelic losses and DNA methylation at DNA mismatch repair loci in sporadic colorectal cancer. *Carcinogenesis* 1998; 19:1925-9

[175] Da Costa LT, Liu B, El-Deiry WS et al. Polymerase δ variants in RER colorectal tumours. *Nature Genet* 1995; 9:10-1

[176] Muta H, Noguchi M, Perucho M et al. Clinical implications of microsatellite instability in colorectal cancers. *Cancer* 1996; 77:265-70

[177] Samowitz WS, Slattery ML, Kerber RA. Microsatellite instability in human colonic cancer is not a useful clinical indicator of familial colorectal cancer. *Gastroenterology* 1995; 109:1765-71

[178] Furlan D, Tibiletti MG, Taborelli M et al. The value of microsatellite instability in the detection of HNPCC families and of sporadic colorectal cancers with special biological features: an investigation on a series of 100 consecutive cases. *Ann Oncol* 1998; 9:901-6

[179] Brown SR, Finan PJ, Cawkwell L et al. Frequency of replication errors in colorectal cancer and their association with family history. *Gut* 1998; 43:553-7

[180] Jass JR, Cottier DS, Jeevaratnam P et al. Diagnostic use of microsatellite instability in hereditary non-polyposis colorectal cancer. *Lancet* 1995; 346:1200-1

[181] Heinimann K, Scott RJ, Buerstedde J-M et al. Influence of selection criteria on mutation detection in patients with hereditary nonpolyposis colorectal cancer. *Cancer* 1999; 85:2512-8

[182] Salovaara R, Loukola A, Kristo P et al. Population-based molecular detection of hereditary non-polyposis colorectal cancer. *J Clin Oncol* 2000; 18:2193-2200

[183] Jacoby RF, Marshall DJ, Cole CE et al. Microsatellite instability in colonic adenomas as a clinical indicator of hereditary cancer syndromes. *J Tum Marker Oncol* 1995; 10:73-81

[184] Frayling IM. Microsatellite instability. *Gut* 1999; 45:1-4

[185] Cravo ML, Fidalgo PO, Lage PA et al. Validation and simplification of Bethesda guidelines for identifying apparently sporadic forms of colorectal carcinoma with microsatellite instability. *Cancer* 1999; 85:779-85

[186] Vasen HF, Mecklin JP, Watson P et al. Surveillance in hereditary nonpolyposis colorectal cancer: an international cooperative study of 165 families. *Dis Colon Rectum* 1993; 36:1-4

[187] Love RR, Morrissey JF. Colonoscopy in asymptomatic individuals with a family history of colorectal cancer. *Arch Intern Med* 1984; 144:2209-11

[188] Fleischer DE, Goldberg, SB, Browning TH. Detection and surveillance of colorectal cancer. *JAMA* 1989; 261:580-5

[189] Vasen HF, Nagengast FM, Khan PM. Interval cancers in hereditary non-polyposis colorectal cancer. *Lancet* 1995; 345:1183-4

[190] Rodriguez-Bigas MA. Prophylactic colectomy for gene carriers in hereditary nonpolyposis colorectal cancer. Has the time come? *Cancer* 1996; 78:199-201

[191] Järvinen HJ, Mecklin JP, Sistonen P. Screening reduces colorectal cancer rate in families with hereditary non-polyposis colorectal cancer. *Gastroenterology* 1995; 108:1405-11

[192] Baba S. Hereditary nonpolyposis colorectal cancer. An update. *Dis Colon Rectum* 1997; 40 (Suppl):86-95

[193] Sankila R, Aaltonen LA, Järvinen HJ et al. Better survival rates in patients with MLH1-associated hereditary colorectal cancer. *Gastroenterology* 1996; 110:682-7

[194] Myrhoj T, Bisgaard ML, Bernstein I et al. Hereditary non-polyposis colorectal cancer: clinical features and survival. Results from the Danish HNPCC register. *Scand J Gastroenterol* 1997; 32:572-6

[195] Fujita S, Moriya Y, Sugihara K et al. Prognosis of hereditary non-polyposis colorectal cancer (HNPCC) and the role of Japanese criteria for HNPCC. *Jpn J Clin Oncol* 1996; 26:351-5

[196] Bertario L, Russo A, Sala P et al. Survival of patients with hereditary non-polyposis colorectal cancer: comparison of HNPCC and colorectal cancer in FAP patients with sporadic colorectal cancer. *Int J Cancer* 1999; 80:183-7

[197] Percesepe A, Benatti P, Roncucci L et al. Survival analysis in families affected by of hereditary non-polyposis colorectal cancer. *Int J Cancer* 1997; 71:373-6

[198] Farrington SM, McKinley AJ, Carothers AD et al. Evidence for an age-related influence of microsatellite instability on colorectal cancer survival. *Int J Cancer* 2002; 98:844-50

[199] Jernvall P, Mäkinen MJ, Karttunen TJ et al. Microsatellite instability: impact on cancer progression in proximal and distal colorectal cancers. *Eur J Cancer* 1999; 35:197-201

[200] Horii A, Han HJ, Shimada M et al. Frequent replication errors at microsatellite loci in tumours of patients with multiple primary cancers. *Cancer Res* 1994; 54:3373-5

[201] Masubuchi S, Konishi F, Togashi K et al. The significance of microsatellite instability in predicting the develpment of metachronous multiple colorectal carcinomas in patients with nonfamilial colorectal carcinoma. *Cancer* 1999; 85:1917-24

[202] Kat A, Thilly WG, Fang WH et al. An alkylation-tolerant, mutator human cell line is deficient in strand-specific mismatch repair. *Proc Natl Acad Sci* USA 1993; 90:6424-8

[203] Fink D, Nebel S, Aebi S et al. The role of DNA mismatch repair in platinum drug resistance. *Cancer Res* 1996; 56:4881-6

[204] Friedman HS, Johnson SP, Dong Q et al. Methylator resistance mediated by mismatch repair deficiency in a glioblastoma multiforme xenograft. *Cancer Res* 1997; 57:2933-6

[205] Aebi S, Fink D, Gordon R et al. Resistance to cytotoxic drugs in DNA mismatch repair deficient cells. *Clin Cancer Res* 1997; 3:1763-7

[206] Fink D, Nebel S, Norris PS et al. The effect of different chemotherapeutic agents on the enrichment of DNA mismatch repair deficient tumour cells. *Br J Cancer* 1998; 77:703-8

[207] Carethers JM, Chauhan DP, Fink D et al. Mismatch repair proficiency and in vitro response to 5-fluorouracil. *Gastroenterology* 1999; 117:123-31

[208] Tokunaga E, Oda S, Fukushima M et al. Differential growth inhibition by to 5-fluorouracil in human colorectal carcinoma cell lines. *Eur J Cancer* 2000; 36:1998-2006

[209] Meyers M, Wagner MW, Hwang HS et al. Role of hMLH1 DNA mismatch repair protein in fluoropyrimidine-mediated cell death and cell cycle responses. *Cancer Res* 2001; 61:5193-5201

[210] Grem JL, Danenberg KD, Behan K et al. Thymidine kinase, thymidylate synthase, and dihydropyrimidine dehydrogenase profiles of cell lines of the National Cancer Institute's Anticancer Drug Screen. *Clin Cancer Res* 2001; 7:999-1009

[211] O'Connor PM, Jackman J, Bae I et al. Characterization of the p53 tumor suppressor pathway in cell lines of the National Cancer Institute Anticancer Drug Screen and correlations with the growth inhibition potency of 123 anticancer agents. *Cancer Res* 1997; 57:4285-4300

[212] Hemminki A, Mecklin JP, Järvinen H et al. Microsatellite instability is a favorable indicator in patients with colorectal cancer receiving chemotherapy. *Gastroenterology* 2000; 119:921-8

[213] Elsaleh H Powell B, McCaul K et al. p53 alteration and microsatellite instability have predictive value for survival benefit from chemotherapy in stage III colorectal carcinoma. *Clin Cancer Res* 2001; 7:1343-9

[214] Samimi G, Fink D, Varki NM et al. Analysis of MLH1 and MSH2 expression in ovarian cancer before and after platinum drug-based chemotherapy. *Clin Cancer Res* 2000; 6:1415-21

[215] Fedier A, Schwarz VA, Walt H et al. Resistance to topoisomerase poisons due to loss of DNA mismatch repair. *Int J Cancer* 2001; 93:571-6

[216] Magrini R, Bhonde MR, Hanski ML et al. Cellular effects of CPT-11 on colon carcinoma cells: dependance on p53 and hMLH1 status. *Int J Cancer* 2002; 101:23-31

[217] Pichierri P, Franchitto A, Piergentili R et al. Hypersensitivity to camptothecin in MSH2 deficient cells is correlated with a role for MSH2 protein in recombinational repair. *Carcinogenesis* 2001; 22:1781-7

[218] Jacob S, Aguado M, Fallik D et al. The role of the DNA mismatch repair system in the cytotoxicity of the topoisomerase inhibitors camptothecin and etoposide to human colorectal cancer cells. *Cancer Res* 2001; 61:6555-62

[219] Gupta M, Fan S, Zhan Q et al. Inactivation of p53 increases cytotoxicity of camptothecin in human colon HCT116 and breast MCF-7 cancer cells. *Clin Cancer Res* 1997; 3:1653-60

[220] Koi M, Umar A, Chauhan DP et al. Human chromosome 3 corrects mismatch repair deficiency and microsatellite instability and reduces N-methyl-N'-nitro-N-nitrosoguanine tolerance in colon tumour cells with homozygous hMLH1 mutation. *Cancer Res* 1994; 54:4308-12

[221] Berry SE, Kinsella TJ. Targeting DNA mismatch repair for radiosensitization. *Sem Radiat Oncol* 2001; 11:300-15

[222] Berry SE, Garces C, Hwang HS et al. The mismatch repair protein, hMLH1, mediates 5-substituted halogenated thymidine analogue cytotoxicity, DNA incorporation, and radiosensitization in human colon cancer cells. *Cancer Res* 1999; 59:1840-5

[223] Brown KD, Rathi A, Kamath R et al. The mismatch repair system is required for S-phase checkpoint activation. *Nat Genet* 2003; 33:80-4

[224] Taketo MM. Cycloxygenase-2 inhibitors in tumorigenesis. *J Natl Cancer Inst* 1998; 90:1529-36

[225] Sheng H, Shao J, Morrow JD et al. Modulation of apoptosis and Bcl-2 expression by prostaglandin E2 in human colon cancer cells. *Cancer Res* 1998; 58:362-6

[226] Tsujii M, Kawano S, Tsuji S et al. Cyclooxygenase regulates angiogenesis induced by colon cancer cells. *Cell* 1998; 93:705-16

[227] Boolbol SK, Dannenberg AJ, Chadburn A et al. Cyclooxygenase-2 overexpression and tumor formation are blocked by sulindac in a murine model of a familial adenomatous polyposis. *Cancer Res* 1996; 56:2556-60

[228] Rao CV, Rivenson A, Simi B et al. Chemoprevention of colon cancer by sulindac, a nonsteroidal anti-inflammatory agent. *Cancer Res* 1995; 55:1464-72

[229] Cruz-Correa M, Hylind LM, Romans K et al. Long-term treatment with sulindac in familial adenomatous polyposis. *Gastroenterology* 2002; 122:641-5

[230] Baron J, Cole B, Sandler R et al. A randomized trial of aspirin to prevent colorectal adenomas. *N Engl J Med* 2003; 348:891-9

[231] Sandler R, Halabi S, Baron A et al. A randomized trial of aspirin to prevent colorectal adenomas in patients with previous colorectal cancer. *N Engl J Med* 2003; 348:883-90

[232] Xu XM, Sansores-Garcia L, Chen Xm et al. Suppression of inducible cyclooxygenase 2 gene transcription by aspirin and sodium salicylate. *Proc Natl Acad Sci USA* 1999; 96:5292-7

[233] Gupta RA, Dubois RN. Colorectal prevention and treatment by inhibition of cyclooxygenase-2. *Nat Rev Cancer* 2001; 1:11-21

[234] Hallak A, Alon-Baron L, Shamir et al. Rofecoxib reduces polyp recurrence in familial polyposis. *Dig Dis Sci* 2003; 48:1998-2002

[235] Rüschoff J, Wallinger S, Dietmaier W et al. Aspirin suppresses the mutator phenotype associated with hereditary nonpolyposis colorectal cancer by genetic selection. *Proc Natl Acad Sci USA* 1998; 95:11301-6

[236] Burn J, Chapman PD, Bishop DT et al. Diet and cancer prevention. The concerted action for polyp prevention (CAPP) studies. *Proc Nutr Soc* 1998; 57:183-6

INDEX

#

A

B

C

H

I

J

K

L

M

N

O

P

Q

R

S

T

U

V

W

Y